SPORTS TRAINING PRINCIPLES

Published by A & C Black (Publishers) Ltd
37 Soho Square, London W1D 3QZ

Fifth edition 2007
Fourth edition 2002
Third edition 1997
Second edition 1989

First edition published 1980 by Lepus Books, an imprint of Henry Kimpton
(Publishers) Ltd

Copyright © by Frank Dick 1980, 1989, 1997, 2002, 2007

Cover photograph of male athletes at starting line of race courtesy of
© Getty (Terje Rakke)

All illustrations redrawn by Dave Saunders

ISBN 978 0 7136 8278 6

A CIP catalogue record for this book is available from the British Library.

Other books of interest from A & C Black

Abdominal Training (Second edition)
by Christopher M. Norris
This is the definitive guide to core stability – developing, safely and effectively, the condition of the trunk muscles – a crucial component of fitness for a variety of sports.

The Complete Guide to Core Stability (Second edition)
Matt Lawrence
The definitive 'core stability' training handbook for fitness leaders and other fitness professionals. This book looks at what core stability is, the muscles that are involved and the benefits gained from improving your core stability.

The Complete Guide to Sports Nutrition (Fifth edition)
Anita Bean
This highly successful book will show you how improved nutrition can help to enhance performance, boost energy levels, achieve faster and better training results, and reach higher competitive standards.

The Complete Guide to Endurance Training (Third edition)
Jon Ackland
This book will teach endurance athletes, such as long-distance runners, cyclists, swimmers and triathletes how to make the right training decisions, train smarter and achieve better results. Includes 58 specific programmes to get you started.

The Complete Guide to Strength Training (Third edition)
by Anita Bean
This unique combination of effective training methods and cutting edge nutritional guidance delivers a comprehensive programme suitable for the beginner and advanced trainer alike.

The Complete Guide to Stretching (Third edition)
Christopher M. Norris
This book provides an accessible overview of the scientific principles that underpin stretching and flexibility and offers more than 70 exercises designed to increase range of motion across the entire body.

Food for Fitness (Third edition)
by Anita Bean
A concise sports nutrition guide, an invaluable menu planner and a comprehensive recipe book, all rolled into one. Written to complement **The Complete Guide to Sports Nutrition**.

CONTENTS

PREFACE

It has always fascinated me that athletes are able to produce almost identical times over their racing distance, yet their training plans seem extremely diverse. This fascination naturally led me to enquiry, and I began with a study of the relevant aspects of anatomy, physiology and psychology.

In presenting my interpretation of these aspects, I wish to acknowledge, both with respect and gratitude, the counsel of several authorities: Dr H. Robson (Loughborough University) and Dr Siggerseth (University of Oregon), who were my lecturers in anatomy and kinesiology; Tom Craig (formerly physiotherapist to Glasgow Rangers Football Club), who wrapped much 'meat around the bones' of part 1. Dr Soderwall (University of Oregon), Dr Clyde Williams (Loughborough University), and Dr Craig Sharp (West London Institute of HE), guided me through the complexities of physiology, which I present as part 2. Professor Miroslav Vanek (Charles University, Prague), Peter Hill and Jean Carroll (both formerly of Dunfermline College of Physical Education), and Dr Pamela F. Murray (Royal Air Force, Cosford) provided new insight to the world of psychology, as set out in part 3. Bridging anatomy, physiology and psychology is the theme of applying each science to the growing child, a concept made much clearer for me by Dr Ivan Szmodis (Central School of Sports, Budapest).

The sciences of anatomy, physiology and psychology are essential basics in pursuing this enquiry, but are as far from being an explanation as bricks are to being a house. Part 4 might then be thought of as the 'cement', giving these bricks context.

So many associates have helped me in this area of study that it would be impossible for me to list them all here. However, I would like to record my deep indebtedness to them and to mention especially: Dr Geoff Gowan, Basil Stamatakis, Tony Chapman, Ron Pickering, Wilf Paish, Friedhelm Endemann, Stewart Togher, Vladimir Kuznyetsov, Peter Radford, Sandy Ewen, Gerard Mach, Carlo Vittori, Wilson Young, Gordon Forster, Denis Watts, Harry Wilson, Alex Naylor, Bill Bowerman, Dr Elio Locatelli, Seppo Nutilla, Peter Coe, Max Jones, Carlton Johnson, John Issacs, Erkki Oikarinen, Rita Englebrecht, Dr Ekkart Arbeit, and Norman Brooke for their thoughts and comments on strength, speed, mobility and endurance.

It would be very difficult to say exactly when I first began to draw together the detail of the final part of this book. Whenever it was will coincide with the origins of that fascination referred to earlier. I see Part 5 as the design or blueprint, and it is my opinion that every coach I have ever met (from several sports) is responsible for its content.

It has also become very clear to me that central to the education and development of any coach is what he can learn from the athletes themselves. I owe each one of the athletes I have coached an immense debt in this respect.

Although the book began to grow several years before pen was put to paper in the autumn of 1975 for the first edition, the nature of its contents means the subject matter requires regular review. The second edition did, in fact, consider again certain aspects of strength, speed and endurance training, and, in particular, focused more tightly on the area of regeneration in the section 'Training v straining'.

In the third edition, three colleagues contributed their specialist knowledge to take the components of training theory, as set out here, to a new level. Dr Craig Sharp (West London Institute) reviewed and edited part 2, while Professor Miroslav Vanek (Charles Institute, Prague) and Dr Pamela F. Murray (researcher, Royal Air Force, Cosford) wrote and introduced new material for part 3. I am very grateful for their continued professional and authoritative input.

In the fourth and fifth editions I have enhanced the content relating to process in parts 4 and 5, with the help of Andy Roxborough (UEFA Technical Director), Josef Vengelos (UEFA), Ian McGeechan (former Chief Coach Scotland RU), Dr Ekkart Arbeit, Dr Elio Locatelli (IAAF Technical Director), Dr Peter Bonov, Dr Dane Korica, Dr Ron Maughan, Peter Kesne and Dr Wolfgang Ritzdorf.

As a student, it was put to me that each one of us is exposed to thousands of facts and opinions and that any ideas we think of as our own are, in fact, simply an interpretation of these facts and opinions. My objective here has been to present my understanding of the principles which may help you establish your presentation of training theory to the advantage of the athletes in your charge. I hope you discover this to be the case.

Throughout this book athletes and coaches are, in the main, referred to individually as 'he' rather than 'he or she'. This has been agreed with the publisher as an expedient only.

Finally, I would like to acknowledge with sincere gratitude, the excellent work of three secretaries in typing this text from really bad handwriting! Janet Leyland (1980), Jackie Brown (1989, 1997, 2002), Anna Stanforth (2002) and Elvie-Jo Shergold (2007).

INTRODUCTION

'Those who are enamoured of practice without science are like a pilot who goes into a ship without rudder or compass and never has any certainty of where he is going.'
(Leonardo da Vinci)

Coaching is mainly an art and, like the artist, the coach must have two attributes. The first is creative flair, that marriage of aptitude and passion which enables him to draw an athlete's dream towards realisation. The athlete, moved to express himself within a social mosaic, chooses to do so in pursuit of competitive excellence in sport. The coach creates order and direction for that expression.

The second attribute is technical mastery of the instruments and materials used. The athlete is the instrument and the material with which the coach works. Structurally, he is a system of levers, given movement by the pull of muscle, and obedient to the laws of physics. Functionally, he is a dynamic integration of adaptive systems. But more than that, he is a reasoning being.

A gardener who works to create ever greater beauty in a plant, does so on the basis of his knowledge of the plant's behaviour in certain conditions. His art lies in the adjustment of these conditions. The coach may have the advantage over the gardener in that the athlete, unlike the plant, can perceive his total environment, rationalise situations, compare present with past, predict the consequences of actions and rapidly adapt his behaviour within his personal framework of attitude, values and motivation. At first sight, the active involvement of the athlete makes the coach's task seem simpler than that of the gardener. After all, 'two heads are better than one'! Yet the infinitely variable behaviour, which might result from even one simple adjustment to the athlete's environment, confirms the extraordinary complexity of the coach's art. The coach must clearly understand the purpose of each practice and its relevance to the total scheme of preparation, yet comprehend fully the role of sport as but one part of the life of a growing and changing person. So the coach is not only in the technical business; he is in the people business.

To accept the full weight of this responsibility, the coach, in these the early years of the 21st century, must move towards a deeper appreciation of those sciences which relate to the athlete. This is not to say that pragmatism is dead; there will continue to be situations where the coach 'knows' a practice is correct, according to his 'feel' for coaching athletes. This is, of course, part of the coach's art and it should stimulate rather than inhibit pursuit of explanation. Many established practices may work (and for good reason) but, until underlying principles are defined, what basis do we have for developing further practices or for communicating experience in coaching to *all* sports?

And there are at least two reasons why we should feel confident that coaches will continue to increase their effectiveness in delivering their art. First, there is the certain knowledge that the sciences which influence performance are accelerating the intelligence resource coaches need to ensure athletes fulfil their performance potential. Next, there is irrefutability to the words of Arie de Geuss:

'*Probably the only sustainable competitive advantage we have is the ability to learn faster than the competition.*'

So we enjoy an advantage in a world where the performance-related database is expanding exponentially. That world is one of constant change where, on the one hand, we are exposed to change and learn to adapt to it, and on the other we learn to impose change.

In drawing together the substance of the following pages it has not, then, been my intention to create an apotheosis of sports science. The various changes will, I hope, contribute to the coach's sources of reference, form part of a basis for understanding current coaching research, and offer a framework of training principles for an ever-expanding source of practices designed to help the athlete in preparation for excellence in his sport. *Sports Training Principles* has been written to provide a launching platform for your lifelong learning as a coach.

The coach is most certainly not 'enamoured of practice without science', but I would not wish to make him a bookworm, equipped only with sports science jargon. His art is to weave his understanding of related sciences into the fabric of coaching an athlete. It is a practical art, based on careful appraisal of all relevant knowledge. I hope this book will contribute to your interpretation of this fine art.

PART 1

RODS TO LEVERS

An athlete may be thought of, structurally, as a series of connected rods. The design of each connection will determine the nature and range of movement between adjacent rods and, consequently, their potential function. These connections are the joints, the rods, and the bones. Combined, they form the *skeletal system*. The movement at any given joint is made possible by the pull of muscle on bone across the joint. The total arrangement of muscle and its attachment to bones forms the *muscular system*. Part 1 looks at these two systems, and the *mechanical laws* which they must obey, to effect an appreciation of the athlete's aggregate movement potential for the expression of energy.

So, part 1 serves as an introduction to the sciences of anatomy, kinesiology and biomechanics. These sciences are fundamental to the coach in the design and selection of exercise on the one hand, and technique development and analysis on the other.

1 THE WORKING PARTS

AXES

It is easy to understand how a wheel spins about an axle, and at right angles to that axle. If the athlete had wheels instead of arms and legs, the axles being located at the shoulders and at the hips, it would again be easy to understand why the wheels would rotate or spin at right angles to the body and on the same plane as the direction in which the athlete was moving. If the axles are now faded out in the mind's eye and the arms and legs are considered as rotating like wheels – not round and round, but forwards and backwards like pendulums – it appears that the body is equipped with invisible axles, or axes, and that the movement at the joints is rotation. However, whereas the wheel may rotate on one plane only, the body's joints permit greater freedom of movement.

Our bodies are three dimensional. There are three axes of rotation – vertical, transverse and anterior-posterior – for the body as a whole and, in principle, at each joint. We will now look at the axes and consider them in the light of the whole body movement and the movement at various joints (fig. 1).

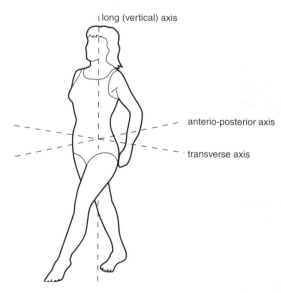

FIG. 1 The body's axes

Vertical axis

The vertical axis is the long axis of the body and is that about which the figure skater spins, or the ballet dancer pirouettes.

If the body is tilted to lie parallel with the ground, i.e. horizontal, rotation is still possible about the long axis (e.g. the child rolling sideways downhill or the straddle jumper rolling round the bar). Although horizontal, the rotation is described as about the body's vertical axis. In describing rotations, it is important to identify clearly the axes under consideration as if the person is standing. Very little confusion arises when discussing the whole body in flight, but occasionally problems arise with a particular joint action. For example, just as the long axis of the body is referred to as the vertical axis, so also is the long axis through a joint. Hence the actions of turning out one's feet like Charlie Chaplin, twisting one's head and shoulders to the rear, and turning off a tap (with elbow extended) are all examples of rotation about the long/vertical axis. Taking the last example, however, consider the arm held out to the side (abducted) and swung forwards, as in a discus throw. This rotation is about the vertical axis through the shoulder, while long axis rotation of the arm which will influence the attitude of the discus, will, in this case, be about the transverse axis through the shoulder. The moral of the story is to *be precise in defining axes.*

Transverse axis

The transverse axis is that described in the 'wheels for limbs' reference above. These particular axes would apply to shoulder and hip. Examples of rotation about these axes in the athlete are kicking a ball, the pulling action of the arms in swimming, and the piking to extension movements of the gymnast. Returning to the vertical axis situation mentioned above, rotations about the transverse axis become rotations about the vertical axis when the arm is abducted. For example, the actions of underarm bowling and the forehand in tennis are similar in terms of movement at the shoulder joint, although different muscles may be involved due to changing angles of pull on levers. Consequently, when considering transverse axis rotations, one must also consider rotations with an abducted limb. These include the pull-through of the hurdler's trail leg into the line of running, and the golfer's swing.

The transverse axis of the body as a whole is that about which the trampolinist or springboard diver rotates in a front or back somersault. The high jumper who uses the flop technique rotates about the vertical axis at take-off and about the transverse axis in bar clearance.

Anterior-posterior axis

The cartwheel somersault of an acrobat is a useful visual image of an athlete rotating about the body's anterior-posterior (A-P) axis. This axis is from front to back and is seen in joint actions where, for example, a rider presses her knees against the flanks of her mount. A soldier standing at ease, then responding to a command to stand to attention, would be rotating the leg on the hip about the A-P axis. Similarly, arms raised sideways or returned to the side are rotating on the shoulder about the A-P axis. Other examples are the hip/spine movements of the side-step or body swerve in football, the tilting of the pelvis in recovering the hurdler's trail leg, and certain expressions of lateral movement in dance.

JOINT ACTIONS

Related to the axes of rotation outlined, there are the specific actions of flexion, extension, adduction, abduction and rotation. An understanding of these actions affords fuller appreciation of movement and technique.

Flexion

Flexion is the rotating of one lever about another in such a way that the angle between these levers is reduced. Bringing hand to shoulder is an example of flexion at the elbow. The soccer player who can keep the ball in the air by using his knee is doing so by flexing his thigh on his hip and, simultaneously, flexing his lower leg on his thigh. The spine too may be considered as a lever or a series of levers. As a guide, any movement which curls the athlete into a tucked shape or round, like a ball, is flexion of the spine.

Two more types of flexion are described, at the shoulder and the ankle. Flexion at the shoulder is the raising forward of the arm above the head, as in swimming backstroke arm recovery. Plantar flexion is pointing the toe, standing on tiptoe. Dorsi flexion at the ankle is turning the toes up towards the knee (as in Aladdin's shoes!). Horizontal flexion at the shoulder is in such actions as bench press, discus arm, forehand in tennis, and shot put arm.

Extension

Extension might be thought of as the opposite of flexion and is the rotating of one lever away from another. Thus the angle between the levers increases towards 180°. If greater than 180°, the action is referred to as hyperextension. At the moment of delivery in shot put, the arm is completely extended (straightened) at the elbow. As the basketball player leaves the floor for a jump shot, extension takes place at the hip, knee and ankle. As the volleyball player jumps to block an opposition spike, then elbows, wrists and fingers are extended. In a hollow-back somersault, the extreme arching of the spine is hyperextension.

Extension of the arm on the shoulder is the opposite action to that described for flexion and is demonstrated in the overhead smash shots in tennis, squash and badminton, also in javelin arm and in the powerful pull phases of the arm action when swimming butterfly, freestyle or breaststroke. Extension at the ankle is the action of plantar flexion, making the line of the lower leg/foot straight, or even convex. Ballet dancers and gymnasts are capable of the latter. Horizontal extension at the shoulder is seen when the athlete, standing in the crucifix position, presses the arms backwards, or when in reverse flies in weight training.

The actions of flexion and extension are considered as rotations about the transverse axis of a given joint, and the body's tendency to a total flexion or extension is also about this axis.

Adduction

Adduction is the drawing of a lever towards the mid-line of the body, e.g. moving the legs from standing astride to standing with the legs together, or in returning the arms from a position in which they are out from the side back to the side. Thus the action of bringing the legs towards each other in breaststroke leg action is one of adduction, as is gripping the body of a horse with one's knees when riding.

The action of adduction may take a lever past the mid-line, e.g. in crossing one's legs or in sweeping a soccer ball across the body from one side to the other. Obviously, to perform such an action, the leg would have to be either slightly extended or flexed on the hip to permit passage of one leg beyond the obstruction of the other.

Abduction

Abduction is the opposite movement to adduction and is therefore the movement of a lever *away* from the mid-line. Raising an arm to the side and moving the legs from being together to legs astride are examples of abduction. The shot-putter emphasises the abduction of his putting arm and the hurdler abducts the trailing leg to ensure clearance of the barrier.

The actions of adduction and abduction are normally considered to take place about the A-P axis.

Rotation

All movements of levers are rotations, but the expression 'rotation', when considered with the anatomical actions of flexion, adduction, abduction and extension, is taken to mean long-axis rotation. When Charlie Chaplin turned his feet outwards, the action was outward or lateral rotation. When he turned them inwards, so that he was pigeon-toed, the action was inward or medial rotation. Lateral means 'to the outside or outwards', medial means 'to the inside or inwards'. Abduction, then, could be described as a lateral movement and adduction as a medial movement.

The action of rotation is normally understood to take place about the vertical axis, but, again, care must be taken to define the axes precisely.

BASIC STRUCTURE

Bone

The rods are the athlete's bones and they become levers via the joints. The structure of each joint will dictate its function potential, hence the contrast between the mobility of the shoulder complex of joints and the stability of the hip joint; the difference between cervical intervertebral movement and the lumbar intervertebral movement; and the functional variable available to the elbow as opposed to the knee. While it is not essential that bone names be memorised, it is useful to know their relationship to each other (fig. 2).

FIG. 2 The skeleton

Deltoid (middle and posterior fibres)
Triceps brachii
Brachioradialis
Wrist/fingers flexors/extensors
Adductor magnus
Vastus lateralis
Biceps femoris
Semimembranosus
Semitendinosus

Trapezius (upper, middle and lower fibres)
Infraspinatus
Teres minor
Teres major
Latissimus dorsi
External obliques
Gluteus medius
Gluteus maximus
Tensor fascia latae
Vastus intermedius
Gastrocnemius
Soleus

Deltoid (Anterior fibres)
Triceps brachii
Biceps brachii
Brachialis
Brachioradialis
External obliques
Adductor longus
Vastus lateralis
Rectus femoris
Vastus medialis
Dorsi-flexors
Toe extensors
Evertors
Invertors

Trapezius
Pectoralis major
Latissimus dorsi
Serratus anterior
Rectus abdominis
Internal obliques
Transversus abdominis
Gastrocnemius (medial head)
Soleus

FIG. 3 The muscles

Muscle

Muscles, by converting chemical energy into mechanical energy, pull on the bones and bring about the actions already described. The specific action of a muscle will be defined by the levers it connects and the position and angle of attachment (fig. 3). In several instances, a muscle crosses two joints and is therefore responsible for two separate actions. The efficiency of each action will be critically affected by the stability status of each joint.

Tendon

Tendon attaches muscle to bone. The Achilles tendon, for example, attaches the calf muscles responsible for ankle extension to the large bone at the rear of the heel (the calcaneus). On gripping this particular tendon between forefinger and thumb, the extreme toughness of this tissue is at once apparent. Due to this strength, the tendon itself is seldom injured. However, the connections of tendon to muscle or tendon to bone are more vulnerable to injury.

Ligaments

The ligaments are bands of white fibrous tissue connecting bones about a joint. They may be considered as guardians of the joint's stability as they are extremely resistant to distortion and stretching. Certain types of mobility work are geared to passive stretching of ligaments to permit a greater freedom or range of movement. However, it must be borne in mind that such work restricts their role as stabilisers. Once stretched, the ligament will maintain its new length, having plastic rather than elastic properties (fig. 4).

Periosteum

The connective tissue surrounding the bone is periosteum. In the grown organism it has a supporting function and when strong tendon, ligaments or muscle are attached to a bone, the periosteum is incorporated with them. This is the final connection of muscle to bone. While it is obviously a strong connection, it is nevertheless vulnerable to injury when strained. Stress may accumulate or occur as a result of fatigue and strong muscle contraction, or in maximal contraction when imbalance has caused an unnatural alignment of the joint. In the growing organism, periosteum protects a layer of tissue containing the 'bone-growing' cells. It is an unstable material and extremes of muscular fatigue or force of contraction must be discouraged.

Synovia

Most joints of the body are completely surrounded by a capsule lined with a synovial membrane. This membrane lines the whole of the interior of the joint

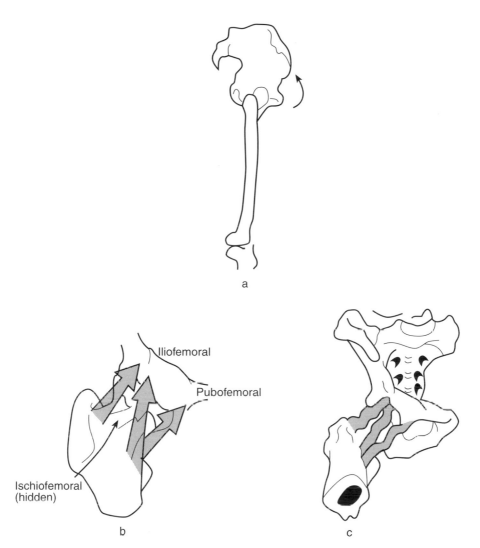

FIG. 4 The ligaments of the hip (from Kapandji, 1988). As the child develops from the quadruped posture to the erect posture, and the pelvis tilts upwards and backwards (a), all ligaments become coiled round the neck of the femur, in the same direction. Extension winds these ligaments tighter (b); flexion unwinds, and slackens them (c). The stretching of these ligaments in the quadruped to upright posture demonstrates plastic, rather than elastic, properties of ligaments.

except the actual ends of the bones which meet in that particular joint. The membrane releases a constant small flow of a lubricant called synovia or synovial fluid. Exercise appears to increase the amount of fluid released, while injury to the joint encourages an extremely rapid flow.

Cartilage

Cartilage may be thought of as a shock-absorbing or reducing agent. In the knee, cartilage discs not only cushion the impact of movement between the two bones, but also serve to ensure perfect contact between them. Fibrocartilage discs act as cushions between the various bones or vertebrae which are stacked one upon the other in the spine. Finally, the ends of each bone meeting at a joint are protected by *articular* cartilage.

It should be remembered that cartilage has no blood supply and consequently cannot repair itself once damaged. However, it would appear that synovia provides cartilage with nutrients and it has been shown that with exercise the amount of available fluid increases. This flow increases the efficiency of joint movement.

THE UPPER LIMBS

Reflection on the number of movements and actions performed by the upper limb complex will point to its primary characteristic – mobility. Mobility depends on combinations and permutations of actions at four joints. These joints will be considered in order from that nearest the spine to that farthest from the spine. The technical terminology to describe part of an appendage nearest to the spine is proximal, and that more distant is distal.

Shoulder

The following shoulder actions are possible about the axes indicated.

Transverse axis: *flexion* – arm raised forwards; *extension* – arm pulled downwards or backwards. These opposing actions can be seen clearly in the arm movements in running. The plane in which these movements take place is the *sagittal* plane (fig. 5a).

Anterioposterior axis: *abduction* – raising the arm out from the side; *adduction* – returning the arm from a position of abduction to the side. These actions are in the *frontal* plane (fig. 5b).

Vertical axis (arm parallel with spine): *rotation outward* (*lateral*) – clockwise movement of the straight right arm, e.g. turning a tap off; *rotation inward* (*medial*) – anticlockwise movement of the straight right arm, e.g. turning a tap on.

Vertical axis (arm abducted): *horizontal flexion* – starting from a position with arm held out from the side (abducted), the arm is brought forward towards the

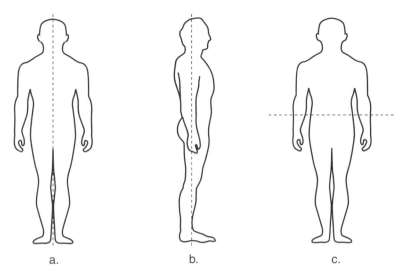

a.   b.   c.

FIG. 5 The primary planes of the body: (a) separation at the sagittal plane; (b) separation at the frontal plane; (c) separation at the horizontal plane

midline. This is seen in the discus arm action, in bench press, or in wrapping the arms about the body to keep warm; *horizontal extension* – the reverse to horizontal flexion. These actions are in the *horizontal* plane (fig. 5c). Combinations of these actions permit immense adaptability, e.g. slipping an arm into a coat sleeve, combing the hair at the back of the head, scratching the opposite shoulder blade from above or below, throwing in a ball at soccer, and even dislocations on the gymnastic rings.

Application examples of shoulder mobility

Arm action in high jump: a coaching point often quoted for high jump arm action is 'thumbs in, elbows out'. By turning in the thumbs the arms are medially rotated and this in turn slides the winglike scapulae (shoulder blades) round the rear wall of the rib (thoracic) cage. As this happens, the joint between the humerus and the part of the scapula which receives it (glenoid fossa), is brought forward allowing greater range of extension.

Discus arm: in discus, the abducted arm must be supported by the powerful abductor muscles and the discus aligned by controlled inward rotation of the arm, yet the action which applies force to the discus is one of fast horizontal flexion over as great a range as possible. The limited degree of inward rotation must cause the scapula to be a restricting agent to a great range of horizontal extension, but this is preferable to the outward rotation employed by the beginner who struggles to keep the discus securely gripped by the distal phalanges of his throwing hand at the limit of extension. If the athlete continued this outward rotation, his arm would assume the starting position for javelin throw. Many top discus throwers hang the discus low and behind the hip as if they were attempting to place the throwing hand in their hip pocket. Here the arm is kept inwardly rotated until the athlete moves into his throwing position, when the discus is then allowed to swing the arm out to an increased range of movement. Tennis strokes at below shoulder level involve similar principles.

Javelin arm: the arm in the javelin throw is withdrawn prior to the actual throw, as in the outward rotation of the arm, the horizontal extension of the shoulder (arm abducted), the backward movement of the shoulder girdle, and rotation about the long axis of the spine. A fundamental adjustment must then be made to allow the thrower to pull along the length of the javelin and forcefully project it. This involves even greater rotation and a consequent sliding of the entire shoulder under the javelin. In fact, what is involved is a rapid positional change from extreme horizontal extension to extreme flexion. There is a clear relationship between this action and that of the tennis serve, the forehand smash in racquet sports, the volleyball spike, the soccer throw in, and the arm action in butterfly and freestyle swimming.

Elbow

At the elbow joint, two axes of rotation are evident.

Transverse axis: *flexion* – hand brought to the same shoulder; *extension* – elbow straightened. These opposing actions can be seen clearly in activities such as chinning the bar (flexion) and push-ups (extension).

Vertical axis: *pronation* – forearm is rotated medially to a palm down or overgrasp position; *supination* – forearm is rotated laterally to a palm-up or undergrasp position. These actions are applied when using a screwdriver to screw or unscrew with the right hand. The clockwise action of screwing on a nut is supination, while the anticlockwise action of unscrewing a nut is pronation. The right-handed pole vaulter supinates the right forearm and pronates the left in gripping the pole. The tennis player serves with pronation but supinates for backhand shots.

Elbow mechanics

Flexion efficiency depends on the position of the forearm, i.e. pronation or supination, and the position of the arm relative to the shoulder. Extension efficiency depends on the position of the arm relative to the shoulder. The relative efficiency is illustrated in strength measurements listed in table 1.

position	extension force	flexion force
Arm stretched above shoulder	43 kg	83 kg
Arm flexed at 90°	37 kg	66 kg
Arm hanging at side of the body	52 kg	51 kg

TABLE 1 Elbow extension and flexion force compared in three different positions (Kapandji, 1982)

From this we can deduce man's suitability to climbing and certain implications of limb alignment for vaulters and apparatus gymnasts. Considerable difference can be measured at 90° of flexion when the forearm assumes varying points of rotation between supination and pronation (table 2). The difference has been explained by Provins and Salter (1955) as (1) biceps are stretched but poor leverage, (2) brachioradialis is the same, (3) brachialis is the same, and (4) pronator teres is at greatest length and leverage.

position	strength force	standard deviation
Supination	19.64 kg	3.82
Mid-position	21.60 kg	4.05
Pronation	13.41 kg	2.00

TABLE 2 Isometric flexion strength relative to elbow joint position (adapted from Rasch, 1968)

This will obviously make a difference in how chinning the bar and biceps curls are performed, and how high bars, poles, etc., are gripped. It should also be pointed out that in gripping a bar in pronation, with the object of performing biceps curls, the weight of the bar will place considerable stress on the extensor muscles of the wrist as the bar is raised. As the stress increases, the wrist will be pulled to a position of flexion, thus stretching the extensors of the fingers and forcing the flexors to release their grip on the bar. The total effect is similar to the action performed in unarmed combat when attempting to disarm an opponent who holds a weapon. The hand containing the weapon is seized, the wrist forced into flexion, and the weapon is dropped.

Returning to extension of the elbow, the triceps are at their greatest mechanical advantage and are stretched when the arm is abducted. However, it must be realised that there is a problem since the action at the elbow and the shoulder are really opposing each other. Immediate connection should be clear, keeping the elbow high in shot. There is another little muscle involved in extension and that is the anconeus. Its main function is to pronate as the elbow extends, e.g. in javelin long axis spin and in imparting spin to tennis shots.

Wrist

The wrist is a very adaptable complex of joints, offering rotation about three axes.

Transverse axis: *flexion* – palm of hand is moved towards the forearm; *extension* – back of hand is moved towards the forearm. These actions are immediately recognisable in the final wrist flick in shotput (flexion), or the whipcracking action of a badminton backhand (extension).

Anterioposterior axis: *adduction* – small finger side of hand is moved towards the forearm; *abduction* – thumb side of the hand is moved towards the forearm.

The former is seen when chopping wood with a hand axe, the latter in the final flicking action of the wrist when imparting spin to the discus.

Vertical axis: there is a limited amount of rotation about the long axis which contributes to the total manipulative capacity of the fingers. It must be constantly borne in mind that the force efficiency of this joint is limited, but must be developed if an accumulated force from leg, hip, trunk, shoulder and elbow are to be transferred to an implement held in the hand. This is particularly the case with a heavy implement such as shot, where wrist or finger injury can terminate an athlete's ambitions for an entire season. It is also pertinent for lighter implements such as javelin, racquet or golf club.

Fingers

All other joints of the upper limb complex combine to allow the discrete manipulative capacity of the fingers to function efficiently. The grab of a mechanical digger cannot perform its tasks efficiently if the arm has not been driven to the most efficient functioning site. Similarly, the control of shoulder, elbow and wrist are basic to the working of the fingers. These small joint complexes make fine movement possible by rotation about two axes for the four fingers and thumb.

Transverse axis: *flexion* – the beckoning action of curling the finger towards the palm; *extension* – the straightening of the finger to point or indicate. The fingers are flexed in all gripping activities like holding a bar, bat or a throwing implement. Actions of extension are mainly seen as a return from flexion, but static extension may be held as, for example, in karate.

Anterioposterior axis: *abduction* – spreading the fingers; *adduction* – bringing the fingers and thumb together as in the characteristic 'karate chop' position. The fingers are abducted to grip a discus or give maximum area to present to a basketball or water (swimming). Adduction is used when the talon grip is used in javelin. The upper limb joint complexes afford immense movement potential, from the foundation of mobility. This is demonstrated from subtleties of finger and wrist actions in the pianist and strings musicians; to the touch of the racquet player or bowler in cricket; to the power of throwers, gymnasts and weight lifters. Conditioning enhances that potential by building on mobility and motor coordination programmes.

In addition, the thumb is capable of *opposition*. This action is the bringing of the thumb across the palm to the small finger.

SPINE

The bony axis of the trunk is the spine, or spinal column. The spine is at once a single rigid lever and a series of levers. As a single lever it can sustain great burdens, or accept the powerful extension of the lower limbs, in connection with the upper limbs, to propel an object or the body itself. As a series of levers it is capable of immense mobility and can absorb the shock of impact from above or below. Thus the spine offers the body an extremely wide range of movement by virtue of its adaptability. The spine may be likened to a series of cotton reels joined end to end with a piece of string passing along the central tunnel. Each cotton reel represents a *vertebra*: man is a vertebrate because he has a backbone, a worm is invertebrate because it has none.

Vertebrae and discs

The vertebrae gradually increase in size from neck to tail. This is because each vertebra must bear the weight of all parts of the body above it. The farther down the spine, the greater the weight, hence its solid structure. In the hole in the middle the spinal cord passes through, like a vast bundle of wires in a telephone cable. This is the communications system linking brain and body. Damaging this cable will cut off communications to parts of the body below the level of the damage, hence the terrible consequences of spinal injury and the classification system according to the level of injury in paraplegic sport.

The discs are the cushions between vertebrae and damaging them brings considerable pain and discomfort. This is caused not so much by the pressure of bone on bone, but by pressure on the cord, or branches of the cord. These would normally leave the main cable via the gap between the two vertebrae kept free by the disc in question.

Shape of the spine

The analogy of a column of cotton reels is slightly inaccurate because the spine is not straight when viewed from the side or behind. The spine has a characteristic series of curves, the evolution of which is interesting.

Babies at birth have only one curve, that which gives the body the appearance of a comma (fig. 6a). The cervical (neck) curve is formed by the strong intermittent pull of the infant's muscles on the spine as he begins to sit up and hold up his head. It is emphasised further in the tilting back of the head to see where he is crawling to, or in looking for his next meal (fig. 6b). Once he is on his feet, the pelvis (hip bone) is pulled forwards and downwards by ligaments attached to the bone of the thigh (fig. 4). This action, combined with the body's weight bearing down on the lower spine as he pulls himself erect, pulls the lower spine forwards, completing the final curve of the spine (fig. 6c).

Movements in the spine

The tension of ligaments joining vertebrae, and the shape of vertebrae at different levels of the spine, dictate the movements of which the spine is capable. (Exceptions are the two vertebrae upon which the head rests; the atlas and axis vertebrae.) Rotation is possible about three axes in the spine, rendering a most mobile complex of joints.

Transverse axis: *flexion* – the curling forwards of the head towards the hips. It takes place in all regions of the spine, but is most free at the cervical and lumbar regions. The contribution of head and hip movement to the overall picture of spine flexion is worth noting. Tension of extensor muscles and solid restrictions, such as the ribs or excess weight about the middle, are the main limiting factors to spine flexion. Flexion is seen in front somersault or in the rock-back position in pole vault. The shoulders may readily become rounded, encouraging flexion of the spine at its upper third. This shows in a stoop and can be brought about by tiring or weakening of the extensors, occupational postures, or overconditioning of flexors. The ease with which this may happen creates a problem in weight bearing on the shoulders, where instability is introduced

a   b

c   d

FIG. 6 The developing spine: (a) the newborn baby has one spinal curve – making the basic shape something similar to a comma. This curve will remain in the thoracic region; (b) the young child has already introduced a second curve in the cervical region; (c) once upright, the third curve is developed in the lumbar region as early as three years, becoming obvious by eight years and assuming characteristic adult shape around 10 years (d).

and injury may result due to exceptional pressure for which this part of the lever system is ill-prepared; *extension* – the straightening of the spine. It takes place most freely at the cervical and lumbar spine, but is restricted in the thoracic spine. The expression of hyperextension is used to describe a degree of extension which moves far beyond normal postural extension. This movement is very evident in arching positions in gymnastics, such as the hollowback somersault, and so on. The total maximum range of flexion of the spine from sacrum to skull as a whole is approximately 110° and extension 140° (Kapandji, 1995). These values will, of course, vary considerably with age and ability levels.

Anterioposterior axis: *lateral flexion* – the curving of the spine to either side, as in reaching the right fingers towards the right ankle while looking straight ahead. It is possible at all levels, but is greatest at the junction between thoracic and lumbar spine. The tilting of the pelvis to recover the trail leg in hurdles involves a degree of lateral flexion, as do twisting movements involved in the complex patterns of agility displayed in diving, or in body swerve in field games, slalom skiing, etc. The total maximum range of lateral flexion from sacrum to skull is approximately 75–85° (Kapandji, 1995). Again, there are variations related to age and ability.

Vertical axis: rotation/twisting along the length of the spine is most free in the cervical region and through the thoracic region, but is negligible in the lumbar spine. This particular property of the spine is very important and both strength and mobility must be worked at. The athlete attempts to take the spine to extremes of rotation in order to 'compress the spring' in throws, hence the 'wound-up' position in discus and javelin, or in the preparation phases of tennis strokes, golf swing, etc. The total maximum rotation from sacrum to skull is approximately 90° (Kapandji, 1995), with variation according to age and ability levels.

The spine is the critical conduit of structure and function in movement potential. Its musculature development is focused on as the pillar on which all posture depends, so core strength protection holds priority in coordinating programmes. There must be sensitivity to even the smallest imbalances. The capacity to respond rapidly to compensate and the strength to counter threat to integrity of structure in this complicated joint complex is critical. Developing movement potential through mobility work and complex motor skills cannot be progressed at the expense of maintaining core strength.

THE LOWER LIMBS

Although the complex of lower limb joints offers a limited movement potential compared with the upper limbs, they are extremely stable. Indeed, this stability is fundamental to the two basic functions of the lower limbs: support of the body's weight, and locomotion.

Hip

It is very important to remember two details when considering hip joint movement. First, some of the muscles which are involved in joint actions at the hip are also involved in joint actions at the knee (fig. 7). Second, the pelvis (hip) is jointed not only with the femur (thigh) but also with the spine. This means that there must be very careful analysis of movement in any technical sport. The correct alignment of pelvis and spine is critical if maximum advantage is to be gained from the contribution of muscle actions at the hip joint (with femur), knee, ankle and foot. The following actions are possible about the axes indicated.

Transverse axis: *flexion* – the thigh is raised forward towards the chest. A limiting factor in this action is the state of flexion or extension at the knee. This is due to the 'hamstrings' group of muscles bridging two joints. When both hips are flexed, there is a tilting upwards and backwards of the pelvis, flattening the

FIG. 7 Effect of two-joint actions on two-joint muscles: rectus femoris (dotted line) and hamstring group (solid line) (from Kapandji, 1988)

lumbar curve. Tilting the pelvis in this way aids hip flexion; *extension* – the thigh is pulled backwards. A limiting factor again is the state of flexion or extension at the knee. This is due to the rectus femoris bridging two joints. The forwards and downwards tilting of the pelvis helps extension. Hyperextension is brought about by exaggerating the lumbar curve. In effect, then, this does not alter the degree of extension between femur and pelvis but does considerably influence the angle between femur and the erect or extended spine above the lumbar region.

Anterio-posterior axis: *abduction* – the drawing apart of the thighs as in moving to stand with legs astride. The movement is limited by the adductor muscles, the iliofemoral and pubofemoral ligaments, and the bony structures themselves. The active maximum is 90°, while passive gives a greater angle only when combined with flexion and the forward tilt of the pelvis; *adduction* – the drawing together of the thighs as in gripping the flanks of a horse. This obviously must be combined with flexion or extension if a thigh is to be adducted past the mid-line of the body. The maximum degree of adduction beyond the mid-line is approximately 30°. The position of greatest instability of this joint is when the hip is well flexed and adducted, e.g. when sitting with the legs crossed.

Vertical axis: *rotation outward (lateral)* – the action of moving towards splayed feet (ballet dancer) is limited by the iliofemoral and pubofemoral ligaments and, consequently, by the state of flexion or extension of femur on pelvis; *rotation inward (medial)* – the action of moving to stand pigeon-toed. This is limited by the ischiofemoral ligament and therefore by flexion or extension at the hip. Inward rotation is the easier, due to the slackness of the ischiofemoral ligament in movements combining flexion/abduction/inward rotation. This particular situation is the root of a problem for the beginner hurdler, who habitually drops the trailing knee to give an abbreviated first stride away from the hurdle.

outward rotation	hip	inward rotation	
60°	flexed	35°–45°	
30°	extended	30°–40°	

Knee

This joint must effect a mechanical compromise to reconcile two mutually exclusive requirements: great stability in extension when body weight and lever lengths impose stress, and great mobility in flexion when the joint must adapt to irregularities of terrain, changes of locomotive speed and direction, and in control of foot movements as in soccer, dancing, etc.

Satisfying these two requirements completely is almost impossible. Despite the ingenious mechanical devices incorporated in the joint, the poor degree of interlocking of surfaces (an essential for mobility) exposes the joint to immense risk of strain and injury. The following actions are possible about the transverse and vertical axes.

Transverse axis: *extension* – straightening the knee. The knee is considered extended when the thigh and lower leg form what is virtually a straight line. Only a very slight increase (5°–10°) is possible beyond this point and may be produced by passive extension, i.e. when standing on a decline. Extension beyond this is abnormal. Extension of the hip aids extension of the knee by stretching the rectus femoris; *flexion* – the action of bringing the heel towards the buttock. The possible range depends on the state of flexion/extension at the hip joint and also whether the knee flexion is active or passive.

active	hip action	passive
140°	flexed	160°
*120°	extended	†110°–140°

*Due to weakened hamstring and stretched rectus femoris, but follow through can bring heel to buttock
†Due to stretch of rectus femoris

Vertical axis (leg in natural alignment with body): *rotation* – this is only possible when knee is flexed, and the degree of rotation varies with the degree of knee flexion until the knee is flexed at 90°; *outward* – the foot is turned outwards, with knees bent as in commencement of the breaststroke leg kick; *inward* – the foot is turned inwards with knees bent, as in the initiation of rotation in javelin and discus.

outward rotation	knee flexion	inward rotation
32°	30°	20°
42°	90°	30°

There is also a phenomenon known as automatic rotation. At the completion of knee extension the lower leg rotates outwards on the femur. Conversely, if the knee is extended while the foot is anchored on the floor (as in standing) then the first action described is seen as the femur rotating inwards on the lower leg. The injury potential in field games such as football and rugby is clear, for example, when there is forced outward rotation of femur on lower leg, while it is naturally rotating inward in extension.

Ankle

Several expressions are used uniquely in describing ankle joint actions. These actions are possible about the transverse, anterio-posterior and vertical axes when the joint is not weight bearing (e.g. when the foot is not in contact with any surface).

Transverse axis: *plantar flexion (flexion)* – this is the action of pointing the toes. To complicate matters, this action is referred to as ankle extension when rising up on the toes (i.e. when the ankle is weight bearing). The main muscles responsible for plantar flexion have greatest efficiency when the knee is extended and the ankle is in dorsi flexion; *dorsi flexion (extension)* – the action of turning the toes up towards the knee. There is less rotation possible in dorsi flexion than there is in plantar flexion.

Anterio-posterior axis: *inversion* – the action of turning the medial (big toe) side of the foot upwards towards the inside of the knee. Inversion injuries (i.e. where the trauma is sustained on the lateral side) account for 80% of all ankle injuries; *eversion* – the action of turning the lateral (small toe) side of the foot upwards towards the outside of the knee.

Due to the demands for directional change in the majority of games, the latter two actions are extremely important. Lateral changes of direction will ultimately require departure from the running surface via inversion or eversion. Moreover, these actions facilitate adaptation to a terrain.

Vertical axis: as indicated above, rotation is more free in plantar flexion than in dorsi flexion; *outward* – the turning of the foot outwards; *inward* – the turning of the foot inwards. Once again, these actions are critical in changing direction and in adjusting balance in variable terrain.

Foot

In discussing the ankle joint actions, especially those of inversion and eversion, the actions of the foot have already been introduced. Man's foot has been the unfortunate victim of the progress of civilisation, and its properties are gradually being lost. Our ancestors may well have been able to oppose their big toes in the same way that we can oppose our thumbs. However, the toes may be flexed, extended, adducted and abducted in much the same way as fingers.

Due to the complex of 26 bones, the foot is well equipped both in strength and mobility to adapt to any type of terrain. This adaptability is obviously fundamental to efficient locomotion. The foot is the first and final contact with the surface of the ground, and a lack of ability to accept loadings of momentum on any given surface will result in dissipation of effort or possible injury.

Kapandji's observations (1988) are worth noting: 'The town dweller always walks on even and firm ground with his feet protected by shoes. There is therefore little need for the arches of his feet to adapt to new terrains and the supporting muscles eventually atrophy: the flat foot is the price paid for progress and some anthropologists go so far as to forecast that man's feet will be

A = Head of first metatarsal
      (ball of big toe).
B = Head of fifth metatarsal
      (ball of small toe).
C = Tubercles of the calcaneus
      (base of heel).

A, B & C are the three
supports for three arches
in each foot. (8a.)
A–B is the anterior arch.
B–C is the lateral arch.
C–A is the medial arch.

Fig 8a.

When both feet are placed together,
a fourth arch is created, half by the
right foot, half by the left. (8b.)
All four arches together constitute
the plantar vault.

Fig 8b.

FIG. 8 Plantar vault

reduced to mere stumps. This thesis is borne out by the fact that in man in contrast to the ape the toes are atrophied and the big toe can no longer be opposed.'

This stage is still a long way off and even civilised man can still walk barefoot on a beach or on the rocks and grip with his toes. There can be little doubt that the small muscles of the foot can and should be developed to maintain the integrity of the plantar vault, inter alia (fig. 8) and, as a consequence, retrieve its adaptive capabilities.

The lower limbs joint complexes afford immense potential from the foundation of strength. We are a long way from exhausting that potential. Control of the toes to hold brushes in painting; of the feet and ankles in flamenco and the modern variants of Celtic dancing; and of total lower limb complexes in soccer, skiing, and ice skating, demonstrate this in the area of motor coordination. Gymnasts, acrobats and limbo dancers demonstrate this in the area of mobility. Weight lifters, ski jumpers, throwers and ballet dancers demonstrate this in the area of strength. Mobility and motor coordination embrace lower limb joint complex movement potential by building on strength.

To summarise chapter 1, an understanding of the extraordinary movement potential of the lever system is fundamental to the design of the technical models demanded of sports disciplines, and to the selection of exercises for effective technical development and technical performance. Chapters 3, 6 and 11 build on this understanding which is then translated through parts 4 and 5 into practice.

FIG. 9 Examples of exercises demonstrating the total movement potential of the body's system of levers: circuit training; active mobility; passive mobility; basic weight training; related strength exercises and specific strength exercises

FIG. 9 Continued

MALE/FEMALE BODY VARIATIONS

Before leaving this section, male/female variations are worth noting. Due to the extreme width of the female pelvis compared with the male pelvis, the angle between femur and tibia is generally greater for women than for men. This is clearly a disadvantage when force of knee and hip extension is required and highlights the high injury potential not only at knee and hip, but at the junction of sacrum and ilium, and pubic symphysis which are less stable in women than in men, particularly in the two or three days premenstruation.

The female shoulders are also narrower than in men and the lateral angle radius/ulna on humerus is greater, providing a weaker force application potential in 'pulling' and 'pushing' activities. The length of the female spine is approximately 86% that of the male spine and this, combined with a greater distribution of weight towards hips/thighs, gives women a relatively lower centre of gravity and therefore an advantage where potential stability and/or balance is required.

SUMMARY

Whole body movement, and the movement at each joint, can be described in terms of rotations about axes. These movements are classified as actions in specific anatomical terms. In any given activity, several combinations of joint actions, made possible by a specific programme of muscle contractions, will take place. The interplay of these actions will dictate the final efficiency as an expression of energy.

In the first instance, the range of a joint action will be a function of that joint's structure. Secondary limiting factors are imposed by the soft tissue structures bridging and surrounding the joint. A working knowledge of all the body's structures must then be seen as basic to an appreciation of the body's total movement potential and to analysis of technical models. It is convenient to study body movement with reference to three areas.

(1) The upper limb complex is designed for mobility and is the final link in a force sequence for many activities. By its nature, it is the fastest link in the force sequence and training is aimed at ensuring that the contribution of this link is synchronised in its application of speed, force, range, and final technical 'touch' after other joint complexes have provided their contributions.

(2) The spine is variously a complex of joints providing a remarkable range of movement in some activities and a powerful pillar linking lower and upper limb complexes in others. Both strength and mobility must be developed to ensure that demands of stability and mobility can be met.

(3) The lower limb complex is the initiator of a force sequence in many activities. Great force must be generated by the complex, frequently with only instantaneous

ground contact. Moreover, it must offer sufficient mobility to permit rapid adjustment to any given terrain. Consequently the lower limb must provide mobility, stability and the capacity to express force at speed.

It must be stressed that although the coach considers each joint action in analysis of a given movement, no action should be thought of in isolation, but as part of the total movement, both in terms of force contribution and timing.

2 STRUCTURAL CHANGES IN THE GROWING CHILD

STAGES OF GROWTH

It takes approximately 20 years for all the morphological, physiological and psychological processes of development to bring the newly born child to maturity. The unfolding of his development is a long but necessary period, during which time growth cannot simply be seen as an increase in height and weight, but as a gentle ebb and flow of differentiating and integrating forms and functions.

The child, in his various stages of growth, is not a mini-adult. It must be clearly understood that from stage to stage in his growth, the child varies in the proportion of individual body parts in terms of length, volume and weight. Each part grows at a different rate, ranging from twofold expansion (head) to fivefold expansion (legs), between birth and maturity (figs. 10, 11). Implicit in this is that certain skills may require considerable adjustment of the neuromuscular processes from year to year, according to shifting emphasis of growth. Consequently, as the athlete grows, it seems advisable to maintain principal elements of technique training throughout the year, relating the solutions to short-term technical challenges to long-term technical models.

Several authorities have attempted to classify the stages of development (see table 3).

Stage	Characteristic growth landmarks	Age Male	Female
Newly born	Healing of the umbilicus		
Infant	Up to appearance of first milk teeth	0.5	0.5
Crawling age	Up to learning to walk	1–1.5	1–1.5
Small child	Up to appearance of the first permanent tooth	6	6
Early school age (pre-puberty)	Until first signs of maturity. Beginning of growth spurt, rapid genital development, first breast development	11	9

TABLE 3 Stages of growth against age and gender (adapted from Grimme, 1953)

Stage	Characteristic growth landmarks	Age	
		Male	Female
Puberty	Period between appearance of pubic hair and first menarche or development of male sperms	14	14–15
Adolescence	Puberty and end of physical growth	22	18
Age of achievement	Period of optimal capacity	variations in these stages cover a great range but are normal	

TABLE 3 Continued

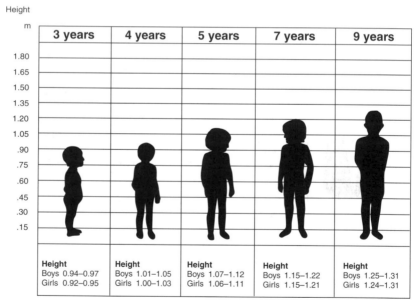

FIG. 10 Growth of the child. Average height progression, showing the 'parting of the ways' after approximately nine years, in terms of relative height increase, and absolute height. Modified from *Family Health Guide* (Reader's Digest, 1972).

Height
m

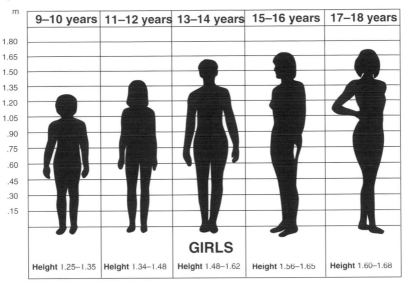

9–10 years	11–12 years	13–14 years	15–16 years	17–18 years

GIRLS

| Height 1.25–1.35 | Height 1.34–1.48 | Height 1.48–1.62 | Height 1.56–1.65 | Height 1.60–1.68 |

Height
m

9–10 years	11–12 years	13–14 years	15–16 years	17–18 years

BOYS

| Height 1.25–1.37 | Height 1.36–1.48 | Height 1.47–1.61 | Height 1.59–1.74 | Height 1.66–1.81 |

FIG. 10 Continued

FIG. 11 Alterations in body proportions during growth (from Bammes, 1964)

Skeletal development

With the exception of the skull and collar bone (clavicle), all the bones in the body are formed from cartilage. The process starts from before birth and concludes with final ossification of the skeleton between 18 and 22 years of age. Bone lengthens by growing at the junction between the main shaft and the growing end which is known as the epiphysis. In the long bones (i.e. the arms and legs), most growth takes place at one end only. This is extremely significant when one considers that the thigh bone, for example, grows mostly at the knee end, which is exposed to considerable training loads. Ossification is the destruction and breakdown of cartilage and its replacement with bone tissue. This process is accompanied by the setting down of an increasingly thick layer of bone around the cartilage (perichondral ossification) and from within the cartilage (endochondral ossification).

The growing bone has a greater proportion of softer material in the basic substance, which is essential for compressive and tensile strength. This, and the sponge-like nature of immature bone material, which is still in the process of developing adaptability to loading, means that the growing bone is more elastic but has less bending strength. This is a major cause of the reduced load-bearing capacity of the child's skeleton.

Hormones affect the process and rate of skeletal development, but functional loading may also influence the process. Most research has considered the role of hormones, but a considerable volume of research would indicate that controlled loadings will favourably influence skeletal growth. Research in this area has suggested that: (1) intermittent submaximal loading (80–90% maximum) stimulates height growth (Tittel, 1963); (2) excessive loading in quality or quantity inhibits height growth (Schede, 1963); and (3) muscle pull, above all, is the functional stimulus for the growth in thickness of the bone (Harre, 1973).

It is my opinion that, in the early growth stages, working the child to a point where loading cannot be repeated due to fatigue and/or insufficient strength is fundamentally working against the most favourable conditions for healthy growth. However, insufficient motivation on the part of the child may terminate activity long before this point is reached.

Craig (1972) has suggested that, by developing a systematic general training programme of exercise for all muscle groups, sufficient balance is achieved to relieve bones of possible continuation and/or accumulation of stressors which can exist where the bone is required to accept a loading for which it is not ready. Such accumulation must be avoided, as Craig has noted: 'the cumulative effect of the repetitive trauma of such stressors will cause injury, which may not manifest itself until later athletic life'. Caution, then, should be exercised in encouraging the growing athlete to attempt loadings near his 'motivated limit', i.e. limits arrived at through strong external motivation.

Tendencies of growth

We can see from figures 12a and 12b that, over time, there is a pattern to the increase in weight and height. By plotting this we can identify anomalies in growth and development, and select athletes on the basis of specific anthropometric criteria for a sport or discipline.

There is reference in several papers to phases of extension (growing up) and phases of abundance (growing out) as factors of some importance in the training of athletes. Such changes, then, are not a matter of continuous increase. Several attempts have been made to relate these phases to athletic events and performances (table 4).

The changes in relative body dimensions have been mentioned earlier in connection with the possible variations in the development of athletic skill and ability. The amazing complexity of this shift in relative dimension is probably best illustrated in a piece of work conducted on elite swimmers between eight and 14 years of age in the former German Democratic Republic (GDR) as figure 13 shows. Looking to the future, tables may be constructed to show indices of age-specific, strength-weight ratios as this might give a clear guide as to which physical characteristics (age-dependent, or specific growth rate dependent) are temporarily regressive (table 4).

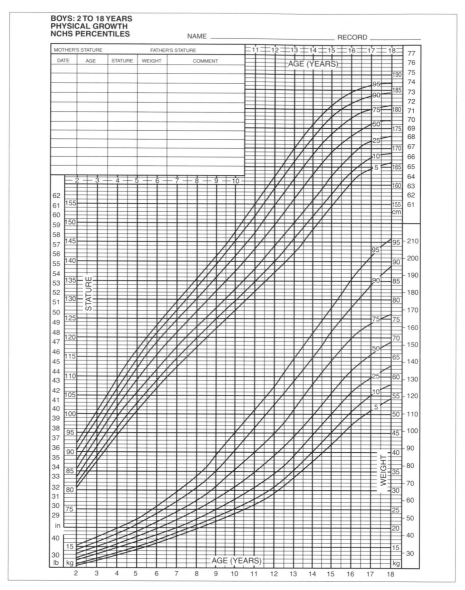

FIGS 12a Boys' Physical Growth Percentiles

Against this background it is important to avoid the temptation to ignore the less proficient in favour of the superior athlete in his early teens. Superiority may well be due to early physical development which frequently leaves an athlete's peers unable to meet him on equal terms. The spread of growth in these years is considerable. Attention must therefore be given to those youngsters who are able to perform skills efficiently, and compete with considerable success, but have yet to develop. In short, a judgement of body size based solely on age is unreliable, but can

FIG 12b Girls' Physical Growth Percentiles

be made reliable if it is seen against the individual's stage of maturity. Early, late and normal developers must be seen in 'performance perspective'.

The total time of pubescent growth lasts longer for boys, although girls start earlier by 1½–2 years. The 14-year-old girl is already approximately 97% final height, and at 18 years of age is 96% final leg length. On the other hand, the 14-year-old boy is approximately 85% final height, and 80% final leg length at 18–22 years of age.

feature		norm value		mean value		spread	mean of 5 best	
		value	age	value	age		value	age
Class 7 x	Height cm	151.6	13	159.2	14.5	150.9–167.3	160.3	16
+ 12.8 yrs	Weight kg	40.7	13	43.0	13.5	34.4–51.6	54.5	15.5
	Thigh length mm			429		409–447	444	
	Lower leg length mm			358		336–378	380	
Class 8 x	Height	157.8	14	167.1	15.5	160.9–173.2	169.3	16
+ 13.8 yrs	Weight	45.7	14	50.0	15.0	43.4–56.6	52.2	15.5
	Thigh length			448		430–466	460	
	Lower leg length			376		352–397	386	
Class 9 x	Height	163.6	15	173.0	16	168.1–177.9	175.3	16
+ 15 yrs	Weight	50.7	15	56.6	16	50.9–62.3	60.1	16
	Thigh length					450–478	469	
	Lower leg length					374–408	400	

TABLE 4 Comparison of body measurements of young middle distance athletes with the average values for the former German Democratic Republic (adapted from Harre from Marcusson 1986).

SUMMARY

The period up to and through the adolescence years of rapid growth is not only one of preparation for serious competition in the later peak performance years in the 20s and 30s, it is also a period of preparation for high pressure competition in the growing years. Clearly this is the case in sports such as gymnastics and, to a variable extent, swimming, but it is also true where an early and exceptional level of talent takes an athlete beyond his peers and finds him competitive in top level sport. As a consequence, the coach must understand the athlete's patterns of growth. From these patterns it seems logical to establish the fundamentals of techniques before the pubertal growth spurt, as pubescence and adolescence create disproportionate relationships between body parts. In some instances, a technical model is established to meet the short-term objectives of junior arenas, then changed later. In others the model will be progressively modified in stages to suit the demands of short-, medium- and long-term performance objectives. Training loads should be progressed via numbers of repetitions and/or speed rather than by increasing resistance, which should not go beyond an estimated 80–90% maximum. Epiphyses are almost certainly damaged if this advice is ignored. Loading which compresses the spine, as in several orthodox weight lifting exercises, must not be employed until the spine has stopped growing and/or has been protected by developed spinal musculature. Prediction of height growth patterns is possible and is used in several countries to select athletes according to anthropometric trends in given disciplines.

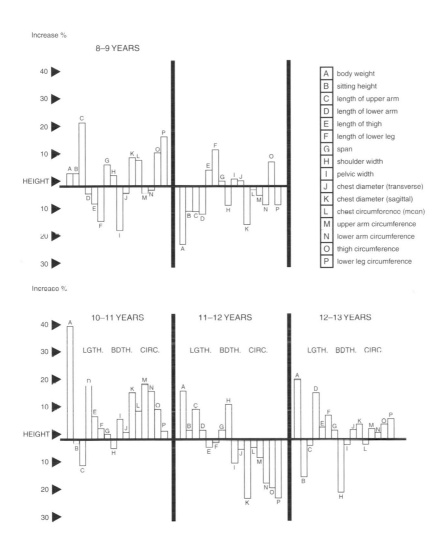

FIG. 13 Relative rate of growth of body parts (from Harre, 1986)

3 BASIC MECHANICS

A detailed knowledge of 'laminae and particles' is not required by the student of training theory, but he should attempt to achieve some working knowledge of those terms which are most frequently used in analyses. To this end, the following is presented.

DEFINITIONS

Motion

Motion is simply a change of position, but should be defined as a change relative to another body, a fixed point, etc. For example, the femur flexes on the pelvis; the basketball player breaks past his opposite number, and so on. Some types of motion are not easily observed because they are too slow (e.g. the opening of a flower) or because they are too fast (e.g. the beating of a fly's wing). Cinematographic analysis is often used to study motion in sport. Such study may range from an analysis of team play to the analysis of an athlete's technical efficiency.

Rest is the status of an object when its position, with respect to some point, line, surface, etc., remains unchanged. It is important to know that in any given activity there is no movement at some joints while there is at others. Where there is no movement the muscle activity is referred to as *static* and where there is movement the muscle activity is *dynamic*.

A study of motion and rest, relative to limbs or bodies, etc., forms the basis of mechanical analysis: *linear motion* is motion in a straight line. This is also referred to as translatory motion (e.g. running 60 m); *angular motion* is the motion of rotation. This is also referred to as rotary motion (e.g. a front somersault); *curvilinear motion* is motion which involves linear and angular motion (e.g. a cartwheel or a hammer thrower advancing and turning across the circle).

Centre of gravity

The centre of gravity is a body's centre of weight. In other words, it is that point about which the body is balanced relative to all three axes. When a body is in flight, any rotation takes place about the centre of gravity. When describing rotation in flight, direction of rotation about an axis is defined as clockwise or anticlockwise.

Vertical axis (long axis of the body): the athlete is standing on the clock face, i.e. a pirouette to the right is a clockwise rotation (fig. 14b).

Transverse axis (axis through the hips, left to right): the athlete has the clock face on his left, i.e. a front somersault is a clockwise rotation (fig. 14a).

Anterio-posterior axis (axis from front to back through hips): the athlete faces the clock, i.e. a cartwheel to the right is clockwise rotation (fig. 14c).

The centre of gravity represents the intersection of these axes, which in the athlete's body is roughly half way between umbilicus and pubic crest and 3 cm in front of the spine. Provided the imaginary perpendicular from this point to the ground falls within the athlete's 'base' (e.g. feet), he will not fall over. The relationship of this perpendicular to the body's point(s) of support is critical in the study of sports technique.

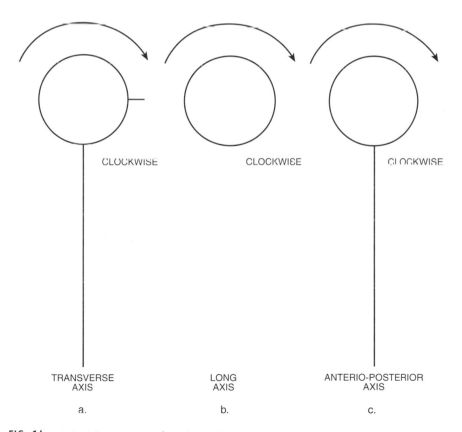

FIG. 14 Basis for defining rotation about the body's axes

Force

Force is anything which produces motion or changes of motion. It could also be seen as a push or pull, a tendency to distort, and so on. As applied to work or movement analysis, three factors must be considered: (1) magnitude of force, i.e. its size (e.g. 400 joules); (2) direction of the force, i.e. in which direction the force is applied (e.g. vertically); and (3) point of application of force, i.e. where the force is being applied (e.g. at the athlete's foot) as figure 15 shows.

Work is the overcoming of a load or resistance and is measured as the product of force x distance moved. In most cases, the force producing work in moving the athlete's limbs is the contraction of muscle. This usually results in a shortening and thickening of the muscle without a change in volume. The product of the force with which it contracts, and the range through which the force is applied, is the measure of the mechanical work performed by the muscle. Some confusion must arise when the muscle contraction is static (isometric). The force provided by the contracting muscle is applied through 0 range – producing mechanical work of force x 0 = 0. In this case there appears to be no mechanical work performed, but energy has certainly been expressed as physiological work which might be measured in terms of heat energy. It becomes convenient, then, to measure mechanical work according to its energy cost.

Energy cost

One joule of work is that performed in raising 1 newton, 1 m. One newton is the force acting on the mass of 1 kg at normal acceleration of gravity. One joule may also be expressed as 0.239 calories. One calorie is the amount of heat required to raise 1 g water, 1°C. The basic unit for most purposes is a kilocalorie (kcal) which is 1000 calories (4186 joules). The energy costs of various activities can be calculated and standardised as an aid to studying the balance of energy input (nutrition) against energy output (work). For example, sitting at ease = 1.6 kcals/minute, while walking at 8.8 kph on flat ground = 5.6 kcals/minute. (See also table 6, p. 51.)

The athlete's body weight should remain constant if the calorie input (diet) equals the calorie output (activity).

Machines

A machine is a device for performing work. Among the simplest machines are the pulley, the lever, the wheel and axle, the inclined plane, the wedge and the screw. All complex machines comprise simple machines which, in the case of the athlete are almost always levers. Machines are concerned with two forces – that put into the machine (effort, or internal force, or force) and that which the machine attempts to overcome (resistance, or external force, or load).

A lever is a rod turning about a fixed point (axis). In the athlete, the levers are bones. The forces are expressed by the contracting muscles pulling on the bones,

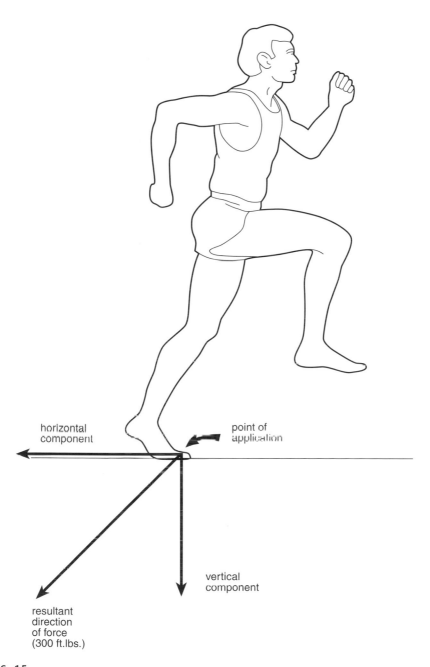

horizontal
component

point of
application

vertical
component

resultant
direction
of force
(300 ft.lbs.)

FIG. 15 Force application in long jump

CLASS 1

CLASS 2

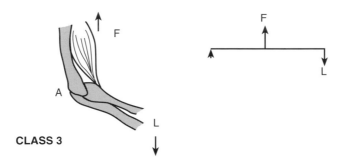

CLASS 3

FIG. 16   Classes of lever

Class 1   Triceps extending forearm on arm; gastrocnemeus, soleus
and plantaris plantar
flexing – when foot is off the ground

Class 2   Gastrocnemeus, soleus and plantaris
plantar flexing – when the foot is on the ground

Class 3   Biceps, brachialis, brachioradialis and pronator teres flexing
the forearm on the arm

and the loads vary from other bones or the athlete's own body weight, to external loads such as barbells, discoi, oars, water, kinetic energies, etc.

The efficiency of the lever depends on certain mechanical factors. Of primary importance are the exact position on the lever of the application of force (F), the location of the load (L), and the axis in question (A).

The relative positions of these points dictates the 'class' of lever and, while it is not essential that these are memorised, an understanding of how these levers work may help in technical analysis (fig. 16). Broadly speaking, class 1 is built for equilibrium, class 2 for saving force, and class 3 for speed and range of movement. The distance from F to A is known as the force arm, and the distance from L to A as the load arm. Any lever system will balance when:

$$\text{force} \times \text{force arm} = \text{load} \times \text{load arm}$$

In table 5, what force is required to make each system balance in a class 1 lever system? From the figures in table 5, the following can be seen.

(1) The force required to move the lever is indirectly proportional to the length of the force arm.

(2) Only when the two arms are equal in length will the force equal the load.

(3) By adding to the length of the force arm, the force may be reduced to almost nothing.

(4) The effect of the load follows the same rules as those which determine the effect of the force.

(5) The force necessary to operate the class 1 lever depends upon the relative length of the lever arms.

With small adjustments these observations also apply to class 2 and class 3 levers.

force	x	force arm	=	resistance	x	load arm	answer
F	x	2	=	10	x	18	F = 90
F	x	8	=	10	x	12	F = 15
F	x	16	=	10	x	4	F = 2.5
F	x	8	=	10	x	2	F = 2.5

TABLE 5 Equilibrium exists where force x force arm = load (resistance) x load arm

This brief expansion on the 'mathematics of levers' is not advanced purely for academic interest. It may help, for example, in creating new possibilities for strength training where the total available resistance is relatively low. By thoughtful use of levers, or pulleys, the effect of this low resistance can be increased.

Before moving on from levers, the value should be noted of bony devices which provide greater mechanical advantage of muscle pull. They achieve this by increasing the length of the lever arm, changing the direction of force application, and so on. There are several examples, but few illustrate this better than the patella (kneecap). The force of muscle pull may be thought of as having two components. One provides rotation of one lever on another and the other pulls along the length of the levers, and by so doing provides joint stability. If the direction of muscle pull is almost parallel with the levers concerned, the stabilising component is very great and the rotational component small. The converse is true if the direction of muscle pull is more angular. The patella changes the direction of application of force of the knee extensors by providing a greater angle of insertion of the patellar ligament into the tibial tuberosity. This change of direction raises the effective force of the knee extension by increasing the component of rotation and decreasing the stabilising component.

LAWS OF MOTION

There are three laws of motion – inertia, acceleration and reaction.

The law of inertia

A resting or moving body will remain in that state until a force alters this situation. By this law, both motion and rest are states of resistance or loading. The amount of resistance to change of state (inertia) is dependent upon the mass of the body concerned and its velocity. Velocity is the relationship of the distance covered to the time taken – *and it has a direction* (45 kph south). Inertia has legion examples in sport, ranging from starting in rowing or sprinting, to raising an opponent in wrestling, to tackling in rugby.

The law of acceleration

Acceleration is directly proportional to the force causing it and inversely proportional to the mass of the body involved. Acceleration is the rate of change of velocity. This implies increase or decrease in the distance covered in a given period of time but, in addition, since velocity has direction, acceleration must also be implied in a rate of change of direction. Thus centripetal acceleration is that continuous change of direction which permits an athlete or cyclist to move round a curve.

The law of reaction

For every action there is an equal and opposite reaction. When stepping onto a chair or box, one is supported by the counterforce offered by the chair or box. If the counterforce is less, one will fall through! When flight is considered, as in jumping, and a body part moves in one direction, then some other part or equivalence of force must act in the opposite direction.

Gravity

One force which will act on the body at all times is that of gravity. When an athlete launches himself or an object into flight, as soon as flight is commenced, there is a force which causes a reduction in upward velocity at a speed of 981.274 cm/sec^2. The centre of gravity of the object or athlete will be seen to trace a course – a parabola (fig. 17). It should be noted that whether or not the athlete rotates or moves parts of his body while in flight, the parabola of the athlete's centre of gravity is dictated by the angle and speed of take-off. Should the implement have aerodynamic properties then, of course, the flight path will not be a parabola.

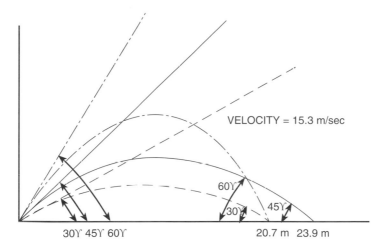

FIG. 17 Once launched, the centre of gravity of athlete or implement must follow a parabolic path in flight. Here, this is seen in the path of the object projected at various angles at 15.3 m/sec.

Momentum

Momentum is the quantity of motion and is therefore the product of mass x velocity. The body is frequently put in motion, or assisted in motion, by transfer of momentum from a part of the body to the whole body, as in the free leg and arms in the high jump. Momentum may be linear or angular.

Mass

Mass is the quantity of matter. It is given dimension from weight/gravity.

Moment of inertia

Moment of inertia is the distribution of a body's mass, i.e. its size. If a gymnast tucks himself into a ball, his moment of inertia is small about the transverse axis. If he extends into a star shape, his moment of inertia is large about the transverse axis. Moment of inertia might well be thought of as the rotating body's radius.

Angular momentum

Angular momentum is the product of the moment of inertia x angular velocity, i.e. revolutions per minute. The importance of understanding angular momentum should not be underestimated because it has a considerable number of applications in sport. This concept may be illustrated by assuming that an imaginary gymnast is rotating at 5 revs/minute with a radius of three units. His angular momentum is (3 x 5) = 15 units. Now, assuming there is no deceleration due to friction, air resistance, and so on, the momentum will remain at 15 units. If the athlete now reduces the radius to one unit, the momentum remaining the same, his angular velocity is now 15 revs/minute. An understanding of this may enable sophisticated control of rotation in flight.

Related in part to this is the fact that the reaction of the body to a long lever will be greater than to a short one. In throwing movements involving rotation of the body, the longer the lever, the less will be the force but the greater will be the instantaneous linear speed at the end of the lever. This is also relevant in all striking activities, ranging from golf to soccer.

Finally, when considering rotation, it is worth bearing in mind that it is seldom about one axis only. Also, in several sports, there can be the sudden intervention of an outside force when a body is already rotating. When this happens, the principle of precession applies. When a body is rotating clockwise about one axis, and a force intervenes to make it rotate clockwise about a second axis, the reaction is for the body to rotate clockwise about the third. If the intervening force in this situation makes it rotate anticlockwise about the second, the reaction is anticlockwise about the third (fig. 14).

SUMMARY

There has been no intention here to present an exhaustive review of mechanics, but more realistically to establish some understanding of basic terminology used in mechanical analysis. It must be remembered that in dealing with mechanical laws, the athlete is biomechanical and flexible; he is not a machine, but a man. The excellent and more detailed mechanical information available to students of physical education and coaches in specific texts must always be interpreted with this in mind.

Because the neuromusculoskeletal complex is a self-regulating system operating within a framework of mechanical laws, even a well-established technical model may be compromised. Muscular imbalances, poorly-monitored practice and fatigue, for example, may produce compensatory biomechanical adjustments which, over a period of time, create less effective technique and, as a consequence, underperformance. Ideally, technical performance should be regularly monitored via biomechanical analysis using digital video. There is a growing resource of software programs specifically designed for this purpose. Throughout his career, Jack Nicklaus, the legendary golfer, annually worked with a professional over a two-week period to 'realign my swing'. Compensations must be determined to reestablish technical models which are stable and robust.

SUMMARY OF PART 1

When analysing movement or investigating new possibilities of technique, it is tempting to focus attention on a single joint action or on one mechanical principle. However, it is basic to all study of movement that it is the most efficient compromise which must be sought. Moreover, one must be constantly aware of a joint action relative to other joint actions, a joint action relative to whole body movement, and all actions relative to mechanical laws. Consequently it is suggested that the student of techniques in sport should establish a technical model for a given discipline or sport. This technical model will represent the most efficient compromise. It will embrace broad principles of movement, such as upward tilting of the pelvis for all activities where vigorous extension of the leg(s) is required to give vertical force (e.g. in most lifts, throws and jumps), or the sequence of joint action and force direction in all arm strike activities. These broad principles are, in the main, based on common sense and a knowledge of anatomy and mechanics. However, many principles have grown simply from experience and observation. For example, it is debatable whether coaching points such as 'keep your eye on the ball' in racquet games, cricket, volleyball and baseball, or 'keep your head down' when playing a golf shot or kicking a ball, grew from an extensive knowledge of anatomy or mechanics!

Whether principles grow from theory or from experience, one is always drawn to the same conclusion that our system of levers must be considered in its entirety when creating technical models and, thereafter, suggesting coaching advice. The sciences of kinesiology and biomechanics have grown from applied anatomy and mechanics. The coach, who wishes to create a deeper reservoir of information as a basis for establishing technical models and for studying their development, should take time to study these sciences.

Formerly when coaches wished to experiment beyond existing technical models, it came down to trial and error and the occasional casualty. Today, new models specific to athlete can be trialled via computer generated hologram imagery. Varying degrees of adjustment to speed, range, direction, force and synchronisation of one or several joint actions may be built into the model and performance outcomes analysed.

REFERENCES FOR PART 1

Collective Authors (1972) *The Family Health Guide.* Reader's Digest, London

Craig, T. (1972) *Prevention is the Only Cure.* 3rd Coaches' Convention Report

Harre, D. (1986) *Principles of Sport Training.* Sportverlag, Berlin

Kapandji, I. A. *The Physiology of the Joints.* Churchill-Livingstone, London, Vol. 1 (1982) Vol. 2 (1988) Vol. 3 (1995)

Marcusson, H. (1961) *Das Wachstrum von Kindern und Jugendlichen in der Deutschen Demokratischen Republic.* Akademie Verlag, Berlin

MacKenna, B. R. & Callender, R. (1998) *Illustrated Physiology.* Churchill Livingstone, Edinburgh

Provins, K. & Salter, N. (1955) Maximum torque exerted about the elbow joint. *Journal of Applied Physiology* 7, pp 393–398

Rasch, P. J. & Burke, R. K. (1968) *Kinesiology and Applied Anatomy.* 3rd Edn. Lea & Febiger, Philadelphia

Rasch, P. J. (1989) *Kinesiology and Applied Anatomy.* 7th Edn. Lea & Febiger, Philadelphia

Tittel, K. (1963) *Beschreibende und Funktionelle Anatomie Des Menschen.* Jena, Fischer (Hueter, Volkmann, Jores)

BIBLIOGRAPHY

Clarke, H. H. (1967) *Application of Measurement to Health and Physical Education.* 4th Edn. PrenticeHall Inc., New Jersey

Collective Authors (1975) *Abstracts of the 5th International Congress of Biomechanics.* S.V.U.L., Helsinki

Cooper, J. M. & Glassow, R. B. (1972) *Kinesiology.* C. V. Mosby, St. Louis

Dyson, G. H. G. (1977) *The Mechanics of Athletics.* 7th Edn. University of London Press

Fleishman, I. E. (1964) *The Structure and Measurement of Physical Fitness.* PrenticeHall Inc., New Jersey

Hay, J. G. (1973) *The Biomechanics of Sports Techniques.* PrenticeHall Inc., New Jersey

Hopper, B. J. (1973) *The Mechanics of Human Movement.* Crosby, Lockwood, Staples, London

Jeffries, M. (1976) *Know Your Body.* BBC Publications, London

Kelley, D. L. (1971) *Kinesiology: Fundamentals of Motion Description.* PrenticeHall Inc., New Jersey

MacConaill, M. A. & Basmajian, J. V. (1969) *Muscles and Movements: A Basis for Human Kinesiology.* Williams & Wilkins Co., Baltimore

Margaria, R. *(1976) Biomechanics and Energetics of Muscular Exercise.* Clarendon Press, Oxford

Nourse, A. E. (1972) *The Body*. 3rd Edn. TimeLife International, Amsterdam

Scott, M. G. (1963) *Analysis of Human Motion*. 2nd Edn. AppletonCenturyCrofts, New York

Spence, D. W. (1975) *Essentials of Kinesiology: A Laboratory Manual*. Lea & Febiger, Philadelphia

Tricker, R. A. R. & Tricker, B. J. L. (1968) *The Science of Movement*. Mills & Boon, London

PART 2

THE LIVING MACHINE

The analogy is often made of athlete and machine. The 'machine' in this case must develop increased efficiency of *energy expression* and *energy production* in the athlete's pursuit of competitive advantage. Moreover, the 'machine' is actively involved in the development process.

In part 1, the *skeletal* and *muscular systems* were seen as the basic structures which give final expression of energy when programmed to do so via the *central nervous system* (discussed in part 3).

In part 2, the production of energy to give those structures movement is considered in detail, as is the collective involvement of several other systems. The *digestive system* processes the nutritional content of the athlete's diet to produce not only energy for bodily function, but also the various materials necessary to maintenance, repair and growth. The *oxygen transporting system* combines the *respiratory* and *circulatory* systems in its role of carrying oxygen and fuel to the working muscle where chemical energy is converted to mechanical energy. To permit all systems to function with least possible embarrassment, there must be a dynamic stability of the body's internal environment. This is afforded by the *fluid systems* and *endocrine system*.

Dr Craig Sharp advised on part 2.

4 NUTRITION

The connection between the foods we eat and our functional capacity has been the subject of considerable interest for at least 3000 years. Biblical injunctions concerning the diet are numerous and, in other religions and cultures, food taboos and rituals may often be traced to this connection.

One of the first accounts of how meat might influence muscular work was recorded in Greece around the 5th century BC. The normal diet of the time was vegetarian but two athletes turned carnivorous and the result was evidently an increase in body bulk and weight. Thereafter, the belief that meat would make up for loss of muscular substance during heavy work gained considerable ground. Even today, the intrusion of scientific half-truths has reinforced this belief and many athletes will not go without meat during preparation for competition. The reason for the popularity of such half-truths and beliefs may be summed up by Astrand (1967): 'The fact that muscles are built of protein makes it tempting to conclude that ingestion of excess protein stimulates muscle growth and strength.' While lack of certain foodstuffs may bring about a decrease in functional capacity, or even illness, it has yet to be proved that excessive consumption of foodstuffs will increase functional capacity.

The energy value of food is measured in kilocalories (kcal) (see p. 38). Foods vary in their calorie content: 1 g carbohydrate yields 4 kcal, 1 g lipid yields 9 kcal, 1 g protein yields 4 kcal. A detailed account of the day's activities can help establish the athlete's daily kilocalorie expenditure. For quick reference, the energy cost of various activities is often standardised (table 6). In sport, not only should we ensure appropriate kilocalorie intake, but also quantity of carbohydrate, protein and lipid (table 7).

Energy needs depend on activity, age, gender and body build. Most energy is used when the muscles are working during breathing, digestion, circulation, exercise, etc. A balanced diet should provide correct nutrition and, ideally, the same amount of energy that is expended in activity. Foods are classified according to their nutritional value:

Macronutrients

- Carbohydrates provide the body with energy.
- Lipids provide stored energy.
- Proteins supply material for growth and repair of body tissues.

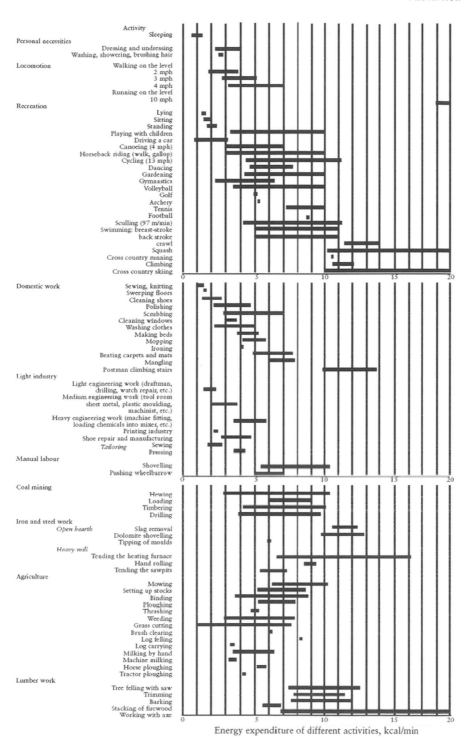

Energy expenditure of different activities, kcal/min

TABLE 6 Energy expenditure of different activities (from Astrand and Rodahl, 1986)

Micronutrients

- Mineral elements contribute towards growth and repair and essential body chemistry.
- Vitamins regulate the body mechanisms.
- Phytonutrients support the immune system.

Water

- Water is essential in all body functions (74% lean body mass; 65–75% body volume).

The majority of foods only become usable after their complex structure has been broken down into simpler forms. This process begins in the mouth when food is cut and ground up by the teeth and mixed with saliva. Digestion of most foods begins at this stage, due to the presence of enzymes. The stomach, a muscular bag which contracts rhythmically, continues the churning and digestive process by adding its own enzymes in the juices it secretes, and there are others later in the digestive corridor in the duodenum (part of the small intestine).

sport/discipline	k calories gm/kg/day	carbohydrate gm/kg/day	fats gm/kg/day	protein gm/kg/day
% contribution of macronutrients to daily kcal intake of athletes	100%	65–75%	15–25%	10%
Speed elastic strength: e.g. sprints, jumps, gymnastics, racquet games, volleyball, baseball, related field sports roles	3,500– 5,000	8	15%	1,5– 2,0
Strength endurance: e.g. middle distance, swimming, rowing, skating, downhill skiing, related field sports roles	4,000– 6,000	8–10	20%	1,5– 2,0
Strength: e.g. weight lifting, throws, wrestling, related field sports roles	6,000– 8,000	6–8	25%	2,0– 2,5
Endurance: e.g. long distance, langlauf, 90 mins+ efforts	4,000– 7,000	10	25%	1,5

TABLE 7 General picture of athletes' diets

MACRONUTRIENTS

Carbohydrates

As their name suggests these are compounds of carbon, hydrogen and oxygen. Carbohydrate is the principal constituent of the normal diet and, generally speaking, it meets most of the body's energy requirement. Carbohydrates occur in several forms – the simple sugars or monosaccharides, and the complex sugars, i.e. disaccharides, trisaccharides, etc. Simple sugars are often regarded as 'empty calories' and the recommended balance in the diet should be 60–65% complex sugars to 40–35% simple sugars.

Simple sugars

Major monosaccharides
The most common in normal diet are the hexoses (six carbon atoms).

Glucose: as the end product of carbohydrate digestion, glucose is the main form of carbohydrate used by the body and is the major fuel required to provide energy. It occurs naturally in sweet fruits.

Fructose: similar to glucose in terms of its carbon, hydrogen and oxygen composition, fructose is apparently absorbed more readily than glucose and, being independent of insulin, is not associated with the 'rebound hypoglycaemia' sometimes caused by too rich sugar foods, such as sweets and chocolate. Its value as a fuel, then, might be countered by its implications for coronary heart disease and the possibility of acidosis caused by increased blood lactate when consumed in large quantities. It is found in honey, sweet fruits and maize.

Galactose: though similar to glucose, galactose is found in different sources, mainly yeast, liver and human milk.

Complex sugars

Disaccharides (fig. 18)

Sucrose: this sugar is found most commonly in the diet. It's found in maple syrup, treacle, white, brown and demerara sugar. Digestion breaks it down to glucose and fructose. Sucrose is a valuable energy source but, unfortunately, it encourages the activity of oral bacteria responsible for tooth decay.

Lactose: during digestion lactose, which is the starch found in milk, is broken down to glucose and galactose. Milk has a very high nutritional value, although recent research has indicated an apparent 'lactose intolerance' in some individuals.

Maltose: this sugar is found in malt extract. Malt is the product of heating and drying germinated barley (a necessary link in the brewing and distilling processes).

FIG. 18 Disaccharides

Digestion breaks maltose down to glucose only. Malt extract is a most valuable source of energy for the athlete.

Trisaccharides and tetrasaccharides

These sugars occur less frequently in foods than monosaccharides and disaccharides. The trisaccharides are found in peas, beans, and in both root and green vegetables. The tetrasaccharides are found in such foods as the meat substitutes used by vegetarians. Little importance is attached to the trisaccharides and tetrasaccharides as energy suppliers and, since they are difficult to break down and may cause indigestion, their intake is not recommended for the athlete.

Polysaccharides

Starch: the principal energy source and the product of cereals. It might be thought of as the stored energy of vegetables. The digestive system breaks down the starches to maltose, which itself is broken down to glucose. Sources of starch are legion, ranging from bread to rice to pasta. Heating breaks down the starch molecules to smaller compounds called dextrins.

Glycogen: this sugar is to animals what starch is to vegetables. It is referred to as 'stored glucose' in the athlete, and is found in the liver and muscle. When released it is a readily available fuel source as glucose in muscle. It is the glycogen reservoir that the liver accesses in its vital function of maintaining levels of blood glucose, which is the *only* fuel for the brain.

Cellulose: Though of very little food value to the body, cellulose gives plants their rigid structure and provides essential fibre in the diet. Western diets tend to be low in fibre; a fact that is of some concern to nutritionists, for it is a most vital component of diet. Intestinal health is dependant on a regular flow of nutrients and expulsion of waste. Fibre in the diet ensures this. Fruit and vegetables are key resources, as are high-fibre bran breakfast cereals. Natural bran is favoured here as it expands on its journey through the digestive system, whereas most other breakfast cereals shrink.

The body is well-equipped with regulatory mechanisms which discourage the immediate absorption of food substances once saturation level has been reached. However, this mechanism can be bypassed according to Saltin and Hermansen (1967) who advanced the 'glycogen overshoot' theory. It is believed that this has considerable significance for the long duration endurance athletes who must have high reserves of energy. Applying this theory one week before a major competition, the athlete depletes glycogen stores by hard training and then is deprived of carbohydrate for four or five days. On the final days before the major competition, the athlete takes a very rich carbohydrate diet. The result is that the amount of available glycogen in the body is much higher than would normally be the case (fig. 19). This may not, however, be an ideal situation for the long endurance athlete (see p. 62). Such 'carbo-loading' still has an important place in distance running, but now it is programmed as a 'non-stop' boost,

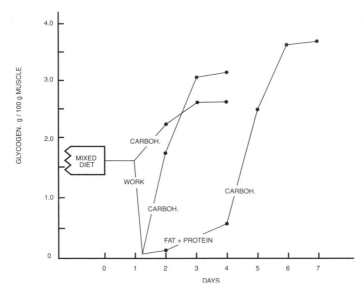

FIG. 19 Glycogen 'overshoot'. Different possibilities of increasing the muscle glycogen content. For further explanation see text (from Saltin and Hermansen, 1967).

i.e. during the final three days of the taper, the carbohydrate intake is substantially increased (but not the total calories).

FATS (TRUE CHEMICAL NAME = LIPIDS)

Fats, like carbohydrates, are composed of carbon, hydrogen and oxygen, but the quantity of oxygen is considerably less in fats. Fats are certainly the most concentrated source of energy of all foodstuffs, yielding twice as many kilocalories, weight for weight, compared with carbohydrates. The provision of stored energy is probably their most important role in nutrition. However, they are also valuable in maintaining body temperature in, for example, the subcutaneous fat layer of sea or lake swimmers, and protecting vital organs (e.g. kidneys) with layers of fat or adipose tissue, as well as contributing in the provision of those fatty acids essential to health and in providing a transport medium for the fat-soluble vitamins.

Lipids, as fats (solid) and oils (liquid) are broken up into tiny globules by bile salts secreted by the liver. These act on fats like a detergent on an oil slick and in this form the fats may more readily react with chemicals similar to those involved in carbohydrate digestion. Even the substances of fat digestion which have not been completely broken down may pass through the gut wall to be carried, in lymph along the lymphatic system, to a point in the region of the chest where they are emptied into the blood.

The liver plays a most important role in the metabolism of fats. It may convert available glucose into fat and then into other usable substances in the body. Our fat stores, then, may be derived from excessive carbohydrate intake, or from fats and oils (figs 20 and 21).

H_2 – hydrogen; O – oxygen; CO_2 – carbon dioxide; P – phosphate; ADP – adenosine diphosphate; ATP – adenosine triphosphate.

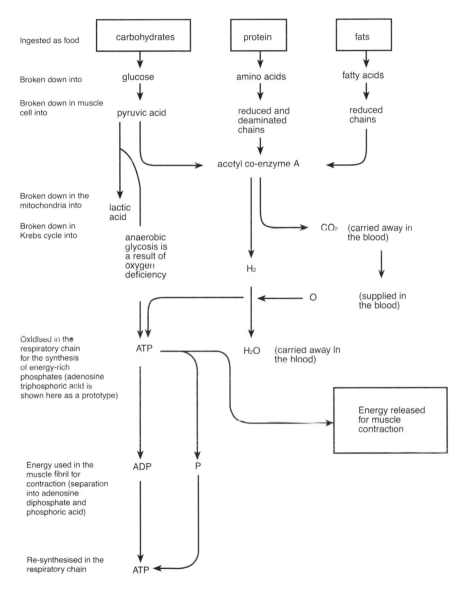

FIG. 20 Metabolism of nutrients and their conversion into ATP, which when broken down to ADP provides energy for muscle contraction (the conversion of food into energy)

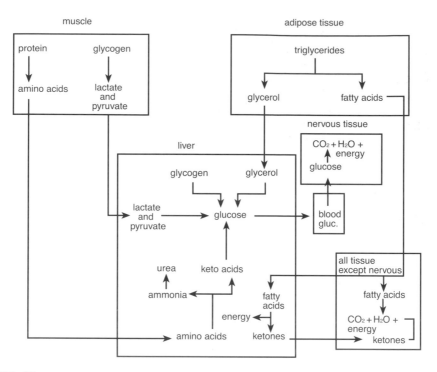

FIG. 21 Summary of metabolism of stored foods as a source of energy (i.e. in fasting) (from Vander, Sherman and Luciano, 1970)

Fats belong to a much larger biochemical family known as lipids. The family is described below, but not all members have nutritional significance.

Triglycerides (Acyl glycerols): Triglycerides are also converted from dietary carbohydrates so the quality and quantity of dietary carbohydrates have a substantial consequence on the body's fats profile. The most common of these is triacylglycerol, or triglyceride or 'neutral fat'. Most edible fats and oils consist of compounds of glycerol (commonly known as glycerine) plus fatty acids. The main reason why, say, lard differs from nut oil or cream, lies in the different types or proportions of fatty acids which combine with glycerol. When three fatty acids combine with glycerol, the compound is triglyceride (fig. 22).

Fatty acids may consist of long chains of carbon atoms which have two hydrogen atoms attached to each carbon atom (fig. 23). When all the carbons in a fatty acid chain are linked by single bonds, the fatty acid is said to be *saturated* with hydrogen bonds. If the chain contains one (mono) or more than one (poly) it is *unsaturated* (fig. 24).

Triglycerides occur in vegetable fats and oils, animal fats, fish oils and dairy fats. The main difference between animal fats and dairy fats, on the one hand, and vegetable fats and oils, and fish oils on the other, is that, except for palm oil

FIG. 22 Triglycerides. Such fats are called triglycerides because the compound glycerol in each molecule is attached to three fatty acid units.

PALMITIC ACID

STEARIC ACID

FIG. 23 Chemists refer to such fatty acids as saturated due to the presence of pairs of hydrogen atoms along the whole length of the chain. The two saturated fatty acids here are present in the harder fats, such as lard.

LINOLENIC ACID

ARACHIDONIC ACID

FIG. 24 The existence of 'gaps' in the pairs of hydrogen atoms characterise the unsaturated fatty acids. The two unsaturated fatty acids shown here are present in fish oils.

and coconut oil, the latter have a much higher proportion of unsaturated fatty acids. It is well known that high blood cholesterol levels are associated with coronary heart disease and that the cholesterol level can be reduced by eating foods rich in unsaturated fatty acids. This is of considerable interest with reference to the health of the heart and circulating system/network. Table 8 illustrates the saturated/unsaturated fatty acid situation in several fats and oils.

Cholesterol has acquired something of a bad reputation recently. It is important to understand that cholesterol is an essential component of the body's chemistry. For example, steroid hormones secreted by the adrenal cortex are derived from cholesterol. Cholesterol can, however, become a problem if its content in the blood exceeds a healthy amount. Consequently, it is becoming normal practice to monitor the blood from as early as age 30 and certainly annually from the age of 40. Monitoring involves blood analysis as set out in table 8.

Total cholesterol	<5.0 mmol/l	(desirable)
	5.0–6.0 mmol/l	(borderline)
	>6.0 mmol/l	(high)
LDL cholesterol	<3.0 mmol/l	(desirable)
(low density	3.0–4.0 mmol/l	(borderline)
lipoprotein)	>4.0 mmol/l	(high)
HDL cholesterol	0.9–1,5 mmol/l	(desirable)
(high density	<0.9 mmol/l	(low)
lipoprotein)		
HDL % of total	>20	(desirable)
	<20	(low)
Triglycerides	<2.3 mmol/l	(desirable)
	2.3–4.5 mmol/l	(borderline)
	> 4.5 mmol/l	(high)

TABLE 8 Blood cholesterol analysis

HDL is regarded as 'good' cholesterol due to its role in protecting against disease, so higher scores are generally good. This score can be improved by increasing aerobic exercise, monounsaturated fats, fish oils and moderate alcohol, or by reducing or eliminating saturated fats, particularly hydrogenated fats and the less healthy carbohydrates.

LDL is regarded as 'bad' cholesterol because when it oxidises it lines the arteries. Oxidation of LDL results from free radicals in foods. Antioxidants (betacarotene, vitamin C, vitamin E and selenium) attract free radicals and so help prevent this oxidation process. The level of LDL can be reduced by eating antioxidant foods listed above. Fibre and soya protein can also lower LDL. Generally, foods to cut back on or to avoid are poor quality carbohydrates and foods with a high cholesterol content.

Phospholipids: again the glycerol 'backbone' is present in this compound but only two fatty acids are attached, plus phosphate and a base containing nitrogen. The latter situation bridges the worlds of fats and proteins and, as a rule, the fatty acids are unsaturated. The phospholipids have important functions to perform in the body, ranging from fat absorption to the insulation of nervous tissue with the myelin sheath. They are not only manufactured by, and exist in, the body itself, but are also in the foods we eat. For example, lecithin is present in egg yolk and soya beans. Yakovlev (1961) has emphasised the inclusion of lecithin in the post-competition diet to aid recovery.

Sphingolipids: these compounds contain fatty acid, phosphate, choline, a complex base (sphingosine), but no glycerol. The sphingolipids are closely associated with tissues and animal membranes.

Glycolipids: there is neither glycerol nor phosphate in this compound. Instead there is a monosaccharide galactose, plus fatty acid and sphingosine. The glycolipids are found primarily in photosynthetic tissue (i.e. the leaves of plants).

Eiocosanoids: arachidonic acid, a 20 carbon fatty acid (fig. 24) is the central building block for these derivatives which include vasoactive substances such as prostaglandin and prostacyclin. Eiocosanoids are critical to a number of body functions including immune response, inflammation and airway resistance.

Steroids

The basic structure of all steroids is formed from four interconnected rings of carbon atoms (fig. 25). The steroids include cholesterol, vitamin A, bile salts, testosterone and oestrogen.

FIG. 25 Four interconnected rings of carbon atoms form the basic structure of all steroids

Fats in foodstuffs are primarily triglycerides, combined with small amounts of free fatty acids, phospholipids (such as lecithin) and the salts of cholesterol. Eating animal fats may cause problems associated with saturated fatty acids, but they do provide one of the most valuable sources of vitamins A and D. So, if margarine is used instead of butter, it must be composed of vegetable oils only and enriched with vitamins A and D.

The final breakdown products of fat metabolism are free fatty acids which, like glucose, are fuel for muscular activity. Recent research shows these fatty acids are the preferred fuel for the long duration endurance athletes (fig. 26). Williams (1975) has pointed out that since this is the case, the application of the glycogen overshoot theory may not be in the athlete's interest in training. It may be better to 'train' the free fatty acid energy pathway by training in a 'fasting' state, therefore encouraging the use of free fatty acids as a fuel. However, before competition, glycogen loading is good sense even for the 5000 m (Newsholme, 1994).

The right balance of dietary fats and oils is essential to good health. These fats and oils are sources of the four soluble vitamins (A, D, E, K) and they are also required to absorb them. They keep the skin healthy and regulate body functions.

The right balance is as follows:

2/3 monounsaturated fatty acids e.g.

- extra virgin olive oil
- avocado
- rapeseed oil
- almonds
- pecans
- peanut oil

1/3 polyunsaturated (omega 3 and omega 6) and saturated.
Each of these three (omega 3; omega 6; saturated) represent 1/9 of the daily fats and oils intake. So:

1/9 omega 3 e.g.

- fish oils
- soya bean
- flax oil
- walnut

1/9 omega 6 e.g.

- sunflower oil
- corn oil

- sesame seed oil
- blackcurrant seeds

1/9 saturated e.g.

- fatty red meat
- egg yolk
- shell fish
- dairy products
- poultry skins
- hydrogenated fats (present in many margarines and cooking fats)

PROTEINS

It has been pointed out that carbohydrates and fats consist mainly of carbon, hydrogen and oxygen. Protein differs in that nitrogen is an essential part of its structure and neither carbohydrate nor fats can replace protein in the diet without eventual damage to the organism.

Protein molecules are formed by linking smaller units called amino acids, which are the end product of protein digestion (fig. 20). Differences between proteins depend on the identity, number and arrangement of amino acids. Chains of amino acids are polypeptides. If there are less than 50 amino acids, this is a peptide; if more, it is a protein. There are 25 amino acids, 20 of biochemical import and, of these, 10 are known as essential amino acids. They are 'essential' because the body cannot normally manufacture these amino acids at the rate required for proper functioning. The 10 essential amino acids are arginine, histidine, isoleucine, leucine, lysine, methionine, phenylalanine, threonine, tryptophan and valine.

The amino acids go via the blood from gut to liver to general circulation. The liver, again, has an important regulatory function in that it acts as a 'buffer' for amino acids, just as it does for glucose and fats. That is, if the concentration is high in the blood, the liver absorbs a large quantity into its cells. Conversely, in times of shortage, the liver releases its store. It would appear that there is a peak of circulating amino acids approximately two hours after a protein meal. Apparently, then, it is helpful, both for maintenance and repair of muscle tissue, to train at this time. It certainly does not seem advisable to train within the two hour period, or so late afterwards that the body has begun to starve, except of course in the case of the long duration endurance athletes as previously suggested. The liver is also responsible for preparing amino acids for use as an alternative energy source. However, this is a 'last gasp' mechanism and other sources of energy must be favoured.

The protein value of different foods varies quite remarkably. The disadvantages of the fat associated with meat, as pointed out by heart specialists, must be most

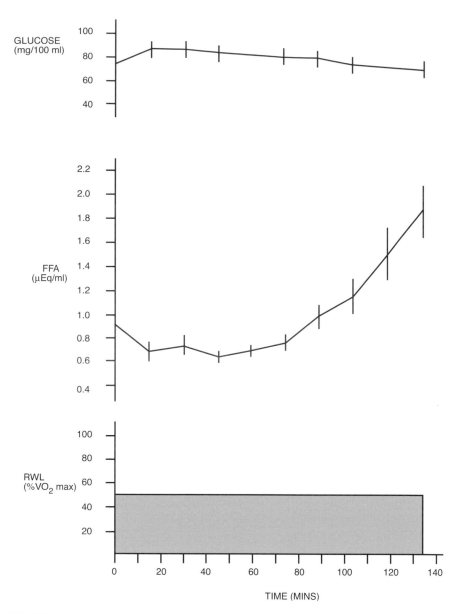

FIG. 26 Free fatty acids appear to become the preferred fuel with increasing duration of exercise (from Williams, 1975)

carefully weighed against the high quality of animal protein and supply of certain vitamins and minerals. When assessing the protein value of the athlete's diet, quality as well as quantity must be taken into account. Some athletes may eat most of their daily protein in the form of potato chips rather than eggs or milk. Nevertheless, in terms of quality, the egg is the most complete protein food (table 9).

	isoleucine	leucine	lysine	phenylalanine	methionine	threonine	trytophan	valine	protein score as measure of excellence
Amino acid combination estimated as ideal for man	270	306	270	180	144	180	90	270	100
Egg protein	428	565	396	368	196	310	106	460	100
Beef	332	515	540	256	154	275	75*	345	83
Milk protein	402	628	497	334	190	272	85*	448	80
Fish	317	474	549	231	178	283	62*	327	70
Oat protein	302	436	212*	309	84*	192	74*	348	79
Rice protein	322	535	236*	307	142*	241	65*	415	72
Flour protein	262*	442	126*	322	78*	174	69*	262	47
Maize protein	293	827	179*	284	117*	249	38*	327	42
Soya protein	333	484	395	309	86*	247	86*	328	73
Pea protein	336	504	438	290	77*	230	74*	317	58
Potato protein	260*	304	326	285	87*	237	72*	339	56
Cassava	118*	184*	310	133*	2*	136*	131	144	22

*Less than the estimated ideal proportion

TABLE 9 Protein value in selected foods (mg per g of nitrogen) (from Pyke, M. 1975)

Because protein foods clearly vary in their quality, and some have negative health implications, it is sensible to prioritise intake.

Higher priority
Whey (the thin liquid part of milk remaining after casein, or curds, and fat are removed). Fish, tofu, soya bean, low fat cheeses and yoghurt, brown rice, oats and mixed vegetables.

Lower priority
Lean beef and other meats, eggs, full fat cheeses, nuts, pulses (beans, peas, lentils), bean sprouts, white rice, maize, potatoes.

For vegetarians, although the protein quality of individual plant foods is lower than foods of animal origin (except soya), by mixing the vegetables and eating cereals, nuts, potatoes, pulses and so on, protein needs will be met; some vegetarians also include whey in their diets.

Not all nutritionists agree with the daily protein intake recommended in table 7. For example, it is suggested the athlete in heavy endurance training would find about 2 g/kg/day satisfactory, with 3 g/kg/day for power/strength competitors (Wootton, 1988). Durnin (1975) has suggested that an intake of around 1 g/kg body weight/day would be quite adequate. Although there remains confusing diversity among nutrition experts, it is reasonable for athletes to keep within the 1.5–2.5 g/kg/day range (Lemon, 1991).

MACRONUTRIENTS AND ENERGY

The macronutrients yield energy originally harnessed by plants and, through them, animals. Carbohydrates and fats are the main energy providers. Proteins have a lesser role, as their main functions are to build and repair. Nutritionists have developed a rating scale that compares the capacity of different foods to increase blood glucose concentrations. This is called the *glycaemic index*.

This index indicates the increase in blood sugar over a two-hour period after consuming 50 g of a food compared with 50 g of white bread or glucose. The latter represents 100%. A food with a glycaemic index of 45 indicates that it increases blood glucose to 45% of the level of white bread.

High GI foods include:
Glucose, sucrose, cane/maple/corn, syrup, honey, bagel, white bread, shredded wheat cereals, potato, cornflakes, raisins, banana, puffed wheat cereals, carrot, white rice, white pasta, pitta bread, refined base noodles, butternut squash, watermelon, pineapple and parsnips.

Moderate GI foods include:
Whole grain bread, pasta and noodles, muesli (no sugar), couscous, long grain brown rice, semolina, sweet corn, rye bread, oats, new potatoes with skin, bran muffins, orange, wild rice, beetroot, spinach, lychees, mangoes, melon, dates, lentils and most beans.

Low GI foods include:
Fructose, yoghurt, peanuts, peas, soy beans, apples, peaches, pears, plums, figs, apricots, grapefruit, cherries, milk and milk products.

Consuming low glycaemic foods 30 minutes prior to exercise permits a relatively low rate of glucose absorption into the body. This eliminates 'insulin surge', yet affords a steady slow release of glucose during the exercise. This is an advantage for endurance activities.

High glycaemic index foods consumed 30 minutes prior to exercise cause increased insulin activity (insulin surge) peaking around 30–45 minutes after ingestion. Blood glucose volume likewise surges then drops off rapidly leaving an inadequate supply to meet exercise demands. This is a disadvantage in endurance activities.

In general nutrition, the emphasis must be on the moderate GI foods supplemented by a mixture which is more generous in low GI foods than high. Pre-exercise meals should be mainly low GI with moderate GI. Post-exercise should be high GI plus moderate GI. During exercise of 60 minutes duration or more, carbohydrates should be high GI. This can be achieved through specially formulated sports drinks that provide glucose and electrolytes as well as rehydration. Some people, on the other hand, are quite happy with a banana or a jam sandwich as their energy top-up and still water for their rehydration.

Knowing the glycaemic index of foods is essential to people either with diabetes mellitus type 1 (the pancreas loses its ability to synthesise insulin) or type 2 (the cells resist the effects of insulin). International travel should always be preceded by a briefing on the glycaemic index of local foods to ensure that the delicate balance of glucose intake for those with diabetes mellitus is maintained.

MICRONUTRIENTS

Vitamins

Vitamins are required for the breakdown of macronutrients. Most are the main components of co-enzymes. While they must be present in our food at a certain minimal level, the argument that megadoses will increase sports performance is yet to be proved. In fact, continued excessive intake of A, D or K may be sufficiently toxic to be life-threatening.

Water soluble

These are the B-complex vitamins and vitamin C.

Thiamine (vitamin B1): this forms part of the enzyme responsible for the breakdown of pyruvic acid in the process of releasing energy from carbohydrates. Its presence in the diet is therefore essential. Increased intake is required where there is a high energy requirement, when carbohydrate is excessive in the diet, when the diet is high in white sugar or white flour (when there is no thiamine already added), when foods relied upon to supply thiamine are heated in alkaline or neutral solutions, and when raw fish constitutes part of the regular diet. Thiamine is water soluble so some of it will be lost to the water in which the food is cooked. This applies, of course, to all water soluble vitamins. Thiamine content is high in foods such as brewer's yeast and wheatgerm.

Riboflavin (vitamin B2): like thiamine, riboflavin is a component of an enzyme in the metabolism of carbohydrates, but there would appear to be no correlation between energy requirements and riboflavin. Research into the relative merits of riboflavin as a dietary supplement is inconclusive. Brewer's yeast, liver and meat extract have a high riboflavin content.

Niacin: this again is involved in enzyme activity in the metabolism of carbohydrates. However, unlike thiamine and riboflavin, niacin may be synthesised within the body through micro-organism activity in the large intestine. High quality protein, such as eggs, which are high in content of the amino acid tryptophan, provide the basis for such synthesis. Supplementing the diet with very high quantities of niacin (2–5 g) reduces the concentration of free fatty acids in the blood. Niacin content is high in meat extract, yeast extract and bran.

Pyridoxine (vitamin B6): this is involved in enzyme activity in protein metabolism, but little has been revealed in research regarding the effects of excess or deficiency. Pyridoxine content is high in liver, green vegetables and in wheatgerm.

Pantothenic acid: as a principal component of co-enzyme A, pantothenic acid is involved in energy production from organic acids. Liver, egg yolk and fresh vegetables contain high levels of pantothenic acid.

Biotin: this, like thiamine and folic acid, is a co-enzyme of cellular metabolism. Specifically, it forms oxaloacetic acid from pyruvic acid and the synthesis of fatty acids. Skin condition, physical and mental alertness appear related to biotin status. It is produced by bacteria in the GastroIntestinal (GI) system. Biotin content is high in brewer's yeast, liver, kidneys, legumes, vegetables and egg yolk.

Folic acid (pteroylglutamic acid): this is a key substance in the formation of red blood cells and consequently is associated with vitamin B12. However, this relationship is not yet fully understood. It is also, like pyridoxine, involved in protein metabolism. Folic acid content is high in foods such as liver, oysters and spinach.

Cyanocobalamin (vitamin B12): this is essential to the maturation of red blood cells and is also involved in white cell and platelet formation. Some athletes involved in high energy demanding sports boost B12 levels by injecting large quantities of the vitamin. The athletes concerned claim certain benefits, but there is no research evidence to support these claims at present. Cyanocobalamin content is high in uncooked liver, kidneys, meat, yeast extracts, dairy products and eggs. B12 is not found in any plants, so vegans have to take it in tablet or liquid form.

Ascorbic acid (vitamin C): this cannot be synthesised or stored by the body and therefore must be supplied by the diet. It performs several roles: it aids repair of damaged tissue and absorption of iron, it maintains healthy gums and decreases susceptibility to minor infections, and it is concentrated in some quantity in the adrenal cortex, although its exact function there is at present unknown. It has been shown that the body's ascorbic acid content falls during periods of intensive training. Moreover, when an athlete is sweating heavily, or is losing body fluids (e.g. during a common cold), ascorbic acid status in the body drops severely. Clearly, steps must be made to maintain this level, but it is not always easy. The normal diet may well supply sufficient ascorbic acid for the athlete's needs, but this is not always the case because vitamin C is easily destroyed or lost. As it is water soluble, it is often washed out of food or dissolved in cooking. Heat, processing and lengthy storage often destroy the vitamin, as does exposure to air and light (e.g. cutting an apple). All of this would appear to suggest some supplement of vitamin C to the diet. During intensive training, athletes have been known to take between 1 and 10 g per day. The lower end of this range seems reasonable but is nevertheless high compared with the UK recommendations of 0.03 g per day and USA recommendations of 0.06 g per day. Ascorbic acid content is high in blackcurrants, green vegetables and citrus fruits.

It should be noted that due to their nature, water-soluble vitamins will simply be passed out in the urine if taken in excess and, since the athlete's needs are almost certainly greater than the recommended minimum for the general public, little harm can come of taking supplementary vitamin B complex and vitamin C, though this is not the case with the fat-soluble vitamins which can accumulate in the body.

Vitamin C, like betacarotene (provitamin A), vitamin E and selenium, is an anti-oxidant scavenging free radicals, the tissue-damaging by-products of metabolism.

Fat soluble

These are the vitamins A, D, E and K.

Retinol (vitamin A): this is only found in animal products. However, some vegetables, including carrots and the leafy green vegetables, contain substances called carotenoids which are converted to retinol during absorption through the small intestine. Being fat soluble and stable in heat, it is not exposed to the same danger of destruction by cooking as are B-complex and C vitamins. However, exposure to oxygen and ultraviolet light can reduce retinol status in foods. Retinol is involved in vision efficiency; carotenoids being found in both rods and cones. It also would appear that bone growth, the health of alimentary and respiratory tracts, and local resistance to infection are all vitamin A dependent. High dosage of vitamin A taken regularly is toxic. Fish liver oils, ox liver and sheep liver all have a high retinol content.

Betacarotene (provitamin A): may be converted into vitamin A at the rate demanded by the body's requirements for the vitamin. It is an antioxidant (see vitamin C). It is found in high quantities in green and yellow vegetables (particularly carrots, kale and spinach).

Cholecalciferol (vitamin D): essential to calcium and phosphorus absorption, cholecalciferol has a key role in development of bone and those physiological areas influenced by calcium, phosphorus and parathyroid gland activity. There are two main types of vitamin D:
- calciferol (vitamin D2), which is formed by the ultraviolet radiation of ergosterol (a steroid found in plants such as yeast and fungi)
- cholecalciferol (vitamin D3), which occurs naturally in substances such as egg yolk, butter and the oils of fish liver. It is also formed by the action of ultraviolet radiation on the oils present on the surface of our skins (i.e. when the skin is exposed to sunlight).

Like retinol, vitamin D in excess is toxic. Vitamin D content is high in foods such as egg yolks and vitamin-enriched produce such as margarine.

Tocopherols (vitamin E): vitamin E inhibits breakdown of those fatty acids that assist in cell membrane formation. It is also involved in forming erythrocytes, DNA and RNA, wound healing and normal neural system function and structure.

It is an antioxidant (see vitamin C). It is found in high quantities in whole grain seed, oils and eggs.

Vitamin K (phylloquinone, menaquinone): while the role of vitamin K is clearly involved in blood clotting, no obvious role is played by the vitamin in enzyme systems. It is very difficult to assess whether or not we require vitamin K in our food or whether sufficient is manufactured within our own bodies. Vitamin K is readily inactivated on exposure to light. Of the vitamin K derivatives, vitamin K1 is found in green vegetables, and vitamin K2 in bacteria.

Phytonutrients/phytochemicals

These are a group of compounds that occur naturally in fruit and vegetables. They have become the subject of debate as they are of benefit to the immune system and are as important to health as vitamins. The bitter taste in some vegetables is due to the presence of these compounds.
The phytonutrients include:

Carotenoids :   watercress, broccoli, spinach, yellow squashes, red peppers, carrot, pumpkin, tomato skin
Indoles: Brussels sprouts and cabbage varieties
Isothiocyanates: broccoli, Brussels sprouts, cabbage varieties.

Minerals

The body requires certain minerals in relatively large amounts. These are listed here as major minerals. Other minerals are needed in relatively small (or trace) amounts. These are listed here as minor minerals.

Major minerals (need more than 100 mg/day)

Calcium: this performs several very important functions in the body, namely:

* the formation of bones and teeth
* the initiation of muscle contraction
* blood clotting
* as part of the composition of blood
* certain enzyme activity.

Vitamin D and protein aid calcium absorption, while phytic acid (see iron), oxalic acid (as in rhubarb and spinach) and fats inhibit calcium absorption. While the well-balanced average diet should supply sufficient calcium, and the body will readily adapt to reduced supplies, the athlete is often advised to drink an extra daily pint of (skimmed) milk or to take calcium tablets in order to ensure that calcium levels do not become too depleted due to strenuous training, especially in the case of women endurance competitors who may suffer from osteoporosis.

Calcium content is high in foods such as dried skimmed milk, whitebait and hard cheese.

Phosphorus: this is found in foodstuffs and in the body as phosphate. It has many functions in the body, chiefly:

* formation of bones and teeth
* energy production (ATP and ADP)
* as an essential component of blood
* as an essential inclusion of certain enzymes and hormones.

The average well-balanced diet will provide ample phosphate for the body's needs. Phosphorus content is high in cheese, brains, meat and fish.

Potassium: like table salt, potassium is a key mineral in the maintenance of the body's internal environment, but its role is mainly within the cell, whereas salt works outside the cell. While most diets offer an ample supply of potassium to meet the body's needs, it would appear that when training is so severe and prolonged that cellular proteins are beginning to break down, then the potassium levels in the body are reduced. However, like so many of the areas under discussion here, the body is well-equipped to increase potassium absorption from foodstuffs in order to restore status quo. Soya flour, dried milk, dried fruit and nuts are high in potassium.

Sulphur: like potassium, sulphur is involved in maintaining acid base balance in the body. It also has a key role in liver function. Sulphur is found in high quantities in dried vegetables, fruits, meats, poultry and fish.

Sodium: performs a balancing act with potassium in the process of action potential across cell membranes; acid base balance, osmolality and body water mineral balance. Sodium rich foods are fruits, vegetables and sodium chloride (table salt).

Sodium chloride (table salt): this is the most important soluble mineral of the diet, and is the main component of the extracellular fluid. Consequently it is very important that the sodium concentration of the extracellular fluid is closely monitored. Athletes losing more salt than usual, due to increased perspiration when in a hot environment, must increase salt intake above that provided by the normal diet. Thus preparations such as 'slow sodium' and various electrolyte drinks are included in special diets for athletes exposed to this situation. Ham, corned beef and cheese all have a high salt content.

Chlorine: is involved in the body's water mineral balance, principally in its combination with sodium as sodium chloride. It also influences membrane potential. Foods rich in chlorine are fruits, vegetables and table salt.

Magnesium: like calcium and phosphorous, is involved in the development of bones and teeth. It also has a critical role in certain types of nerve impulse transmission. Calcium 'switches on' while magnesium 'switches off'. Foods rich in magnesium are wheatgerm and green leafy vegetables.

Minor minerals (need less than 100 mg/day)

Iron: the element of iron is essential for production of haemoglobin carried in red blood cells (erythrocytes). If there is insufficient haemoglobin, the oxygen carrying capacity of the blood is reduced and it is reasonable to assume that the athlete's functioning capacity is also depleted. This condition is known as anaemia and by far the most common (but not the only) cause is lack of dietary iron. In these circumstances, ferrous compounds may be taken as dietary additives. However, the body will only absorb what it needs and reject the surplus. Many endurance athletes have suffered from so-called Sports-Pseudo-Anaemia, which is a condition where the total quantity of haemoglobin in the blood is high but the concentration is lower than normal, due to a relatively greater increase in blood plasma. The reduced concentration will, however, keep blood viscosity low and consequently aid the rate of flow to and from muscle (Williams, 1975). Although, generally speaking, athletes, women and growing children have greater iron requirements than other members of the population, it is inadvisable to supplement normal dietary iron without medical advice. Regular blood counts for athletes are recommended. Vitamin C aids iron absorption and it is thought that protein may also assist. However, where diets are very high in bran cereals content, the phytic acid found in the outer husks of the cereals may prevent iron absorption by forming an insoluble compound. Iron content is high in green vegetables such as spinach, watercress and cabbage, in liver, black pudding, red meat, kidney, and in yeast.

Fluorine: serving a most vital role in the healthy growth of bones and teeth, fluorine, like its fellow halogen iodine, is involved in the functioning of the thyroid gland. Furthermore it is now well established that fluorine protects teeth from decay. Fluoridised drinking water, tea and saltwater fish contain quantities of fluorine.

Copper: is essential to the healthy development of the nervous system, especially in the composition of the protective myelin sheath. It is also a component of certain metabolic enzymes. It is present in meat.

Selenium: functions with vitamin E as an antioxidant. Together with betacarotene and vitamin C they complete the 'antioxidant cocktail'. It is present in seafood, meats and grains.

Iodine: is vital to the efficient production of the hormone thyroxine by which the thyroid gland controls the body's metabolic rate. Consequently, any lack of iodine in the diet must have serious and far-reaching effects. Where soils are rich in iodine, the plants nourished by that soil are rich in it too. In regions where soils have poor levels of iodine, potassium iodide is added to cooking salts to make up for this deficiency. Iodine content is normally highest in foods such as saltwater fish, vegetables and milk.

Chromium: has a key role in glycolysis. It is present in legumes, cereals and organic meats.

Manganese: is involved in bone growth, forms part of certain enzymes and is found in the blood and liver.

Molybdenum: is a co-factor for several enzymes critical to bodily function. It is present in animal fats, vegetable oils, meats and whole grain.

Cobalt: is vital to the formation of vitamin B12. The pancreas contains a high concentration, which is used on demand by the body to synthesise insulin and certain other enzymes essential to digestion of carbohydrates and fats. It is found in leafy green vegetables, liver and other foodstuffs, which are vitamin B12 sources.

Water

The body is 60% water and it is essential to keep it that way! Different parts of the body account for different percentages. So, for example, 80% of blood is water; 75% of the brain; 22% of bone; and 10% of fat stores. We lose a considerable amount of water each day through perspiration, exhaled air and urine. The problem for most people is that their environment, diet and activity cause them to lose more water than they realise. Air conditioning at home, in offices, cars, airplanes, etc; heating systems; warm climates; vigorous exercise; nervous tension, all contribute to dehydration or loss of water. We can add to the problem by consuming alcohol and caffeine.

Feeling thirsty is a reminder to top up but, unfortunately, this occurs only when we are down by around 2%. We need to deal with things much earlier than this. Urine should be clear, like water, not yellow. People who are persistently in a dehydrated state are seriously compromising their performance capacity.

For most people, being hydrated means taking in around 1.5 litres of water per day. Athletes need around 2.5 litres but when competition periods are extended, and/or when hot and/or humid, they may need around 3.5 litres.

These guidelines may help ensure a healthy level of hydration:

- Don't wait until you are thirsty to drink water, drink throughout the day.
- Drink small amounts regularly rather than a large amount occasionally.
- Have access to bottled water throughout the day e.g. in the car, on your desk, in the plane, etc.
- Drink still water rather than carbonated. It is absorbed more easily.
- Drink water before, during and after exercise.
- Don't gulp water; sip it.
- Avoid tap water as it often contains extra chlorine or fluoride.
- If perspiring a lot during prolonged you may be losing a lot of minerals in your sweat. Try one of the drinks such as LucozadeSport that not only rehydrate, but replace minerals and contain glucose to top up the energy reservoir.

Nutritional supplements

Nutritional supplements include a wide and varied range of products. The purpose of these is to improve health; and/or reduce the catabolic consequence of exposure to the challenge of adapting to the general and specific stressors of personal lifestyle; and/or prevent particular pathological conditions. They are useful and sometimes even essential therapeutic aids. Without doubt, they are widely used by athletes, often in the belief that they will enhance performance as ergogenic aids. This is only acceptable if they are:

- safe (of no threat to health)
- legal (within the laws of anti-doping policies)
- effective (on the basis of valid studies).

This said, if such products actually enhance performance, affording competitive advantage, their use would be ethically improper and should be prohibited, even if they are not contravening anti-doping laws. Most athletes will use nutritional supplements to achieve regeneration or recovery so that quality and quantity of training units can be increased per unit of time in order to persistently pursue improved competition performance levels. They would argue that this puts them beyond the edge of the ethical issue since it is training, not nutrition, which is affording them competitive advantage.

As our understanding of nutrition continues to expand and change, new advice is being suggested to enhance our health. So, for example, prebiotics, which are similar to fibre, promote the growth of healthy bacteria in the colon. These are naturally present in asparagus, onions, leeks, garlic, chicory, banana, dandelion leaves, Jerusalem artichokes, barley, rye and wheat. They are also available in commercially produced supplements. Another example is probiotics, such as acidophilus culture in yoghurt-like drinks, which help colon bacteria replace unhealthy bacteria that commonly cause disease. Again, such supplements do not raise ethical issues, but because they are designed to adjust how the body functions, all athletes should check these or, indeed, any supplement with the relevant people or agencies.

There have been increasing numbers of athletes testing positive for banned substances, despite the fact that they have apparently not wittingly taken them. The problem is that some supplements have additives which, on their own, and/or in combination with additives within an athlete's total diet of supplements and/or due to the nature of training workloads, may be converted by the body's chemistry to something quite different. In other words, what has come out is not what the athlete believed had gone in. In light of this, in the interest of avoiding accidents which could have serious implications for the athlete's health and career, the 'package' of supplements in use at any time must be approved by relevant authorities. Manufacturers also have a responsibility to code their products in the context of anti-doping laws to help avoid 'accidents', where athletes and/or coaches have simply not understood the biochemical terms used in product descriptions.

Nutritional supplements include those listed in table 10. These are all legal substances. It is not intended to be a comprehensive list, but covers the more 'popular' areas. There are other areas of supplementation, which are most definitely not on the menu. They are banned substances and their use is considered as 'doping'.

Doping is the use by, or distribution to, an athlete of certain substances which could have the effect of improving artificially the athlete's physical and/or mental condition and so augmenting his athletic ability. –(IAAF definition)

√probable–certain　　　? possible　　　x probably not

supplement	proposed advantage	proven advantage
Amino acids: arginine, lysine, ornithine	Stimulate release of HGH; promotes muscle growth	?
Branched chain amino acids, glutamine	Stimulate release of HGH; increased pain tolerance; accelerating regeneration process	√
Antioxidants: beta carotine, vit. C, vit. E, selenium	Reduce muscle damage from unwanted oxidative processes following high intensity muscle activity	√
Aspartates	Potassium and magnesium in salts of aspartate (a non-essential amino acid) improve performance and reduce muscular and central fatigue	x
Bee pollen	Increases energy levels, enhances physical fitness	x
BetaHydroxyBeta-Methylbutyrate (HMB)	Prevents or retards muscle damage and reduce proteolysis (muscle protein breakdown) associated with high intensity strength training	?
Boron	Increases serum testosterone levels	x
Brewer's yeast	Increases energy levels	?
Carbohydrate	Prevents hypoglycaemia, increases carbohydrate metabolism	
Carnitine	Increases lipid catabolism, spares muscle glycogen	x
Choline	Increases acetylcholine to increase strength or lecithin to decrease body fat	x
Chromium	Potentiates insulin action, promotes muscle growth via enhanced amino acids uptake	x

TABLE 10 Some common nutritional supplements

supplement	proposed advantage	proven advantage
Colostrum	Helps tissue growth and repair. Stimulates immune system	√
Creatine (synthesised from amino acids)	Increases creatine phosphate in muscles; increases energy source and stimulates muscle growth	√
Cyanacobalamine (Vit B12)	Enhances DNA synthesis; increases muscle growth	?
Gamma oryzamol	Increases serum testosterone and HGH level; increases muscle growth	x
Gelatin	Improves muscle contraction	x
Ginseng	Improves muscle contraction (NB: some variants contain high levels of Ma Hoang [Chinese Ephedrine] which would show as pseudo ephedrine [illegal] in a urine sample)	x
Glycerol hyperhydration	Increases intestinal and vascular water; improves thermoregulation and cardiovascular function	?
Inosine	Increases ATP synthesis, increases strength, facilitates regeneration	?
Kelp	High level micronutrient source	x
Lecithin	Prevents fat gain, aids neuromuscular regeneration	?
Liquid (increases hydration via isotonic mineral replacement drinks)	Improves thermoregulation and cardiovascular function	√
Magnesium	Increases protein synthesis or muscle contractility, increases muscle growth and strength	x
Medium chain tryglycerides	Increase metabolic rate, promote fat loss	?
Octacosanol	Supplies energy, improves performance	x
Omega – 3 fatty acids	Maintains cardiovascular efficiency	√
Oxygen (pure) inhalation	Improves intense exercise and speeds recovery from intense exercise	√
Pangamic acid (B15)	Increased delivery of oxygen	x

TABLE 10 Continued

supplement	proposed advantage	proven advantage
Phosphate	Delays muscle fatigue. Increases VO2max and ventilatory threshold	?
Phosphatidy-lserine (PS)	Diminishes ACTH and cortisol release without effecting HGH release, thus modifying the body's neuroendocrine response to stress (bovine derived possibly more effective than soya derived)	√
Royal Jelly	Increases strength	x
Saline infusion	Improves thermoregulation and cardiovascular function	√
Smilax	Increases serum testosterone levels; increases muscle growth and strength	?
Sodium bicarbonate or sodium citrate	Increases blood buffering capacity	√
Spirulina	Rich protein source	x
Ubiquinone (CoQ.10)	Increases oxygen uptake	?
Yohimbine	Increases serum testosterone levels; increases muscle growth and strength; decreases body fat; alpha2 adenoreceptor blocker	x

TABLE 10 Continued

Drug testing programmes operate across the range of sports. They vary in detail from country to country and from one international sporting body to another. In principle, however, they are there to ensure a level playing field for all athletes. Testing is based on the presence of the drug in a urine sample. That presence constitutes an offence, irrespective of the route of administration. Some sports are moving to blood samples rather than urine samples.

The International Olympic Committee (IOC) identifies the various classes and methods of doping.

Doping classes

A Stimulants (to increase alertness, reduce fatigue) e.g. amphetamines (in some tonics), ephedrine (in some cold cures), and caffeine (in tea, coffee, cola)

B Narcotic analgesics (to manage pain) e.g. aspirin (in Veganin – short-term painkiller), codeine (in Benylin and other cold remedies)

C Anabolic steroids (to speed recovery, improve competitiveness, increase muscle bulk) e.g. nandrolone (present in small amounts in some body building supplements), stanozolol

D Beta-blockers (to manage tension) e.g. stenolol, propranolol, oxprendol (normally in medicines for hypertension, cardiac dysrhythmias, etc.)

E Diuretics (to manage [lose] body weight) e.g. Amiloride, benzthiazide, bumetanide (present in proprietary brand diuretics)

F Peptide hormones and analogues

- Human Chorionic Gonadotrophin (similar to anabolic steroids) e.g. Pregnyl (medications related to hypogonadism)
- Corticotrophin (ACTH) (to increase blood levels of corticosteroids) e.g. tetracosactrin, synacthen (medications related to adrenocortical insufficiency)
- Human Growth Hormone (HGH: Somatotrophin) (to increase muscle hypertrophy, reduce effects of ageing process) e.g. Humatrope, Norditropin (medications to encourage growth)
- Erythropoetin (EPO) (to increase erythrocyte volume/aerobic capacity)

Doping methods

A Blood doping (endurance athletes)
Blood transfusion of erythrocytes or related products which contain erythrocytes. The blood can be drawn from the same person (autologous) then reinfused later, or drawn from another person then transfused to the athlete (nonautologous). In some areas of this practice, the blood is drawn following altitude training then reinfused before a key championship event.

B Pharmacological, chemical and physical manipulation
This covers the use of substances and methods which alter the integrity and validity of urine samples used in doping controls, e.g. catheterisation, urine substitution, etc.

C Classes of drugs subject to certain restrictions
Different sports may ban different drugs, or there may be laws outside sport within which athletes must operate.

Alcohol is not prohibited by the IOC, but a governing body may test for breath/blood alcohol levels. Marijuana is not prohibited but may contravene civil laws. Local anaesthetics, if medically justified, may be used, but only local or intra-articular injections may be administered, although *not cocaine* as this is a banned drug. Corticosteroids may only be used for topical use (aural, opthalmological and dermatological; local or intra-articular injections; or inhalational therapy [allergic conditions, asthma etc.]), otherwise, they are banned.

Coaches should be committed to ensuring that athletes understand the critical role that nutrition plays in the performance development process. They must also be aware of the detail of their athlete's nutrition. This is part of the athlete's preparation. Without that knowledge it is not possible to relate performance to training and development. Without that knowledge athlete and coach can unwittingly expose themselves to the terrible consequence of an athlete's positive drugs test result. If the coach feels that his understanding of nutrition is limited, then he must have access to a nutritionist/sports scientist in his support team to interpret the situation for coach and athlete so that there is a joint responsibility which may be exercised in ensuring the athlete's nutrition is safe, legal and effective.

FOOD ALLERGIES

It is strongly recommended that all athletes be tested for sensitivity to the range of substances which may bring about an allergic reaction. Skin test or hair follicle tests may be used to uncover sensitivity to pollen, animal dander and foods – including certain drugs taken for medication. Such sensitivities should not be trivialised; an allergic reaction may be hay fever or asthma at one end of the spectrum, or anaphylactic shock or even death at the other. With athletes experimenting more and more with nutrition and supplementation, and with foreign travel and, therefore, different foods and water becoming a regular feature in our lives, there is greater risk of exposure to a nutritional content to which there could be sensitivity and/or an allergic reaction. Once tests are interpreted, the athlete will know what foods or combination of foods to avoid and carry with him relevant permitted medication should problems arise. Such information must be available to the doctor responsible for the athlete's medical welfare or supervision in his sport.

NUTRITIONAL GUIDELINES FOR ATHLETES (PRE, DURING AND POSTEXERCISE)

Against this general nutritional background the following may help in dealing with the more specific aspects of training and competition:

(1) Nutrition, like most of what we require to be effective in our lives, is a matter of balance. It is best illustrated in this diagram – the food pyramid (fig. 27). It is founded on a base of making sure that we have a daily fluid intake of at least 1.5 litres. After that is it about the ratio of one food type to another.
(2) General points for daily intake

Breakfast: High fluid (especially water)
Cereals (natural bran is best)
Fruit
Easily digested light protein (not fried – especially if there is training in the morning)

Balanced diet

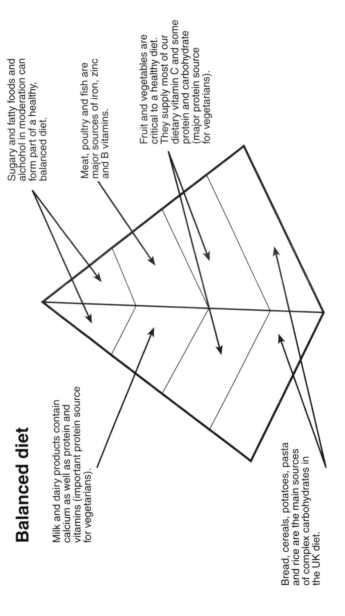

Sugary and fatty foods and alchohol in moderation can form part of a healthy, balanced diet.

Meat, poultry and fish are major sources of iron, zinc and B vitamins.

Fruit and vegetables are critical to a healthy diet. They supply most of our dietary vitamin C and some protein and carbohydrate (major protein source for vegetarians).

Milk and dairy products contain calcium as well as protein and vitamins (important protein source for vegetarians).

Bread, cereals, potatoes, pasta and rice are the main sources of complex carbohydrates in the UK diet.

FIG. 27 Food pyramid

Low and moderate GI carbohydrates if training in the morning
Moderate GI if training or competing in afternoon/evening

Snacks: Fruit, vegetable, cereal bars, water/fruit juice/mineral replacement drinks

Lunch: High fluid (especially water)
High GI carbohydrates if training in morning
Low and moderate GI if training or competing in afternoon/evening
Rich protein – especially egg/cheese, etc. if training in morning
Easily digested light protein if training or competing in the afternoon/evening
Fruit and vegetables
Build in fats/oils

Snacks: Boost carbohydrates – low and moderate GI before evening competition
High fluid intake (especially water)

Dinner: Rich protein if after training or competition
High GI and moderate GI carbohydrates if after training or competing
High fluid intake – especially if there has been a lot of sweat loss in training or competition
Build in fats/oils
Fruits and vegetables

(Try to have dinner normally no later than 19.30)

Supper   Normally this meal is post evening competition
High GI and moderate GI carbohydrates
High fluid intake
Easily digested, light protein
Fruit and vegetables

(Eating late is poor preparation for a good night's sleep – so this is essentially a light meal. However, breakfast the next morning may be boosted with a richer protein intake.)

We each have our own preferences for our daily nutrition routine, so we will have our own variations from breakfast to supper. However, these general principles should be built into our daily routine.

(3) Maintaining recommended daily allowance (RDA) of micronutrients is important for athletes due to the wear and tear of persistent training and competition. Although small, this varies according to age, gender and the impact of combined physical, intellectual and emotional stressors. Status can be checked via cell analysis.

(4) Micronutrient supplementation in the form of antioxidants, multivitamins and mineral tonics is pursued by around 75% of all athletes, although studies do not confirm performance benefit. It is possible that high performance athletes; all athletes involved near the limits of quality and quantity training and competition; athletes operating for long periods in extreme environments; athletes recovering from health problems; and athletes whose total profile of lifestyle stressors is testing the limits of their capacity to adapt and, therefore, causing health problems, will require some level of supplementation. They should seek the advice of a nutritionist in designing a strategy for what and how much to take, and also the frequency of days on/off supplementation.

(5) During and after prolonged periods of exercise where there is a high sweat rate, carbohydrate electrolyte replacement still drinks such as Lucozade Sport, Gatorade and Isostar are recommended rather than water, fruit juices or soft drinks. This is because there is the need to replace sodium and water when fluid loss goes above one litre per hour; sodium assists fluid absorption from the small intestine and prevents fluid loss via urine. Moreover, these drinks contain glucose and sucrose as carbohydrate rather than fructose or glucose polymers, which may irritate the stomach, slowing gastric emptying. Ideal carbohydrate concentration in drinks should be approximately 5–8%, with 20 m Eq sodium and 2.6 m Eq potassium.

(6) Carbohydrate should be taken 3–6 hours before competition, or the maximum quality/quantity exercise which takes athletes to their limit. If it is to be taken within an hour of the competition or exercise, it should be less than 100 gm, within 30 minutes of starting, and be followed by warm-up or light activity.

(7) In trained long-endurance athletes, reducing training and increasing the dietary carbohydrate to more than 10 gm/kg/day for three days prior to competition increases the muscle glycogen stores to their maximum value. This regime is not suitable for those preparing for intense exercise (e.g. for sprints, soccer, tennis).

(8) Where training or competition lasts 90 minutes or more, taking carbohydrate delays fatigue, so enhancing performance. The carbohydrate can be taken during the activity or approximately 30 minutes before the anticipated time of fatigue. Around 30–60 gm/hour carbohydrate is required, whether in liquid or solid form; if solid, it must have a high glycaemic index value, e.g. banana, honey.

(9) In some sports, athletes are required to perform prolonged exertions on consecutive days (e.g. tour cycling), or to perform in high-frequency back-to-back pressure competitions (e.g. World Cup soccer/rugby), or to train several times per day for 6–8 days at a time. Such demands require rapid regeneration by optimising the recovery process, particularly in reference to glycogen synthesis, hydration and muscle tissue repair.

- Glycogen synthesis
  - The optimal rate of replenishing carbohydrate is 0.7 gm/kg/hour, preferably in liquid form of glucose, glucose polymer or sucrose. If solid, it must have a high G.I value. Adding protein to liquid carbohydrate may increase rate of glycogen synthesis.
  - Animal fats intake should be reduced by replacing with vegetable oils.
  - During competition or training periods of more then 90 minutes, glycogen and fluid replenishment is necessary – especially where there is high fluid loss due to heat, air conditioning, etc. Fluids should be ingested at a rate of 1 litre/hour and the carbohydrate concentration kept around 6 gm/litre to optimise carbohydrate and fluid delivery.
  - Post-exercise carbohydrate ingestion should commence within 15 minutes of concluding the activity. To delay can reduce the rate of glycogen synthesis (e.g. delaying for two hours can reduce the rate from 7 mmol/kg/hour to less than 3 mmol/kg/hour). Even under optimal conditions it takes at least 20 hours (5% per hour) to re-establish glycogen stores.
  - When training or competing on consecutive days, muscle glycogen must be replenished between the bouts of activity. This can be done in 24 hours, but if there is muscle damage, for example via eccentric exercise (e.g. high volume or intensity running, jumping, weight training/lifting); or body contact/impact (e.g. rugby, soccer, American/Australian rules football, ice hockey), the glycogen synthesis rate can decrease. This is due to white blood cells (WBC) competing for blood glucose in their endeavours to repair the damaged tissue. This process, however, takes around 12 hours, so early and regular carbohydrate intake through these 12 hours should make sufficient glucose available to the muscle, despite increasing competition from WBC for its use.
  - Active recovery/warm down should be kept at low intensity (less than 35% VO2max) to avoid reducing glycogen stored in fast-twitch muscle.
- Hydration
  - Although, as mentioned under 'water', still drinks are more beneficial than carbonated for rehydration, the difference is not conclusive for electrolyte replacement. As suggested in (5), above, however, there is a case for keeping to still drinks when it comes to glycogen synthesis.
- Muscle tissue repair
  - Highly trained athletes exposed to prolonged periods of persistent training and competition loads have increased protein catabolism. It is very unlikely that protein ingested in their diet falls below the levels indicated in table 7. However, the process of repair/regeneration may require support via taking appropriate protein foods such as eggs, milk, brewer's yeast, fish, meat/poultry, liver, and avoiding poorer protein foods such as rice, soya, gelatin and related foods. Cooking method is also important. So boiled, stewed, grilled and poached foods should replace fried and roasted.

(10) Caffeine in coffee, tea and colas taken in a normal social context will not expose athletes to the risk of a positive drugs test result. A positive test (according to the IOC) would require 12 mg per ml of caffeine in the urine (15 mg per ml – National Collegiate Athlete Association, USA). It is estimated that two cups of brewed coffee (100–150 mg caffeine) or five cups of regular tea (30–75 mg caffeine) or six 12 oz colas (32–65 mg caffeine) will yield urine levels of 3–6 mg per ml.

(11) Alcohol impairs coordination, disturbs fluid balance and interferes with temperature regulation. It cannot be considered a sensible inclusion in an athlete's diet. Post-activity beers may be argued as contributing to fluid replacement (but alcohol dehydrates), or to aid relaxation, yet it can have quite the opposite effect! There are healthier ways to rehydrate and relax. The athlete's body is his vehicle for expressing the performance his training hours deserve. Why abuse it?

(12) Finally, following extensive review of the diets of athletes, it is perfectly clear that the vast majority over-estimate their nutritional requirements. In part, this is borne of the attitude of leaving nothing to chance – 'if something is good for you, more of it is better'. That is simply not true. Over-eating causes more rapid ageing and health risks than a well-balanced diet. In fact, periodic 'fasting' prolongs the life of certain animals, giving them a younger biological age. This practice is also used to 'detox', flushing out the toxic by-products of the food we eat.

The best advice is to keep within the nutritionist's rules for a healthy diet – especially in terms of calories; review nutritional status periodically via nutrition diaries and cell analysis, and stay in the middle weight range for your height and sports discipline.

SUMMARY

With the exception of the days preceding, during or following periods of training at the athlete's limit of load quality and quantity or competition, a regular well-balanced diet should supply his nutritional requirements. Calorific requirement demanded of the athlete's lifestyle should match calorific input from macronutrients; protein content will fall within the range associated with the nature of the sport and growth and repair needs; micronutrients will meet the athlete's needs which are above normal due to the wear and tear of his lifestyle; water intake will ensure that hydration remains at an appropriate level. Special diets may be designed in preparation for the high demands of glycogen stores to fuel the activity; during the activity to replace spent glycogen and reduce the rate of dehydration; and afterwards to restock glycogen stores and rehydrate; to replace reduced levels of micronutrients and speed regeneration and repair. Relevant nutritional supplementation must be considered and responsibly applied following consultation involving athlete, coach, nutritionist and, occasionally, medical adviser. No supplementation should be taken without that consultation and without it being approved as safe, legal and effective. Care should be taken to avoid foods which may have an adverse effect on the absorption of other nutrients (e.g. raw fish, raw egg albumen).

Athletes and coaches must know which substances, products and methods are listed as banned. They must understand *why*, both at the health and ethical levels. They must live within the laws of the IOC anti-doping programme because this is the most comprehensive of all the anti-doping programmes. They must do so not just because they have to, but because they want to.

5 THE OXYGEN TRANSPORTING SYSTEM

DEFINITION, FUNCTIONS AND EFFECTS

The various nutrients available to the body by the metabolism of foodstuffs must be transported to the sites where they are used or stored. This transport is provided by a remarkable fluid which also carries oxygen, hormones and chemicals; is a buffer solution; removes waste products from the tissues; aids temperature control; and helps maintain fluid balance. This fluid is the blood.

Blood

The volume of blood in the body varies from person to person and will increase with training, but it is approximately as follows: men 75 ml/kg body weight; women 65 ml/kg body weight; children 60 ml/kg body weight.

The composition of blood is quite complex, but is summarised by fig. 28.

Cells

Erythrocytes (red blood cells)

Erythrocytes (red blood cells) are formed in the bone marrow at an equal rate to their destruction (haemolysis); this means approximately 2-3 million cells per second. Red cell formation is stimulated by *hypoxia* (oxygen deficiency – see p. 93) and *erythropoietin*, a glycoprotein also known as haemopoietin or erythrocyte stimulating factor (ESF) which is produced in the kidneys. Intravenous injections of renal extracts or glucocorticoids stimulate red cell formation and it has been suggested that testosterone derivatives increase erythropoietin formation.

The average erythrocyte count in men is 5.7 million/mm^3 and in women and children is 4.8 million/mm^3. The red colouring is due to its haemoglobin content, which is a combination of a protein (globin) and a red pigment (haematin). Muscle haemoglobin is called myoglobin. The red pigment contains iron, which readily combines with oxygen. This combination is a very loose affair and the oxygen can be just as easily 'disconnected' or cast free. Herein lies the oxygen transporting property of blood and obvious importance of dietary iron. However, excessive iron will not increase the oxygen-carrying capacity of the blood. Iron absorption is tightly controlled by the body's requirements. When these are met, absorption through the intestine wall ceases and the excess iron is expelled in the faeces.

In men, the average haemoglobin (Hb) content is 15.8 g/100 ml blood, while in

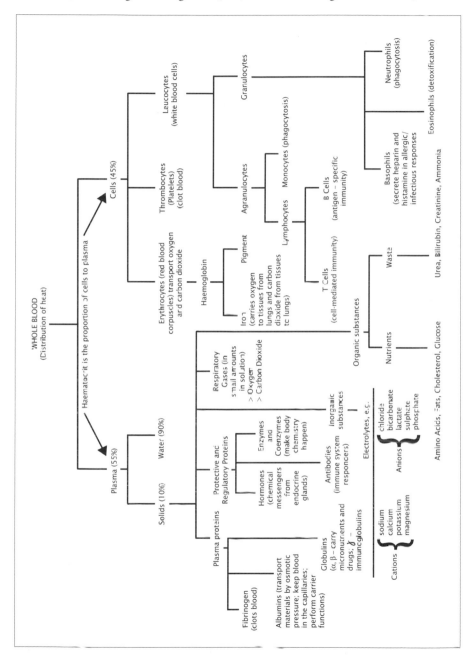

FIG. 28 Summary of blood composition and function

women it is 13.9 g/100 ml blood. To be more precise, normal values may be found within the range 14–18 g/100 ml blood for men and 11.5–16 g/100 ml for women. As 1 g of fully saturated haemoglobin combines with 1.34 ml oxygen, so haemoglobin may be used as an index of the oxygen-carrying capacity of the blood. Occasionally haemoglobin content is expressed as a percentage, but this can be a little confusing since 100% may be normal for one investigator but not for another. Moreover, there appears to be different 'normal' values according to age, gender, nationality, geographic location, and so on. Consequently, one must check the meaning of 100% before evaluating the haemoglobin count of an athlete.

The idea of a normal range seems much less problematic. Information on haemoglobin status is presented in the Edinburgh Royal Infirmary Bioprofile, as in table 11. Reading the haemoglobin line, the athlete appears to be relatively low in the range and consequently we can assume that the oxygen carrying capacity of the blood is also low. The second line tells us why it is low. The Mean Corpuscular Haemoglobin Concentration (MCHC) is an index of the iron status of haemoglobin and here it is clear that the athlete requires some kind of iron therapy suggested by a doctor.

normal range		you
Haemoglobin	Men (14–18): Women (11.5–16)	12.9
*MCHC	32–36	32.2

* Mean Corpuscular Haemoglobin Concentration

TABLE 11 Information sent to an Edinburgh girl who ran 800 m and 1500 m

Training increases the total amount of haemoglobin in the body and this can be assessed by evaluating the red cell volume and haemoglobin count. Periodically the erythrocyte count may rise by 5-10% with sustained work, but this is normally temporary and due to an imbalance of body fluids. However, training has a more variable effect on MCHC and it has been shown that many top endurance athletes have a tendency to iron deficiency (anaemia). This may be due to dietary deficiency, iron loss in sweat, damaged erythrocytes, etc., but may also be part of the adaptive process to ensure a higher speed of oxygen provision to the muscle. Endurance training will increase the blood *volume* by 15-30%, but this hypervolaemia is usually accompanied by a 5-10% fall in erythrocyte and haemoglobin concentration.

Finally, haemoglobin plays an essential part in the removal of carbon dioxide from the tissues to the lungs.

Leucocytes (white blood cells)

The leucocytes (white blood cells) are comprised of the following:

Granulocytes: *neutrophils* – involved in resistance to infection and multiply when there is an infection in the body or when there is local inflammatory reaction brought about by dead or dying tissue. The glucocorticoids increase the number of circulating neutrophils but their ability to migrate into the tissues is reduced, with consequent loss of resistance to infection. The destruction of bacteria by neutrophils is possible because the neutrophils are capable of phagocytosis ('cell eating'); *eosinophils* – collect at sites of allergic reaction and it has been suggested that they limit the effects of substances such as histamine. The level of circulating eosinophils is reduced by the glucocorticoids; *basophils* – have a much smaller share of the leucocyte population (table 12), and relatively little is known of their physiological function. They contain heparin and histamine and may be connected with preventing clotting. Glucocorticoids lower the number of circulating basophils.

Agranulocytes: *monocytes* – like the neutrophils they help remove bacteria and debris by active phagocytosis in the battle against infection. They act against bacteria after the neutrophils, thus forming a second line of defence. The corticosteroids have a similar effect on monocytes and neutrophils; *lymphocytes* – involved in the processes of immunity. They are formed principally from lymphoid tissue. The glucocorticoids decrease the number of circulating lymphocytes and the size of the lymph nodes.

type of cells	average number of cells per micro litre of blood		
neutrophils		5400	
eosinophils		160	
basophils		40	
lymphocytes		2750	
monocytes		540	
erythrocytes	(male)	4.8×10^6	
	(female)	5.4×10^6	
platelets		300,000	

TABLE 12 Composition of the blood's cell volume

It is worth bearing in mind that these defence manoeuvres require an expenditure of energy in addition to the weakness caused when the 'enemy' infection has gained ground. Training is never recommended during this battle unless the infection is very slight. The problem does not end here, however, because even when the battle has been won, the reserves have been depleted and must be allowed to recoup. Consequently the coach must scale down all training until the athlete feels that things are back to normal.

Thrombocytes (platelets)

The thrombocytes (platelets) are very small bodies which are fragments of giant cells called megakaryocytes. When the walls of blood vessels are damaged, platelets adhere to the injury site and secrete materials contained in their granules. This adhesion and secretion is the action of clotting. The number of circulating platelets is increased by glucocorticoids.

The role of the glucocorticoids has been previously mentioned to draw attention to some of the microphysical effects of stressors. Stress increases adrenocorticotrophic hormone (ACTH) activity (see chapter 8), which in turn raises the amount of circulating glucocorticoids. Why this occurs is still unexplained, but these microphysical effects may ultimately cause the major physical problems of high blood pressure, coronary disease, etc. (fig. 29). This is the reason for the concern for the health of 30-45-year-old males constantly exposed to stressors of business, professional life, and so on.

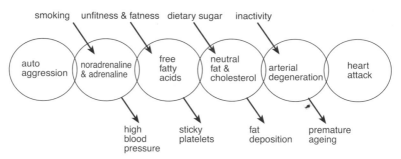

FIG. 29 Factors which contribute to the possibility of a heart attack. Carruthers referred to this situation as 'knitting a heart attack' (from Carruthers, 1971)

Plasma

Approximately 55% of the blood volume is a straw-coloured fluid called plasma. It is made up of over 90% water, and under 10% solids. The solids are made up as follows:

Plasma proteins

These are comprised of: albumins – they carry materials to sites of need or elimination (e.g. minerals, ions, fatty acids, amino acids, bilirubin, enzymes, drugs); globulins – the a1, a2, and ß1, ß2 globulins carry micronutrients and are carriers for drugs. The l globulins are immunoglobins or antibodies which generally protect the body against bacteria, viruses and toxins; fibrinogen – aids blood clotting. (The fluid 'squeezed' from a clot is serum.)

Protective and regulatory proteins

Hormones: (see chapter 8).

Antibodies: produced by the immune system to fight antigens (foreign agents) invading the body.

Enzymes and coenzymes: most chemical reactions occurring in the body are regulated by the catalytic action of enzymes and/or coenzymes. The chemicals which undergo change in an enzymically catalysed reaction are called substrates for that enzyme.

Inorganic substances

These are principally the electrolytes:

Cations (positively charged) – sodium, potassium, calcium and magnesium
Anions (negatively charged) – chloride, bicarbonate, lactate, sulphate and phosphate.

They also include copper, iodine, iron and lead. Lactate is the end product of the lactic anaerobic energy pathway. Normal levels are 1-1.8 mmol/ litre, but in prolonged intensive exercise, this can rise to 20mmol/litre. Due to its ease of diffusion, blood lactate gives a reasonable picture of lactate concentration in muscle. Peak lactic acid concentration in the blood is not achieved until several minutes after activity.

Respiratory gases

Plasma contains small amounts of inspired oxygen and carbon dioxide in sodium and as bicarbonate being transported out of the body via the lungs.

Organic substances

Nutrients: –   amino acids (see chapter 4)
            –   fats and cholesterol (see chapter 4)
            –   glucose (see chapter 4)

Waste: –   urea, from breakdown of protein. This varies in line with protein in the diet.
            –   creatinine, from breakdown of body tissues
            –   ammonia, formed in the kidneys from glutamine brought to it in the blood. This varies with the quantity of acids which are neutralised in the kidney.
            –   bilirubin; during destruction of erythrocytes by the reticuloendothelial system at the end of their 120 day life, haemoglobin is released and both iron and globin are split off and bilirubin is formed.

Other substances are present in minute amounts in plasma, but are not listed here in detail.

Among the properties of blood already listed is its function as a 'buffer solution'. A buffer solution contains a weak acid or alkali and a highly ionised salt of the same acid or alkali. The presence of the highly ionised salt maintains the pH balance of the solution when it is exposed to an influx of acid or alkali substance (see chapter 7, page 117).

Biochemical analysis of blood can probably give the clearest picture of the status of an athlete's body chemistry, short of biopsy techniques. Advancements in technology allow analysis of blood to test over 100 parameters of a given sample of blood in 60 seconds.

To fulfil its tasks, the blood must be:

• pumped around the body (heart)
• contained in tubes/vessels through which it is pumped (blood vessels)

- taken to a source of oxygen (lungs)
- taken to a source of fuel (gut, liver)
- taken to areas where oxygen and fuel are used (tissues)
- loaded with waste (tissues)
- unloaded of waste (lungs, kidneys).

Astrand's and Rodahl's (1986) diagram of circulation helps to give the overall picture (fig. 30).

The heart

The heart is a muscle which, by its contraction, pumps blood round the body to all areas to meet the needs of the moment. For example, at rest, the gut has a lot of blood to cope with digestion and the acceptance of nutrients for transporting to storage or circulation. During exercise the blood is directed to where it is needed, i.e. the muscle for mechanical and physiological work, and the skin for temperature control.

The continuous pumping of the heart also returns 'used' blood, carrying increased carbon dioxide back to the lungs, where the excess carbon dioxide is unloaded and oxygen supplies are replenished. Blood is carried from the systemic circulation through the vena cavae into the right atrium. There is no valve on entry, as thickening and contraction of muscle prevents backflow. It then passes through the tricuspid (A–V) valve into the right ventricle, then through the pulmonary (semilunar) valve into pulmonary circulation – offloading carbon dioxide and taking on oxygen. From the lungs via the pulmonary veins it enters

FIG. 30 Astrand and Rodahl illustrate the circulation 'picture' with great clarity in this extract from *A Textbook of Work Physiology* (1986). The figures indicate the relative distribution of the blood to the various organs at rest (lower scale) and during exercise (upper scale). During exercise the circulating blood is primarily diverted to the muscles. The area of the black squares is proportional to the minute volume of blood flow.

the left atrium. Again, there is no valve. It then passes through the mitral (A–V) valve into the left ventricle, then back into the systemic circulation through the aortic (semilunar) valve then via the aorta. Electrocardiograms (ECGs) are frequently used to assess the status of the heart's contractile mechanisms, but may also be used in laboratory testing work to provide an accurate heart rate assessment. Figure 31 shows the relationship between the ECG, blood pressure, heart sound, and ventricular pressure. The ECG is recorded on a printout form or on an oscilloscope. Changes in the T-wave have been noted when the athlete is experiencing high level stressors in training or competition (Carlile, 1960).

Blood pressure

Blood pressure is also used as a guide to the efficiency of the heart and blood vessels. Normal values are 120 mm/80 mm. This means at systole (i.e. when the heart thrusts its contents from the left ventricle into the aorta which takes the oxygen-rich blood to the tissues) the pressure is 120 mm, and at diastole (i.e. when the left ventricle is being refilled) the pressure is 80 mm. These pressures, especially the systole, rise in the first few minutes of exercise, but gradually fall over the following 30 to 45 minutes. Other blood pressures of interest are those of systole and diastole at the right ventricle which send oxygen-depleted blood along the pulmonary artery to the lungs. These pressures are 25 mm and 7 mm, to avoid damaging the lungs.

When the blood reaches the tissues, the pressure has dropped considerably but is still sufficient to squeeze the fluids through the capillary walls into the tissue. This is because the *hydrostatic* pressure is lower in the tissue than in the capillaries. The

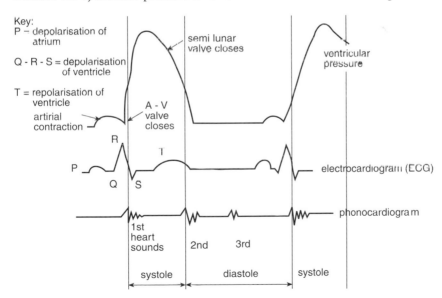

FIG. 31 The relationship between the contraction patterns and mechanisms of the heart, the ECG and the heart sounds (from Guyton, 1966)

return of the fluid to the capillaries is due to *osmotic* pressure generated by albumen in the blood. This may be thought of as a 'thirst' for fluid. The fluid returns to the capillaries and is pressed back towards the heart by hydrostatic pressure. The oxygen required by the tissues is removed from the blood at capillary level and the carbon dioxide formed by the working tissues passes into the capillary to be carried back to the right heart, then on to the lungs. The cycle is then repeated. Any 'spillover' of fluid between capillary and tissue goes into the lymphatic system to be drained off into circulation at another point, or into the body's extracellular fluids.

The volume of blood pumped out with each contraction of the heart muscle is known as the stroke volume. The number of heart beats per minute is called the heart rate. Compared with untrained people, training of the oxygen transporting system at a given workload lowers the athlete's heart rate on recovery from that workload, as well as at rest. The highly trained endurance athlete may have a range from approximately 40 beats per minute to 200 per minute. At the latter rate, the heart is apparently 'failing' because there is insufficient time to fill the volume of the ventricles. As a consequence, the stroke volume is reduced to much less than maximum. (In top male endurance athletes maximum is approximately 220 ml; resting = 80 ml.) As we grow older, maximum heart rate reduces. Astrand and Christensen (1964) suggest 210/minute at the age of 10, 180/minute at 35 years of age and 165/minute at 65 years of age.

Cardiac output is the total volume of blood pumped out by the heart per minute. This is the product of heart rate x stroke volume. Astrand (1986) states that 'cardiac output during standard exercise repeated during a course of training . . . is maintained at the same level'. This implies that stroke volume increases with training (since heart rate decreases).

The blood vessels

The blood vessels are best presented in diagram form, as illustrated in figure 32 showing the complete 'circuit'.

The lungs

The lungs provide the large surface area necessary for the exchange of oxygen (passing into the blood) and carbon dioxide (passing out of the blood). Before it reaches the tiny alveoli, air is warmed, moistened and cleansed as it passes via the nose and mouth through the trachea, bronchi and bronchioles. Finally, exchange of gases takes place between the alveoli and the pulmonary capillaries. Certain measures of lung capacity are frequently used to assess the efficiency of the breathing mechanisms (fig. 33).

- vital capacity is the maximal volume of gas that can be expelled from the lungs following a maximal inspiration
- inspiratory capacity is the maximal volume of gas inspired from the functional residual capacity

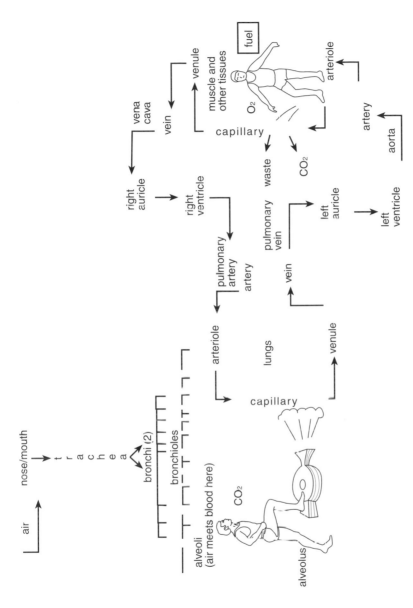

FIG. 32 Schematic diagram of the blood vessels and the passage of oxygen from outside the body, to the working muscle

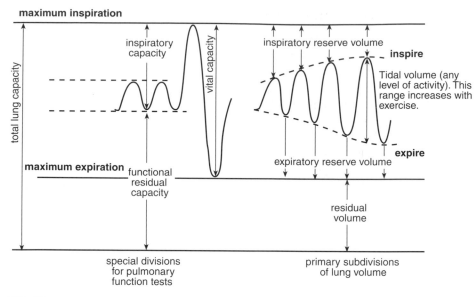

FIG. 33 Diagram of lung volumes and capacities (from Pappenheimer et al, 1950)

- functional residual capacity is the volume of gas remaining in the lungs when the respiratory muscles are relaxed
- expiratory reserve volume is the volume of gas expired from the functional residual capacity
- residual volume is the volume of gas which remains in the lungs even after forced expiration
- total lung capacity is the sum of the vital capacity and residual volume.

In women, the lung volumes are approximately 10% smaller than for men of the same age and size. Training for aerobic endurance may increase vital capacity. Vital capacity decreases with age. Although this is clear in the over 40s, the exact commencement of this decline is normally in the early 30s, but is variable according to the individual concerned.

Vital capacity is greatest amongst endurance athletes – in Stockholm an Olympic medallist in cross-country skiing recorded 8.1 litres.

Gut and liver

It has been pointed out that many of the end products of digestion are absorbed from the intestine into the blood, which carries these products to storage or further processing and then carries required nutrients into general circulation. Concentration of blood flow in this area of the circulatory system is much greater at rest than it is during exercise (fig. 30). Prior to competition, emotional excitement causes an increased flow of adrenaline, an arresting of the digestive process, and a very obvious problem if a meal has been eaten too recently.

The liver performs a number of functions:

- it maintains a supply of glucose to the blood.
- it is the most vital organ of metabolism.
- it is a storage organ, holding glycogen, fat, proteins, some vitamins, and other substances involved in blood formation, and blood itself. These substances are released and reserves replenished as the need arises.
- it synthesises plasma proteins and heparin.
- it secretes bile which is necessary for the absorption of fats and the fat soluble vitamins A, D, E and K.
- it is involved in the formation and destruction of erythrocytes, and in the protection of the body against toxic invaders (e.g. through oxidation of alcohol and nicotine).

The liver has responsibility for making potential energy available to the tissues in the form of glucose. Its efficiency in this role *must* be maximum in exercise. Consequently it is wrong to make demands of the liver to oxidise, say, alcohol, while energy provision is required.

The tissues

The main tissues of interest to those involved in training theory are the muscles, which are dealt with in detail in chapter 6.

Elimination of the waste products of exercise

The principal waste products of exercise are urea, carbon dioxide, water, metabolites other than lactate, and lactic acid itself. The main fate of urea and water is to be filtered through the kidneys and expelled from the body. Carbon dioxide is carried in the blood to the lungs, where it passes into the alveoli and is then expelled from the body. Metabolites other than lactate are disposed of first by oxidation. The oxygen required for this purpose is referred to as that which repays the alactic oxygen debt. Lactic acid is eliminated as follows:

(1) The muscle lactate is disposed of first by oxidation to pyruvate, and then by dissimilation to carbon dioxide and water.
(2) Some of the blood lactate is then taken up by the liver which reconstructs it to glycogen, via the 'cori cycle' (see chapter 7, page 106).
(3) The remaining blood lactate diffuses back into the muscle, or other organs, to be oxidised then dissimilated. Such oxidation of lactate causes formation of carbon dioxide, the fate of which is mostly the reconstitution of blood bicarbonate, before being excreted by the lungs.

It should be noted that lactate cannot be oxidised in the blood stream itself. Moreover, it appears that the reconstruction of glycogen from lactic acid is not possible in human muscle.

MAXIMAL OXYGEN UPTAKE

Maximal oxygen uptake (VO2 maximum) is the body's maximal aerobic power and is defined as 'the highest oxygen uptake the individual can attain during physical work breathing air at sea level' (Astrand, 1970). Oxygen uptake is the difference in oxygen content between the air inspired and the air expired, expressed in ml/kg body weight/minute. In other words it is the amount of oxygen required by the body to fulfil its functions at a given time. Obviously more oxygen will be required in severe exercise and so oxygen uptake will increase. However, a point is eventually reached where the body can take up no more oxygen. At this point the value is referred to as the maximal oxygen uptake.

Evaluation of the athlete's VO2 maximum is the best criterion of his status of aerobic efficiency. In table 13, Swedish statistics give the ranges for certain groups of athletes.

	male	female
400 m	63–69	52–58
800 m–1500 m	74–77	52–58
3000 m	77–82	
Cross country	72–83	55–61
Normals	38–46	30–46

TABLE 13 VO2 max ranges for Swedish athletes according to competition distance (ml/kg body wt/min)

The highest recorded improvements of VO2 maximum are between 15% and 20%. Improvement is made possible by increasing the efficiency of the oxygen transporting system. The principal areas for its possible improvement are as follows:

(1) The heart. Stroke volume can be increased by specific endurance training, as can the capacity to raise the maximum heart rate.

(2) The blood. The oxygen-carrying capacity of the blood can again be increased by specific training. Both total mass of erythrocytes and total haemoglobin may be increased. Ekblom's (1972) 'blood doping' demonstrated the artificial increase of the blood's oxygen-carrying capacity.

(3) The muscle. The difference between the oxygen content of artery and vein (e.g. before and after the muscle accepts fuel and oxygen from the capillaries) is known as the arterio-venous oxygen difference (a-v⁻O2). Increasing the size and number of mitochondria (the oxygen users) of muscle, and the density of capillaries in muscle by specific endurance exercise, will increase the value of a-v⁻O2, as will the increase in myoglobin, the muscles' own internal oxygen transport system.

A relationship between heart rate, % VO2 maximum, and blood lactate concentration is suggested by table 14. However, because heart rate does not increase linearly over the full range of exercise intensity but is close to this over a given range, this relationship can only represent an approximation.

lactic acid mg/100ml blood	% VO$_2$ max.	heart rate	scale of intensity
25	50	130	low
30	60	150	light
70	75	165	high
90	90	180/190	submaximum
100	100	190+	maximum

TABLE 14 Relationship of blood lactate concentration, % VO2 max. and heart rate (adapted from Suslov, 1972)

ACCLIMATISATION TO ALTITUDE

In the mid 1960s the problems of competing at altitude raised questions about the possible advantages of training at altitude. At altitudes, such as that of Mexico City (2.3 km, 7500 ft), there is a reduced partial pressure of oxygen (pO2) due to reduced barometric pressure, thus there is a lower pressure forcing oxygen into the blood in the lungs. The partial pressure at any point is obtained from the formula:

$$pO_2 = \% \text{ oxygen concentration of dry air x barometric pressure}$$
$$-47* *(47 = \text{partial pressure of water vapour})$$

Thus, with a constant oxygen concentration of 20.94% dry air, table 15 shows the pO2 at different altitudes.

Altitude					
m	ft	Pressure, mmHg	kPa	PO$_2$ tracheal air, mmHg	kPa
0	0	760	101.3	149	19.9
500	1640	716	95.5	140	18.7
1000	3280	674	89.9	131	17.5
1500	4920	634	84.5	123	16.4
2000	6560	596	79.5	115	15.3
2500	8200	560	74.7	107	14.3
3000	9840	526	770.1	100	13.3

TABLE 15 Based on dry conditions for average temperature at altitude when the temperature at sea level is 15°C (59°F) and the barometric pressure is 760 mmHg (101.3 kPa). The tracheal air represents inspired air saturated with water vapour at 37°C (98.6°F). There would only be water molecules in the trachea at this point. (Abbreviated from Astramd, Rodahl, Dahl and Stromme, 2003).

m	ft	Pressure, mmHg	kPa	PO_2 tracheal air, mmHg	kPa
			Altitude		
3500	11,840	493	65.7	93	12.4
4000	13,120	462	61.6	87	11.6
4500	14,650	433	57.7	81	10.8
5000	16,400	405	54.0	75	10.0
6000	19,690	354	47.2	64	8.5
7000	22,970	308	41.1	55	7.3
8000	26,250	267	35.6	46	6.1
9000	29,530	230	30.7	38	5.1
10,000	32,800	198	26.4	32	4.3
19,215	63,000	47	6.3	0	.0

TABLE 15 Continued

Hypoxia is more an effect than a fact at altitude because the chemical composition of the atmosphere is almost uniform up to an altitude of over 20,000 ft. Also, at altitude, with the reduced barometric pressure, there is a reduced air resistance, implying an advantage to speed activities. The force of gravity is also reduced, suggesting an advantage where relative strength or maximum strength is critical. Air temperature and humidity are on the whole lower and this increases the loss of water via respiration, causing problems in endurance sports, intermittent but long duration team games, and so on. Finally, ultraviolet radiation is more intense so competition or training during hours when the sun is high should be avoided. The immediate effects of exposure to altitude are:

- increased breathing rate, even at rest
- increased heart rate (tachycardia)
- giddiness
- nausea
- headache
- sleeplessness
- greater arteriovenous oxygen difference
- decreased VO2 maximum
- rapid increase of haemoglobin concentration in first few days.

The total effect of these adjustments is a reduction of work capacity, but the degree of reduction can vary between individuals.

The long-term effects of continued exposure to altitude are:

- increased erythrocyte volume (increased erythropoietin secretion due to hypoxic effect)

- increased haemoglobin volume and concentration
- increased blood viscosity
- continued lower VO2 maximum
- decreased tolerance of lactic acid
- reduced stroke volume of the heart
- increased capillarisation in the muscle.

It is clear that training at altitude is sound preparation for competing at altitude and that altitude performances will improve as adaptation continues.

Although debate continues as to the value of altitude training for enhancing performance at sea level, the balance of practical experience supports the view that there are advantages to a carefully managed programme (see also p. 281).

SUMMARY

Although blood is referred to as the oxygen transporting vehicle, it is also the principal means of transporting to the tissues the fuel and materials essential for maintenance, repair and growth, and of transporting waste from the tissues to disposal sites. The effectiveness of this vehicle is enhanced by increased functional capacity of heart, lungs, blood vessels and blood, combined with more efficient use of oxygen, fuel and various materials at the sites where they are required. Blood also transports heat from muscle to skin.

Increased efficiency of the overall oxygen transporting system implies increased working capacity, which itself implies more value from training units for the athlete and more life in the years of the non-athlete. Specific training will increase efficiency of the system and it is therefore self-evident that both athletes and non-athletes should adopt such training.

Periodic blood analyses are acknowledged to be valuable aids to evaluate body chemistry and are recommended for athlete and non-athlete alike. In addition, it is suggested that VO2 maximum, blood pressure and blood lactate (for a given workload) be similarly tested to establish a broad picture of oxygen transporting system efficiency, relative to the physiological demands of a sport.

The 'anaerobic threshold', or onset of blood lactate accumulation (OBLA point) is also a critical measure. The OBLA point gives an indication of the workload (on cycle, canoe or rowing ergometers, or on a treadmill) at which the body just starts to seriously use anaerobic energy with the probability of a rapid build-up of lactic acid in the blood.

Knowing the heart rate at which this happens can help a competitor to optimise aerobic training by working appropriately just under the OBLA point, i.e. just below the anaerobic threshold. The anaerobic threshold may sometimes be determined without blood sampling – by noting alterations in breathing patterns during a maximum aerobic test.

6 THE WORKING MUSCLE

On arrival at the muscle, the fuel is combusted with or without oxygen as the muscle converts chemical energy to mechanical energy. Before examining the working parts of the muscle, the various 'energy pathways' should be explained.

THE ENERGY PATHWAYS

The energy pathways are each designed to reform (or reconstitute) the compound adenosine triphosphate (ATP). It is the breaking down of this compound which provides energy for cell function. This breakdown may be expressed as an equation (fig. 34), in full, or diagrammatically as the symbolic removal of P from ATP to produce ADP + P.

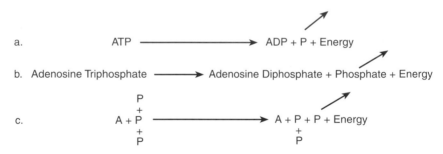

FIG. 34 Breakdown of ATP

The production of this vital compound, which has been referred to as 'the energy currency of life', may be effected by one of three pathways – alactic anaerobic, lactic anaerobic and aerobic.

Alactic anaerobic energy pathway

In the muscle there is a store of a compound, creatine phosphate (or phosphocreatine), which consists of creatine plus a large number of phosphates. If, after ATP is broken down to ADP, a phosphate was added to ADP, thereby reconstituting ATP, then the process of energy production could be continued. A store of phosphates would be required for this, and that is where creatine phosphate comes in. As ATP breaks down to ADP, a phosphate may be drawn from the creatine phosphate store to make ATP. This process may be continued until the creatine phosphate store is exhausted. The hydrolysis of creatine phosphate to resynthesise ATP is regulated by the enzyme creatine kynase.

ATP $\qquad \rightarrow \qquad$ ADP + P + Energy

ADP + P* $\qquad \rightarrow \qquad$ ATP + Creatine

There is approximately three to four times the amount of creatine phosphate as ATP in the muscle. It permits athletes to work at high intensity for 10–15 seconds without lactic acid production. Hence its title as the *alactic* (without lactate) anaerobic (without oxygen) *energy pathway*. Some 25–30 seconds recovery is required for resynthesis of approximately half of the creatine phosphate – ATP energy stores. These energy compounds in the muscle are sometimes known as phosphagen stores and this refers to creatine phosphate plus ATP. Short, intermittent bursts of activity, for example, in football, basketball, hockey, rugby, lacrosse, hurling, fencing, or sprints up to 200 m on the track, will call upon this pathway. Training can develop alactic anaerobic capacity to some extent. This would involve short intervals of maximum effort (5–10 secs) with long rests (one minute).

Lactic anaerobic energy pathway

This energy pathway involves the breakdown of glycogen (glycolysis) in the absence of oxygen, with the resultant formation of ATP plus lactate (lactic acid and associated products). This pathway is therefore referred to as the lactic anaerobic energy pathway. The chemical reaction may be summarised as follows:

Glycogen + P + ADP $\qquad \rightarrow \qquad$ ATP + Lactate

(1 Unit) $\qquad\qquad\qquad\qquad$ (3 Units)

The accumulation of lactate will terminate use of this energy pathway after 40–50 seconds maximum effort. Consequently it is the pathway called upon principally by athletes whose sports demand high energy expenditure for up to approximately 60 seconds, and those in 'multiple sprint sports' such as squash, ice hockey, rugby, lacrosse, hurling, sprint cycling, 400 m track and 100 m swim. Thereafter, there must be a progressive recruitment of an alternative energy pathway. It is known that exposure to lactic anaerobic stressors in training will increase the athlete's ability to utilise this pathway. It should be said that such training must be based on the sound foundation of training to develop the aerobic energy pathway.

Aerobic training produces cellular adaptations which increase the rate of lactate removal, so lactate accumulation commences at a higher level of exercise intensity. For untrained, healthy people the threshold for commencement of lactic accumulation is around 55% VO2 max. A trained athlete can be as high as 75% max. Blood lactate threshold is also known as 'onset of blood lactate acid' (OBLA). The trained athlete can also tolerate 20–30% higher blood lactate levels than the untrained athlete, partially due to a 20% increase in activity of the glycolitic enzyme, phosphofructokinaise.

Aerobic energy pathway

This pathway involves the oxygen transporting system and the use of oxygen in the mitochondria of the working muscle for the oxidation of glycogen or fatty acids. Due to this pathway's dependence upon oxygen, it is referred to as the aerobic energy pathway. This is involved in prolonged work of relatively low intensity and is of increasing importance the longer the sport's duration. Taken to its logical conclusion, only lack of fuel (together with overheating and dehydration) will end an exercise of several hours' duration involving this pathway. The chemical reaction may be summarised as:

1 unit glycogen $+ P + ADP + O_2 = 37$ units ATP $+ CO_2 + H_2O$
1 unit free fatty acids $+ P + ADP + O_2 = 140^*$ units ATP $+ CO_2 + H_2O$
* Approx.

This pathway may be developed by specific training.

It will be seen from the 'rates of exchange' of free fatty acids and glycogen to ATP, that the free fatty acids appear the most favourable currency. However, about 8% more oxygen per calorie is needed if the energy comes from fat sources. The very poor exchange rate of glycogen in lactic anaerobic exercise is only one factor contributing towards the phenomenon known as 'oxygen debt'. The best way of explaining this is to illustrate the situation with an example:

22.4 litres of oxygen are required to remove 180 g lactic acid
180 g lactic acid from glycolysis yields 55 kcal
aerobic glycolysis yielding 55 kcal requires 11.0 litres oxygen

Thus, if the lactic anaerobic pathway is used, 100% interest must be paid on the debt. This is referred to, naturally, as the lactic oxygen debt. There also exists an alactic oxygen debt. The 'bill' here, looks like this:

refill of oxygen stores (blood, myoglobin)	= 1.0 litres oxygen
elevation of temperature and adrenaline concentration	= 1.0 litres oxygen
increased cardiac and respiratory involvement	= 0.5 litres oxygen
breakdown of ATP and creatine phosphate	= 1.5 litres oxygen
total	= 4.0 litres oxygen

So, in addition to the oxygen debt created by the lactic energy pathway, there is an alactic oxygen debt which must be repaid irrespective of the energy pathway used. Repayment of these debts will, of course, rely on an efficient system to aid recovery, which implies a well-developed oxygen transporting system. Consequently it is fundamental to athletes in all sports that the aerobic pathway is trained.

It would appear that the fuelling system for combustion in aerobic exercise varies according to its duration and intensity. In prolonged aerobic exercise the preferred fuel is free fatty acids because the glucose stores (glycogen) are limited compared to the very large fat stores. Unlike glycogen, fatty acids can only be used in the aerobic pathway, whereas in higher intensity exercise involving aerobic and anaerobic pathways, or exclusively anaerobic, the preferred fuel is glycogen.

The contribution of aerobic and anaerobic systems to energy output varies with the duration of the activity concerned. Astrand (1970) has represented this diagrammatically (fig. 35). It must be emphasised, however, that it is not sound to deduce from these statistics that the ratio of training time should vary. The aerobic system is the fundamental basis of all endurance sports and there are few sports which do not make demands of endurance capacity, even if only to ensure quicker recovery within and between training units. A sound aerobic basis will enable the athlete to be exposed to more frequent specific stressors as stimuli for specific adaptation.

The three energy pathways are summarised diagrammatically in figure 37, but before leaving this area, it might be useful to include a brief glossary of expressions often used concerning energy production.

Glycogenolysis: the conversion of glycogen to glucose, mainly in the liver, for use as a fuel.

Glycolysis: the oxidation of glucose or glycogen to pyruvate or lactate, the latter two substances being intermediate steps in energy production.

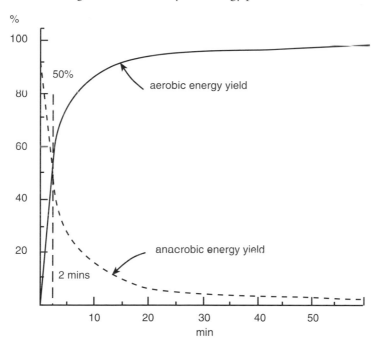

FIG. 35 Astrand's classic representation of % of total energy yield from aerobic and anaerobic pathways, during maximal efforts of up to 60 mins duration, for an athlete of high maximal power for both types of energy production.

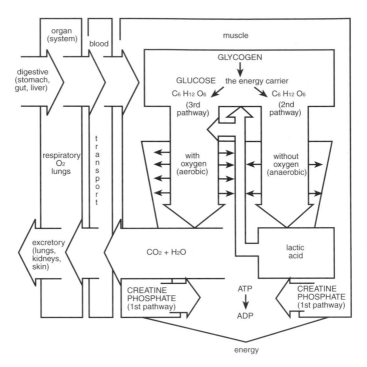

FIG. 36 Schematic summary of the three pathways (from Jäger and Oelschlägel, 1974)

Glycogenesis: the synthesis of glycogen from glucose.

Gluconeogenesis: the formation of glucose or glycogen from noncarbohydrate sources (e.g. glycerol, glucogenic amino acids and lactate).

Tricarboxylic acid cycle: also referred to as citric acid cycle, or Krebs cycle, this is the final common pathway of carbohydrate, fats and protein oxidation to carbon dioxide and water.

Hexosemonophosphate shunt: an alternative system to the tricarboxylic acid cycle and is a side branch of glycolysis. Also known as the pentosephosphate cycle, it produces NADPH which provides reducing power and free energy during anabolic reactions.

Cori cycle: the release of lactate from muscle into the circulation for uptake by the liver and conversion to glucose. Consequently, it is central to lactic-anaerobic energy pathway.

Alanine cycle: the release of alanine (and amino acid) from muscle into the circulation for uptake by the liver and conversion into glucose. It becomes important towards the limits of the aerobic-energy pathway in long-term, high intensity exercise – providing 15–20% of the energy requirement.

Figure 37 gives a general picture of fuel production.

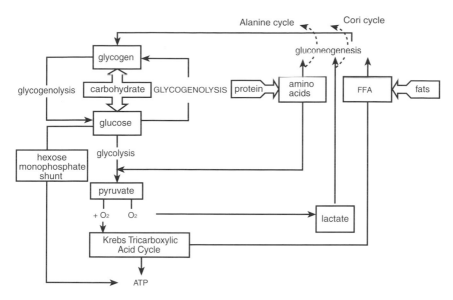

FIG. 37 Summary of the processing of energy fuel sources in the production of ATP

THE MUSCLE

The breakdown of ATP to ADP supplies the energy that is required to cause the muscle to contract, or shorten. By shortening, the muscle pulls on the tendons which are attached to the bony levers. It now remains to explain the mechanisms involved in muscle contraction and in initiating ATP/ADP breakdown.

The muscle consists of many muscle fibres which, if examined under a light microscope, have a striped or striated appearance (fig. 38c). To each muscle fibre is attached the endplate of a motoneuron.

The motoneuron is the nerve cell which finally controls skeletal muscle and the 'endplate' is its attachment to the muscle fibre. A motoneuron and the muscle fibres it supplies is called a motor unit. Occasionally a fibre may be supplied by more than one motoneuron, but as a rule only one motoneuron is involved.

Where very fine movement is required, there may be as few as five fibres to one neuron (e.g. the muscles of the eye). On the other hand, when gross movement is required, as in the thigh, the ratio may be one neuron to several thousand fibres. The motoneuron is housed in the anterior (ventral) part of the spinal cord and signals pass from here along a tendril-like arm, the axon, at the end of which are branches to which are attached the endplates (fig. 39). These in turn are attached to a specific number of muscle fibres. The axon is for the most part surrounded by a myelin sheath, which is 'pinched' at intervals like a string of linked sausages (fig. 39). The pinched areas are known as the *nodes of Ranvier* and due to their presence the nerve impulses can pass quicker along myelinated

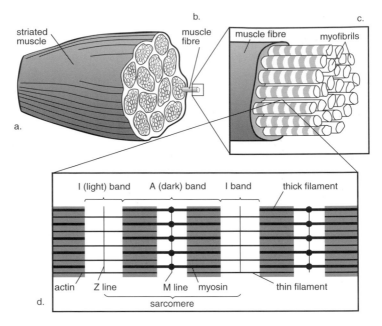

FIG. 38 The striated muscle (a), is composed of muscle fibres (b), which appear striated (striped) under the light microscope. Each muscle fibre is made up of myofibrils (c), beside which lie cell nuclei and mitochondria. The striated appearance of the myofibril arises from the repeated light and dark bands. A single unit of this 'repetition' is a sarcomere (d). This consists of a Z line, an I band, an A band which is interrupted by an Hzone, another I band – then the next Z line. These bands, in turn, arise from the overlapping of actin and myosin filaments (from H. E. Huxley, 1958). The sarcomere is the actual unit of contraction in the muscle fibre, which contains tens of thousands of both sarcomeres and mitochondria (for aerobic energy).

axons than non-myelinated axons. It is believed that this is due to a saltatory conduction (jumping) of the impulse from node to node.

Each muscle fibre consists of bundles of myofibrils beside which lie the nuclei of the muscle cells and mitochondria. The striations noted in the fibre are, in fact, striations of the massed myofibrils. If a closer examination is made of the light and dark bands of the myofibril, the actual contractile mechanism is revealed (fig. 38). The contractile unit, bound by the Z lines, is the sarcomere. As the actin filaments attached to opposing Z lines slide past the myosin filaments towards each other, the Z lines are drawn closer together. The sarcomeres of a single myofibril are joined end to end and all sarcomeres in that myofibril will contract at one time giving a total shortening of that myofibril. Moreover, the 'signal' to contract, which arrives via the axon and endplate at the muscle fibre, causes the whole fibre to contract. Thus, when the signal is sent, contraction of the fibre is brought about by the contraction of all its myofibrils, and the myofibrils contract as a result of the shortening of their sarcomeres.

It should be pointed out that the 'all or none law' applies to muscle fibre contraction. When the signal to contract arrives at the endplate, the whole muscle fibre contracts to the limit of its capacity. On the other hand, when there is no signal the

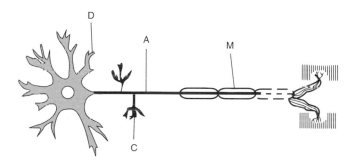

FIG. 39 (top) The motoneuron N, in the spinal cord can be excited (+) directly (1) or via an interneuron (2). Thus, an impulse is propagated in the nerve fibre, and the muscle is stimulated – causing muscular activity. Other nerve terminals can prevent the motoneuron from being stimulated. Schematically, nerve end (3) stimulates interneuron nerve cell (4) which is inhibitory. (lower) Motoneuron; A, axon; C, collateral; D, dendrite; M, myelin (from Schreiner and Schreiner).

muscle fibre assumes its resting length. Thus, there are no gradations of contractile force at the muscle fibre level. Contractile force is graded by the selective involvement of an appropriate number of motor units. The selective involvement is controlled by the central nervous system. This system brings a directive from the cerebrum and this directive is modified or qualified by the proprioceptor mechanisms (fig. 40). Thus, recruitment of the appropriate number of selected motor units for a given task is learned and the muscle concerned is programmed to contract (fig. 40).

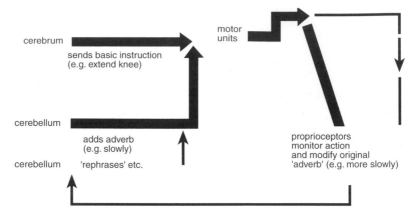

FIG. 40 Control of muscular action

When the impulse to contract arrives at the sarcolemma of the muscle fibre, it passes rapidly to every sarcomere. Within each sarcomere, running longitudinally, there exists a system of tubules known as the sarcoplasmic reticulum. The sarcoplasmic reticulum contains calcium ions and when the impulse arrives the calcium ions are released. This initiates an enzyme reaction with myosin, which causes the breakdown of ATP to ADP, thus releasing the energy to slide the actin and myosin past each other and bring about contraction of the myofibril. The calcium ions are returned to the sarcoplasmic reticulum by active pumping of its membranes. In the meantime, ADP is reconstituted to ATP via the creatine phosphate stores. Here then, among the small pockets of glycogen and scattered mitochondria, is the final product of that process which was started by eating and digesting a meal.

Types of muscular activity

Having gone into such detail in order to explain the mechanism of contraction, it should be said that the researcher rather than the coach is concerned with the microstructure of the muscle. It has become fashionable for the coach to consider the complex detail, described above, under the umbrella term 'the contractile component' of muscle. In popular terminology then, the contractile component is joined both in parallel and in series with 'the elastic component' (fig. 41). That part of the elastic component in parallel comprises such elements as connective sheaths and structural proteins, while that part of the elastic component in series comprises the tendons. The elastic component can be stretched and consequently develop tension due to its elastic resistance to that stretch. This, in effect, is the second mechanism in the muscle's contribution to contractile force. It is effective in those activities which involve voluntary muscle contraction and elastic recoil (e.g. running jumps, hopping, rapid agilities).

There is one other mechanism which may add to the efficiency of the overall force expression of contractile and elastic components. This is the myotonic reflex.

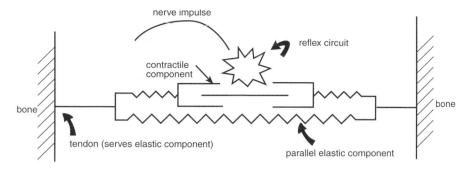

FIG. 41 Schematic representation of the contractile and elastic components plus reflex mechanisms in muscle

Both muscle and tendon are equipped with reflex systems. Approximately 90% of the tendon receptors are accommodated in the musculotendinous junction, while the remainder are in the tendon itself. The stimulus of stretch in this system effects the reflex response of inhibiting the contractile mechanism, thus allowing the muscle to lengthen and therefore relieving the degree of stretch in the tendon and musculotendinous junction. The muscle fibres are equipped with muscle spindle receptors. Their stimulus is the lengthening of the muscle fibre, the response being a stimulus to the muscle to contract, as elicited by the 'knee jerk' reflex.

It is reasonable to assume that in physical activity the reflex response to contract has an overall lower threshold than that to lengthen. The net result of this reflex activity is a more vigorous contraction of a given muscle when it is forcefully stretched (e.g. in the take-off leg in long jump). This 'net reflex' is the myotonic reflex and its existence now provides the athlete with a third contribution to a summated contractile force, although its activation can be harmful, e.g.

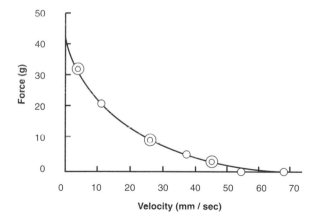

FIG. 42 Force-velocity curve of tetanised muscle at 0°C. Abscissae: force (g wt). Ordinates: velocity (mm per sec). Small circles: experimental points. Large circles: points 'used up' in fitting the theoretical curve. Agreement between theory and experiment is significant only at other points on the curve (Wilkie, D. R. 1956 Brit. med. Bull., 12, 177.) (from Samson Wright's *Applied Physiology*, 1973).

in too vigorous, bouncy, dynamic stretching exercises (as opposed to safer slow stretch). Only when the technical model of an activity is appropriately structured can all three systems (contractile component, elastic component and myotonic reflex) be summated.

The speed of contraction of a muscle will vary inversely with the force opposing it. Thus maximal speed is achieved when the muscle has no force resisting its action and zero speed is achieved when the immovable object is encountered (fig. 42). Maximum strength training is aimed at increasing the quantity of force required before zero speed is reached, while speed training is aimed at acquiring even higher speeds from existing maxima by assisting the movement via motivation, facilitation, learning, etc. If we consider the muscle actions of the athlete in figure 43 it is clear that some muscle actions will be dynamic (cause movement at joints) while others will be static (cause no movement at joints). In any given activity, there is a specific pattern of static and dynamic contraction carefully synchronised to meet the demands of that activity. The specific role of a given muscle within the total scheme of the specific pattern is referred to as *auxotonic*.

static

dynamic

FIG. 43 Static and dynamic work

It should be noted that dynamic and static muscle activity may be subdivided into special classifications. *Dynamic* may be concentric, i.e. overcoming a resistance or load (e.g. quads shortening in raising a squat bar); or eccentric, i.e. yielding to a resistance or load (e.g. quads lengthening in lowering a squat bar). *Static* may be maximum, i.e. meeting an immovable object; or sub-maximum, i.e. the role of the postural muscles in holding the spine in position when standing.

In any activity where muscular contraction arrests eccentric contraction prior to concentric contraction (e.g. when muscle contraction stops you yielding to a load before it will allow you to overcome it), the point at which the eccentric movement stops is known as the point of *amortisation* of muscle. In many technical textbooks the phase during which a limb is being forced to yield prior to this point is referred to as the amortisation phase. Examples of this are in the take-off leg in long jump, in the arms in various agilities in gymnastics, etc. The duration of time in the amortisation phase, and at the point of amortisation, is critical to the efficient contribution of combined force from both contractile and elastic components. It must be emphasised that the eccentric action is *dynamic* in the amortisation phase. If it is passive, then kinetic energy, which has been derived from an approach run or preparatory movement, will be absorbed and the only force available for the ensuing movement will be from the contractile component alone. This is seen when a trampolinist 'kills' the recoil of a trampoline, when a skier 'damps' the undulations of the ski slope and when the testee in the jump-reach test is not permitted a preliminary movement. This whole area should be clearly understood if the coach is to develop specific training exercises for sports demanding this type of muscle activity.

Types of muscle fibre

The study of the muscle's contractile properties usually examines the muscle not only longitudinally, but also through a transverse section. By using muscle biopsy techniques and applying histochemical staining, three categories of human muscle can be identified, based on stain shading – from dark to light with an intermediate shade, depending on the fibre's concentrations of different types or isoforms of myosin ATPase. Slow-twitch (type I) fibres stain dark; fast-twitch (type IIB: also now called type IIX) fibres remain light in colour; the shade of fast-twitch (type IIa) fibres fall between the light and dark.

Other classifications in typing muscle fibres use biochemistry, contractility, fibre structure and function. Table 16 summarises these classifications. Due to their unique characteristics, and their use for specific duration and intensity of activity, fibre biopsy profiles and analysis may provide important evidence of the reactive effect of training loads and the suitability of athletes for specific sports disciplines.

The implication of fibre differentiation is shown in the many studies of muscle fibre population in various groups of athletes (e.g. see Dahl & Rinvik, 1999). Golnick's (1973) classic study illustrates this area of study, showing that specific enzyme activity is involved in speed training (PFK) and endurance training (SDH) and that the percentage of slow-twitch fibres is related to endurance demand. (Table 17).

	Type I	Type II a	Type IIb/IIx
Biochemistry	SO	FOG	FG
Oxidative capacity	High	Medium/high	Low
Calcium capacity	Low	Medium / High	Low
Glycolytic capacity	Low	High	High
Myosin ATPase	Low	High	High
Colour	Red	Pink	White
Contractility	Slow twitch	Fast twitch	Fast twitch
Relaxation	Slow	Fast	Fast
Fibre structure			
Capillaries/mm2	High	Medium	Low
Fibre diameter	Small	Medium	Large
Mitochondrial volume	High	Medium	Low
Function	S	FR	FF
Fatigue resistance	Low	Medium/High	High
Force potential	Low	Medium	High

Key: SO = Slow, oxidative: FOG = Fast, Oxidative, Glycolytic
FG = Fast, Glycolytic : S = Slow Contracting
FR = Fast Contracting, Fatigue Resistant
FF = Fast Contracting, Fast Fatiguing

TABLE 16 Summary of properties of muscle fibre types

athlete	(aerobic) (slow) units of succinate dehydrogenase	% slow-twitch fibres	(anaerobic) (fast) units of phospho fructokinase
Distance runner	8.03	75	15.07
Middle distance runner	5.14	65	26.53
Sprinter	3.95	26	28.34

TABLE 17 Relationship of event to % slow-twitch fibres and enzyme concentration (adapted from Golnick, 1973)

It is very clear, even from our limited understanding of neuromuscular function, that specific training will make many areas of this complex system more efficient. Greater force of muscle contraction can be developed, sophisticated recruitment of motor units may be learned, and energy systems may be trained to meet the specific demands of sports activities.

7 THE FLUID SYSTEMS

HOMEOSTASIS

The body is composed of tissues and the tissues are composed of cells. Each cell has fluid in it (intracellular) and outside it (extracellular, mainly interstitial – in between cells). Provided the various concentrations of substances in the extracellular fluid are controlled, the cells will continue to function efficiently. However, stressors bombard the body and threaten the integrity of the cell-organ-fluid cycle within it. 'Stress' is embarrassment of this cycle, evidenced by greater urgency of activity within the cycle. It is therefore essential that the body maintains a certain constancy of its internal environment to ensure that the composition of extracellular fluid is not threatened. This process is called *homeostasis*. The functions of all organs in the body, with the exception of the reproductive organs, are directed towards the goal of homeostasis. Should the various tissues which comprise each organ fail in their highly specialised contribution towards homeostasis, the cells bathing in the extracellular fluid will be damaged and reduce the organic functioning capacity. The situation may be summarised as follows:

- total body function relies on the efficient functioning of the organs
- the organs' function relies on the efficient functioning of their tissue cells
- the cells' function relies on the constancy of the composition of the extracellular fluid
- the extracellular fluid is given constancy (homeostasis) by the efficient functioning of the organs.

Figure 44 illustrates the total fluid in the body, as well as indicating its relationship to blood composition and volume.

Water, through specific bodily fluids, serves several functions:

- it provides the body's transport and reactive medium
- it is the vehicle for transporting nutrients, gases and for eliminating waste in urine and faeces
- because of its heat stabilising qualities, it absorbs substantial levels of heat with minimal temperature change
- gaseous diffusion only takes place across moistened surfaces
- it affords structure and form to the body.

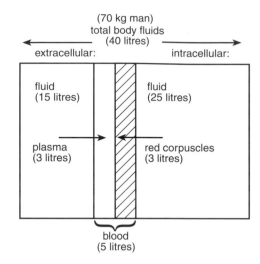

FIG. 44 Distribution of body fluids

SPECIFIC FLUIDS: COMPOSITION AND FUNCTION

Blood

This has already been discussed in some detail (see chapter 5). Approximately 90% of the blood is fluid – most intracellular (e.g. within the blood cells), some extracellular (e.g. the plasma). The latter has a higher amino acid concentration than other extracellular fluid, especially albumin, which is an important factor in keeping plasma inside the capillary blood vessels.

Interstitial fluid

This is that portion of the extracellular fluid outside the blood vessels (e.g. total extracellular fluid, excluding plasma). This fluid includes that in which the cerebrum and spinal cord bathes (cerebrospinal fluid), the fluid in the abdominal cavity, the joint capsules (synovial fluid), the pleural envelope about the lungs, and in the eyes.

Intracellular fluid

This is the fluid inside each cell containing many chemicals and electrolytes responsible for functional efficiency of the cell. Various mechanisms are 'built into' the cell membrane. The mechanisms allow movement of sodium *out* of the cell and potassium and phosphates *into* the cell. Also found in this fluid are glucose, oxygen, carbon dioxide, amino acids and lipids. From previous discussion (see chapter 5), it will be recalled that fuel is combusted with or without oxygen to provide energy for cellular function, leaving substances such as carbon dioxide and lactate which pass through the cell membrane with the assistance of one of the membrane mechanisms already mentioned. These products are then carried in the intra or extracellular fluids of the blood, to be 'blown-off' or oxidised as the case may be. Oxygen travels the reverse route.

Extracellular fluid

This fluid differs from intracellular principally in its electrolyte concentration. These differences of concentration are responsible for electrical potentials across the membrane of the cell. If these electrical potentials did not exist, it would be impossible for nerve fibres to conduct impulses or for muscle to contract. In addition, the extracellular fluid provides a system for the transport of nutrients and other substances. It may help to recall that plasma and lymph are both extracellular fluids.

Lymph

This has already been discussed with reference to the white cells' role in the body's immune system. The walls of the lymphatic capillaries are freely permeable to protein and approximately 95% of protein, lost from the oxygen transporting system each day, is returned via the lymphatic vessels. If these plasma proteins were not returned, death would result in 12–24 hours. Consequently it has been suggested that the single most important function of lymph is its role in returning plasma protein to circulation.

Acid-base balance and pH

Maintaining the acid-base balance of the body's fluids is critical to homeostasis and ensures the optimal metabolic functioning and general regulation of the body's physiology.

Acids ionise in solution, releasing hydrogen ions (H^+). Examples in the body include carboxylic acid, citric acid, and phosphoric acid.

Bases (alkalis) accept H^+ to form hydroxide ions (OH) in aqueous solutions. Examples in the body include sodium and calcium hydroxide.

The pH refers to the concentration of H^+. Solutions with relatively more OH than H^+ have a pH above 7.0 and are referred to as basic or alkaline. Solutions with more H^+ than OH^- have a pH below 7.0 and are referred to as acidic. Distilled water has a pH of 7.0, so $H^+ = OH^-$. Figure 45 is a picture of the pH scale from 0–14, with examples.

Very narrow pH ranges are highly specific to given body fluids. Extreme changes in pH produce irreversible damage to enzymes.

Buffers are chemical and physiologic mechanisms which prevent changes of H^+. There are three buffering mechanisms:

- Chemical buffers – for example, carbolic acid and sodium bicarbonate.
- Ventilatory buffer – the respiratory centre increases breathing rate in response to an increase in H^+ in body fluids.

FIG. 45 Examples of pH values

- Renal buffer – the kidneys continually excrete H^+ to maintain acid-base status of body fluids.

In prolonged high intensity exercise, large amounts of lactate enters the blood from active muscle. At exhaustion, blood pH can approach 6.8. Only after conclusion of exercise does blood pH stabilise and return to 7.4.

Fluid accumulation

Occasionally fluid collects at certain sites in the body. A fluid collection is known as an *oedema*. If this occurs in a potential space (e.g. joint space) it is known as an *effusion*. Several things may cause this. For example, infection can cause a blockage of the lymphatics (drainage system) in a potential space, through the accumulation of dead white cells. Trauma caused by a knock or strain may also cause an effusion, which may be reduced by applying ice packs or cold water to the affected region. Again, hormonal factors can elicit fluid retention. For example, the female hormone oestradiol triggers retention of fluid. Fluctuation in body weight in the course of the female menstrual cycle is mainly attributable to ebb and flow of the body's fluid volume. Oedema, effusion, or fluid retention, may lead to discomfort, e.g. swollen joints, and possible influence on relative strength, as well as reduction of functioning capacity. The phenomenon may even constitute a serious health threat if it exerts pressure on blood vessels. Consequently, medical advice should be sought to discover the cause.

Fluid loss

The kidneys, in addition to filtering approximately 1700 litres of blood in 24 hours and rejecting the blood's waste products in soluble form in the urine, are the key agents in controlling expulsion or retention of body fluid. In other words, they are the principal regulators of the body's fluid volume and concentration. If the body's salt-water balance is disrupted, water must be retained in the body or a greater concentration of salts must be expelled (or both) to restore equilibrium. This imbalance can be caused by internal or external conditions, for example, the high sweat rate required to cool the body by evaporation in a hot environment or through persistent exposure to air conditions or the considerable loss of fluid via sweat, urine, 'running nose', etc., which accompany upper respiratory tract infections such as the common cold. Since a greater proportion of water than salts and electrolytes is lost in the first instance, intracellular and extracellular fluid concentration, and ultimately blood concentration, increases. The consequent increased osmotic pressure causes (1) release of anti-diuretic hormone (ADH) from the posterior pituitary which *increases reabsorption of water* by the tubules of the kidney, and (2) withdrawal from circulation of the hormone aldosterone which is secreted by the cortex of the suprarenal gland and this *decreases absorption of salt* by the tubules of the kidney (fig. 46).

When there is excessive water intake, ADH levels are lowered, another hormone angiotensin is formed locally, and aldosterone levels are raised thus diluting and increasing the volume of urine expelled. When body fluids are being reduced, it is self evident that athletes must increase fluid intake to replace that lost and to relieve the body of the increased burden on its regulatory mechanisms (see also 'water' chapter 4, page 73). Moreover, where periods of sweating are prolonged, not only must fluids be replaced but also electrolytes and salts. Fortunately there are several electrolyte solutions commercially available to the athlete, such as Lucozade Sport, Gatorade and Isotar.

The athlete should be aware of those substances which will increase fluid loss and therefore reduce his ability to combat the stressor of heat. These substances include xanthines such as coffee (caffeine) and tea (theophylline), excess sucrose, alcohol, and drugs involving mercurial compounds, chlorothiazide, Diamox, etc. Certain antibiotics require that the athlete drinks more water. Penicillin, for example, is actively excreted by the tubules of the kidney, and athletes are normally advised to increase fluid intake when taking it. Air-conditioned residential, working and exercising environments, and in air travel can have a profound dehydrating effect.

Intentional dehydration has been attempted by athletes to reduce body weight and therefore increase relative strength. This practice is fraught with dangers, not least of which is the impairment of function due to electrolyte imbalance. If weight must be reduced for some reason, then medical advice must be taken. Of course

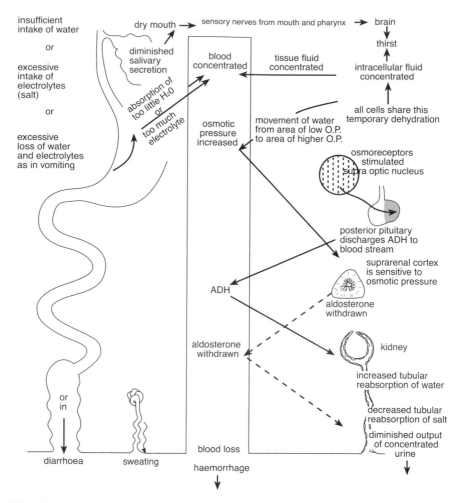

FIG. 46 Regulation of water balance showing measures that restore blood volume and restore body fluids to normal osmotic pressure (from MacKenna and Callender, Illustrated Physiology, 1998).

'dieting' has been pursued, often very successfully, with the view to reducing weight while maintaining or even increasing normal body function. The following observations on the subject should be noted.

(1) Dehydration techniques, using diuretic drugs, are most certainly not recommended for athletes.

(2) Dehydration techniques, via reduction in fluid intake, may only be considered valid if under medical supervision and then only for short periods.

(3) 'Slimming diets' must be considered over an extended period, rather than for rapid weight decrease.

(4) Initial rapid weight loss in dieting is largely due to loss of that water previously required to store the glycogen now liberated to provide energy (3 g water

for each 1 g glycogen). When the stored glycogen is called upon to provide energy, it releases its water which is expelled from the body. Unfortunately, when the 'slimmer' returns to the normal diet, this weight is replaced.

(5) Any diet *must* include all essential nutrients to support the high metabolic demands of the athlete or the relevant metabolic demands of the non-athlete. While an increase in protein intake will increase metabolic rate (to the slimmer's advantage), and a reduction in carbohydrate intake will certainly affect weight loss, it would be fundamentally wrong to avoid carbohydrate completely since muscle and nerve cells rely on carbohydrate for their metabolism. A return to a balanced diet, but scaled down, is the moral of the story.

(6) Some athletes, such as crew members in sailing, of course, wish to increase weight. The ingestion of certain approved drugs can do this, but it is mainly through fluid retention. This cannot be considered a healthy practice, nor should it be recommended for athletes. In the medium term, weight gain may be better pursued by digesting more calories. In the longer term, muscle may be increased.

TEMPERATURE REGULATION

The athlete's problem is maintaining body temperature within the limits which permit him to function efficiently, which is at a body temperature of 37.5°C–38.5°C. In certain conditions the problem is to avoid overheating (hyperthermia). This can be avoided by the loss of body heat to the external environment and the reduction of heat gain from that environment. This will occur when training or competition takes place in a very hot/dry or hot/humid climate. On the other hand, the problem may lie at the other extreme where the athlete must avoid losing body temperature to the external environment and insulate against the low temperature of that environment. This will occur when, for example, sailors are exposed to dampness and extremely low temperatures for long periods of time. This may lead to the condition of exposure or hypothermia.

The balance between heat production and heat loss will be maintained when the sum of the factors to the left of figure 47 equals the sum of factors to the right.

Heat production	Heat loss
1. Basal metabolism	5. Radiation
2. Muscular activity (including shivering)	6. Convection and conduction
3. Effect of body temperature on cells	7. Evaporation (convection)
4. Hormonal effect on cells (thyroxine and adrenaline)	8. Respiration, micturition and defecation

FIG. 47 Factors contributing to the balance between heat production and loss at rest (see overleaf)

(1) Basal metabolism

The metabolic rate is the measure of the rate at which energy is released from foods. It is therefore the rate of heat production by the body, which is measured in kilocalories. Basal metabolic rate is this measurement when the athlete is at his most rested state, i.e. without temperature stressors, etc. It is determined by the inherent rates of chemical reactions in the cell and the amount of thyroid hormone activity in the cells. The basal metabolic rate is generally expressed in terms of kilocalories per square metre body surface per hour. Several factors influence metabolic rate, which is most closely related to the surface area of the skin:

- the basal metabolism of children is greater than that of adults because they are growing as well as coping with day to day lifestyle
- fasting or starvation would appear to decelerate metabolic rate. It has even been suggested that by reducing metabolic rate in this way the ageing process will be slowed down
- protein causes a greater increase in metabolic rate than fats or carbohydrate. On comparing diets of equal calorific value, protein can raise the metabolic rate by 20% over a period of 4–6 hours, while carbohydrate and fats will affect only 5–10% increase.

(2) Muscular activity

Heat production of muscles accounts for 40% of all the body's heat production, even at rest. During severe exercise this can rise to as much as 20 times that provided by all the other tissues put together. This is due to the oxidation of foodstuffs to meet the fuel demands necessary for ATP/ADP breakdown. The metabolic rate, in work of only a few seconds duration, may be over 40 times greater than at rest.

(3) Effect of body temperature on cells

The immediate effect of exposure to high temperature is to increase heat loss via sweating, etc. Metabolism is not greatly affected. If continued exposure elevates body temperature, basal metabolism increases by 7% for every 0.5°C. This would have the net result of further increasing temperature. The immediate effect of exposure to low temperature is an increase in metabolic rate, and shivering further increases heat production. It has been suggested that the metabolic rate can be doubled with the involvement of shivering and that metabolic changes occurring in cold exposure may be hormonally influenced. It is possible to acclimatise both to cold and heat. Should exposure to extremes of temperature continue at a rate incompatible with adaptation to the specific stressor, and without the benefits of acclimatisation, there is a very real risk of hyperthermia or hypothermia.

(4) Hormones

Thyroxine increases the rate of functioning of cell enzymes, thus increasing metabolic rate and heat production. This increase in metabolic rate may also be elicited by adrenaline and noradrenaline. The anterior pituitary gland also influences the metabolic rate indirectly via the thyrotrophic hormone which stimulates the thyroid gland.

(5) Radiation
Radiation is the transfer of heat from one object to another with which it is *not in contact*. Normally, the athlete radiates more heat towards objects cooler than himself, and vice versa. The closer the two temperatures, the less will be the athlete's heat loss. Frequently, athletes express concern that heat is coming from artificial playing areas on which they are training or competing. In many cases this is not really true; in fact the athlete cannot lose all the heat he wishes to that particular playing area. Often, women athletes lose more heat than men by radiation.

(6) Convection and conduction
Heat may also be lost to air and objects with which the body has contact. The cooler the air or object, the greater the heat loss. If air is continually moving past the body, warmed air (from the body's heat) is moved away to be replaced by 'unwarmed' air. The more rapidly the air moves the greater is the quantity of heat conducted from the body. Thus, there exists a combined conduction/convection heat loss due to passage of air over the body surface. Where there is a cool wind and body temperature is to be maintained, athletes should be sheltered or wear wet suits (waterproof oversuit). In water, heat is lost directly by conduction.

(7) Evaporation (convection)
In addition to the small amount of extracellular fluid which continually diffuses through the skin and evaporates, the sweat glands produce large quantities of sweat when the body becomes very hot – up to two litres per hour. This process obviously increases the rate of heat loss through evaporation. As in conduction, air currents play a major role in the removal of heat by evaporation. As the air close to the body becomes saturated, new air arrives to accept the evaporating sweat. Should the air fail to be replaced, then conduction and evaporation avenues of heat loss will be reduced. The situation is more alarming when air is humid because the sweat will not evaporate. Williams (1975) says: 'In hot, dry environments, the limiting factor for heat dissipation is the rate of sweat production, whereas in hot, humid environments it is the capacity of the environment to receive water vapour, i.e. the relative humidity. In the shade outdoors the athlete will therefore be cooler than in the shade indoors, provided the air is moving. On the other hand, when temperature loss is to be avoided, the athlete should keep out of the wind and keep the body surface dry.' Men tend to sweat at higher proportionate rates than women.

(8) Respiration and expulsion of wastes
Approximately 3% of heat lost at 21°C is via these avenues.

Clothing and temperature regulation

Clothing should be considered in light of the foregoing discussion. In a hot environment, cottons, linens and wide mesh (such as string vests) are recommended instead of synthetic fabrics. The latter are, in most variants, less effective in reducing body temperature, being non-absorbent, while the former allow absorption of body moisture and support the evaporation and conduction systems for loss of body heat. This said, advances in technology are reducing the difference between natural and synthetic fabrics. It should also be mentioned that where competition is to be held in hot/dry or hot/humid environments, dry kit should not replace sweat-soaked kit. Wet suits are recommended where the competition environment is cold and, where appropriate, these should be worn between rounds of competitions and during warm-up. In field games and/or winter sports, thought should be given to maintaining a comfortable temperature for continued efficient activity. Above all, both skin and kit must be kept as dry as the occasion permits.

Maintaining body temperature should not be confused with the problems of exposure to strong sunlight. In the latter case, athletes should be as conscious of the need to shelter from the weakening effects of the sun as they are to maintain a body temperature compatible with efficient physical activity.

Acclimatisation to temperature

The body can adapt to the stressors of dry and wet heat. The stressor of high temperature causes a decrease in endurance capacity. Should athletes be required to compete in such conditions they must therefore be exposed to a stimulus for adaptation if performance capacity is to be maintained. The adaptation to external environments, such as altitude, time shift, heat, etc., is known as acclimatisation. Buskirk and Bass (1974) have enumerated the practical aspects of acclimatisation to heat:

(1) Acclimatisation begins with the first exposure, progresses rapidly, and is well developed in 4–7 days.

(2) Acclimatisation can be introduced by short, intermittent exercise periods in the heat, e.g. 2–4 hours daily. Inactivity in the heat results in only slight acclimatisation.

(3) Subjects in good physical condition acclimatise more rapidly and are capable of more work in the heat. However, good physical fitness alone does not automatically confer acclimatisation.

(4) The ability to perform 'maximal' work in the heat is attained more quickly by progressively increasing the daily workload. Strenuous exertion on first exposure may result in disability which will impair performance for several days. Care should be taken to stay within the capacity of the athlete until acclimatisation is well advanced.

(5) Acclimatisation to severe conditions will facilitate performance at lesser conditions.

(6) The general pattern of acclimatisation is the same for short, severe exertion as for moderate work of longer duration.

(7) Acclimatisation in hot/dry climates increases performance ability in hot/wet climates and vice versa.

(8) Inadequate water and salt replacement can retard the acclimatisation process.

(9) Acclimatisation to heat is well retained during periods of non-exposure for about two weeks; thereafter it is lost, at a rate that varies among individuals. Most

people lose a portion of their acclimatisation in two months. Those who stay in good physical condition retain their acclimatisation best of all.

(10) If it is desirable to retain acclimatisation, periodic exposures at frequent intervals are recommended and heat exposures should not be separated by more than two weeks.

Acclimatisation to cold is rather more difficult to study than acclimatisation to heat. This is because man normally protects himself against cold by creating his own miniature subtropical climate with increased and insulated clothing, heated accommodation, etc. 'Local acclimatisation' is known to be possible. For example, when the hands are exposed to cold for short periods over a number of weeks there is an increased blood flow through the hands, enabling them to perform their normal functions without impairment due to cold-induced numbness. While heat will be lost from the body due to local acclimatisation, at least the athlete's functioning capacity will be maintained. This type of acclimatisation is invaluable to sailors, climbers and athletes involved in outdoor winter games or games played in a cold environment. Having said this, the athlete may simply learn how to avoid becoming extremely cold through experience or advice from the technical authorities concerned in the given sport.

Warm-up

Unfortunately there is an astonishing lack of consistency in research conclusions on the physiological value of warm-up. Possible advantages might include:

- increased local muscle blood flow
- increased metabolic rate (7% for 0.5°C increase)
- increased speed of oxygen and fuel transfer to tissues
- increased speed of nerve impulse conduction
- increased speed of contraction and relaxation of muscle
- decreased viscous resistance in the muscle.

Perhaps most of the advantage derived from warm-up is psychological, due to the blend of ritual rehearsal and psycho-physiological preparation unique to each athlete. Even if this is the only advantage of warm-up, it seems ample justification for its inclusion. Pending more conclusive support for the value of warm-up, athletes should be encouraged to pursue the preparation which coach and athlete know to be relevant to the forthcoming competition or training unit. This should not elevate body temperature above 38.5°C.

At the conclusion of a competition or training unit, athletes are frequently encouraged to 'warm down'. This normally involves light but continuous activity, where the heart rate is in the range of 120–140/minute. In pursuit of recovery from exercise-induced stress, the object is principally to raise the metabolic rate and encourage the removal of waste products from muscle through maintaining local blood flow.

SUMMARY

The body's fluid systems comprise blood, interstitial fluid, intracellular fluid, and lymph. Together, they serve two vital purposes. The first is to offer a medium for the transportation about the body of substances essential to normal function. To meet this, a relative stability of fluid volume and concentration must be maintained and this is primarily achieved by a balance between the kidneys and the thirst mechanism. High temperatures, infection and certain dietary inclusions are examples of threats to such stability. The second purpose is temperature control, which is seen as the balance of heat production and loss. A relative stability of body temperature is critical to physical performance. The athlete uses warm-up to attain an optimal temperature for physical performance, using the capacity to adapt to the stressors of dry and wet heat to prepare for competition in climates where such stressors will be evident.

8 THE HORMONES

Hormones are highly specific chemical compounds produced in the specialised cells of the endocrine glands. Unlike, for example, the lymph system, these glands have no ducts and tubes and their secretions are transported normally in the blood. The hormones may exert both generalised and specialised effects on other tissues and organs – functions implied by the word endocrine (*endo*: within, *krinen*: to separate).

Hormones may be divided into two groups – local and general. All general hormones and the most important local hormones are reviewed here. Some general hormones affect all cells, e.g. growth hormone secreted by the pituitary, and thyroxine secreted by the thyroid. Other general hormones affect specific cells, e.g. gonadotrophic hormones secreted by the pituitary affect the sex organs. These substances perform a global function of regulation within the context of homeostasis via the fluid systems.

LOCAL HORMONES

Local hormones affect cells in the immediate vicinity of the organ which is secreting the hormone.

Acetylcholine: acts locally to promote rhythmic activity in smooth muscle (which has no nerve supply), in heart muscle, and in certain epithelial tissue (e.g. oesophagus and trachea). However, this hormone is probably best known in another capacity: acetylcholine occurs in the motor nerves which run from the spinal cord to skeletal muscles. It is the 'transmitter' substance of the skeletal system. Synthesis of acetylcholine occurs in the cytoplasm of the nerve-muscle junction, but is quickly stored in about 300,000 synaptic vesicles and secreted to effect transmission of nerve impulses across a given synapse (fig. 48). Where chemical transmission of nerve impulses is effected by acetylcholine, these fibres are known as cholinergic. Such fibres are found in parts of the sympathetic and parasympathetic systems and in the motor fibres to skeletal muscle.

Histamine: found in higher concentration in lung, intestine and skin, and those tissues which are exposed to the external environment. It would appear that histamine occurs in the tissue mast cells, the basophil cells and platelets of the blood. The exact form in which it is held in these cells is not yet known. Secretion by damaged cells anywhere in the body causes the walls of local capillaries to allow

FIG. 48 Diagram showing processes involved in synthesis release and disposal of acetylcholine at cholinergic nerve terminal and receptor site.

Ach	=	Acetylcholine	NAP	= Nerve action potential
ChA	=	Choline acetyltransferase	*→	= Sites of active transport
AChE	=	Acetylcholinesterase		

by Dr P. F. Heffron, Middlesex Hospital Medical School (from Samson Wright, 1973).

more fluid to pass through them, resulting in oedema. Histamine is released in conditions such as hay fever, and antihistamine drugs are taken to counter the unhappy effects of histamine release.

Prostaglandins: act principally on smooth muscle which contracts or relaxes according to the location, quantity and nature of the prostaglandin involved. They may cause dilation of certain blood vessels and increased heart rate through increased sympathetic nervous action. They may also stimulate or inhibit the release of free fatty acids according to whether the quantity of prostaglandins involved is low or high respectively. The prostaglandins would appear to number approximately 20 and these are divided into two categories: E-Prostaglandins (PGE, or E), and F-Prostaglandins (PGF, or F). Both of these groups occur in the central nervous system where their actions are stimulatory or inhibitory on individual neurons, within or without the central nervous system. The prostaglandins also appear to exert a modulatory role in nerve endings and in hormone secretion. Despite the relative infancy of research, the prostaglandins are noted here because they appear to have a role of considerable importance in the regulation of body function. They were independently identified in 1933–34 by Goldblatt and Euler, but still the world of prostaglandins is far from being completely understood.

Angiotensin: stimulates the secretion of aldosterone from the adrenal cortex, thereby promoting sodium reabsorption by the kidney. Angiotensin is also the most powerful pressor substance known, causing general constriction of the arterioles, and increasing blood pressure. This hormone also promotes secretion of the catecholamines – adrenaline (epinephrin) and noradrenaline (norepinephrin) – from the adrenal medulla. Angiotensin is formed in two parts:

- by the action of renin, secreted by the kidneys of the α2 globulin fraction of the plasma proteins, angiotensin I is formed
- by the action of a converting enzyme on angiotensin I, angiotensin II is formed.

The majority of the 'conversion' takes place as the blood passes through the lungs. The α2 globulin is synthesised in the liver and referred to as *angiotensinogen*. Circulation of angiotensinogen is increased by the glucocorticoids and oestrogen. Angiotensin highlights the interdependence of chemicals in such complex bodily processes as homeostasis. It clearly has a key role in saltwater balance.

Kinins: cause contraction of most smooth muscle. In small quantities they reduce arterial blood pressure due primarily to dilation of blood vessels. By increasing the permeability of the blood vessels, plasma proteins are offered ease of egress. In increased quantities, the kinins facilitate the movement of leucocytes from blood to the surrounding tissues. Finally, it has been shown that the kinins stimulate the sensory nerve endings. It would appear that the plasma kinins are formed by antigenantibody interplay.

5–HT: (serotonin, 5–hydroxytryptamine) is present in the mucosa of the digestive tract, in approximately 90% of blood platelets, and in the central nervous system. 5–HT is a derivative of the essential amino acid tryptophan. The process is stimulated by an enzyme found in the digestive tract, nervous system, kidney and liver. There does not appear to be any evidence that blood platelets can synthesise 5–HT, so it is presumed that they 'collect' this hormone while passing through the digestive tract. 5–HT is a cardiac stimulant and constricts the blood vessels, especially the large veins. Associated with the latter is the raising of both systolic and diastolic blood pressure. It also increases the respiratory rate, acts as an antidiuretic, and stimulates smooth muscle and pain nerve endings in the skin. It is possible that the release of 5–HT from the blood platelets, following injury, causes pain and associated reflex actions in the circulorespiratory system. Serotonin is a neurotransmitter in the brain which may be involved in 'central fatigue' in exercise and possibly in the 'overtraining syndrome'.

Due to their proximity in the brain, it is difficult to separate the roles of those nerve terminals whose transmitter substance is noradrenaline or adrenaline (adrenergic) from those whose transmitter substance is 5–HT (serotoninergic). Consequently there is still some question over their respective physiological effects on mood and behaviour.

The adenosine group (ATP, ADP and AMP): found in all cells and the role of ATP in energy production has already been discussed (see chapter 6). The compounds decelerate heart rate and dilate blood vessels, lowering blood pressure. They also relax smooth muscle. The *cytokines* form a group of about 20 which have important effects on the immune system among other functions.

GENERAL HORMONES

The general hormones are associated with specific glands of origin (fig. 49), and are emptied into the blood to be carried all round the body.

The pituitary gland

The pituitary gland consists of two parts: the *posterior* (neural pituitary or neuro-hypophysis), and the *anterior* (the glandular pituitary or adenohypophysis).

Although the pituitary exerts a 'chairman's' influence over the endocrine system, its role is carefully controlled by a most diligent 'chief executive' – the hypothalamus (see p. 133), which in turn is influenced by the cerebrum.

The posterior part of the pituitary gland appears to be the 'store house' for hormones manufactured in the hypothalamus.

ADH (antidiuretic hormone or vasopressin): key role in saltwater balance has already been discussed (see chapter 7). Secretion increases with increasing exercise.

Oxytocin: produces ejection of milk from the lactating breast.

The 'business' of the 'endocrine society' is to maintain the dynamic stability of the body's functioning capacity.

This is achieved via the discretely controlled secretion of HORMONES. Although hormonal function is highly specific, the presence of insufficient quantities of a hormone will affect the integrity of the entire 'society'.
The hormones may be classified as Local or General.

LOCAL
Specialised tissue secrete these hormones for specific localised effect.

GENERAL
The wide ranging effect of contributions from 'members' of the 'society' are dictated by PITUITARY – 'The Chairman of the Board'.

adenohypophysis
neurohypophysis
hypothalamus – 'The Chief Executive of the Board'.
thyroid
4 parathyroids
thymus

2 suprarenals
– medulla
– cortex
pancreas
– islets of langerhans

2 testes (male)
2 ovaries (female)

The 'members' are located around the body

FIG. 49 The endocrine system (from MacKenna and Callender, 1998)

The posterior pituitary secretes these hormones from storage as required.

The anterior part of the pituitary gland has many functions which may be broadly categorised as:

- control of growth (e.g. bones, muscle)
- control of other areas of the endocrine system (e.g. thyroid, adrenal cortex)
- regulation of metabolism of carbohydrates, proteins and fats.

These functions are fulfilled by six hormones secreted by the adenohypophysis, which are as follows:

Growth hormone (somatotrophic hormone, STH, or human growth hormone, HGH): acts directly on the tissues. The following are some effects of growth hormone secretion:

- increases the mass of skeletal muscle
- increases lipolysis (breakdown of lipids) and increases circulating free fatty acids, offering the latter as a source of energy
- increases bone growth
- promotes transfer of amino acids from extracellular fluid to cells
- increases the size of the thymus
- stimulates RNA formation
- inhibits carbohydrate metabolism.

Secretion of growth hormone is increased by:

- exercise, especially in women because oestrogen increases secretion of growth hormone
- lowered glycogen in the blood (hypoglycaemia), or starvation
- circulating amino acids (especially arginine)
- extreme cold and even emotional excitement or stress
- sleep.

Growth itself is primarily affected by heredity, nutrition, good health and the contribution of other hormones in addition to growth hormone, principally the androgens, thyroid hormones and insulin.

ACTH (adrenocorticotrophic hormone or corticotrophin): causes the rapid secretion of glucocorticoids from the adrenal cortex; rapid conversion of cholesterol and its salts to pregnenolone and thence along the mineralocorticoid, or 17hydroxycorticoid, or androgen and oestrogen pathways; a fall in adrenal cortex ascorbic acid concentrations (though its role in the adrenal cortex is not clear); and stimulation of growth. The secretion of glucocorticoids under normal conditions and stress are both dependent upon ACTH secretion (fig. 50).

ACTH is secreted according to a basic rhythm during the course of the day. The peak secretion would appear to occur during sleep before awakening, whereas the trough would appear to occur towards evening. This rhythm of ACTH secretion is reflected in plasma cortisol (fig. 51) and is referred to as being the diurnal or circadian rhythm.

There is considerable evidence to support the theory that rhythmic control is spread over even longer periods. The rate of ACTH secretion is accelerated by disruption of homeostasis (i.e. stress).

Thyrotrophin (thyroid stimulating hormone TSH, thyrotrophic hormone): stimulates growth and acts directly on the thyroid gland to stimulate thyroxine secretion and acts directly with dietary iodine on the thyroid gland. In children increases in thyrotrophin secretion are produced by cold temperatures, but this effect is slight in adults. Normally the hypothalamus is a controller of thyrotrophin secretion and a decrease in thyroid hormone status also effects an increase in thyrotrophin secretion. Consequently this system is one of negative

FIG. 50 Stress and the glucocorticoids

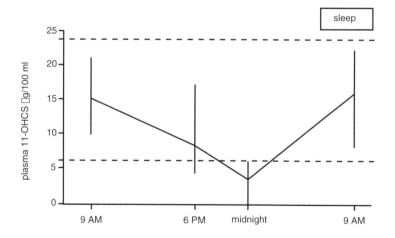

FIG. 51 Mean diurnal variation of plasma 11hydroxycorticoid levels in 24 normal subjects. The vertical lines indicate the range of observations. The horizontal dashed lines show the normal range between 9 am and 10 am. (After Mattingly, D. (1968) in *Recent Advances in Medicine*, 15th ed., ed. Baron, D. N., Compston, N. D., and Dawson, A. M., J. & A. Churchill, London) (from Samson Wright, *Applied Physiology*, 1973).

feedback and is effective both at pituitary and hypothalamus levels. It should also be added that it is thought that stress stimulates secretion of thyrotrophin.

Gonadotrophic hormones

Follicle stimulating hormone (FSH): stimulates ovarian follicle growth in the female and spermatogenesis in the male.

Luteinising hormone (LH or interstitial cell stimulating hormone – ICSH): stimulates ovulation in the female and testosterone secretion in the male. FSH and LH are the pituitary gonadotrophins and their interrelated role is evident in the female menstrual cycle, the central nervous system, and the hypothalamus. It is yet to be clearly shown that a similar periodicity exists in men regarding androgen secretion.

Prolactin (luteotrophic hormone LTH, luteotrophin, lactogenic hormone, mamotrophin, galactin): stimulates secretion of milk and maternal behaviour, inhibits testosterone, mobilises fatty acids.

Endorphins

The endorphins are hypothalomic neurotransmitters and are split from the large prohormone precursor molecule, pro-opiomelancortin (POMC), which is isolated from the anterior pituitary and is secreted into general circulation. Beta-endorphin and beta-lipotrophin increase with exercise and have an opiate, an analgesic effect in response to pain, and this is responsible for the so-called 'exercise high'. Endorphins have also been associated with menstrual cycle regulation and modulating the response of ACTH, prolactin, HGH, catecholamines and cortisol.

THE SECRETING GLANDS

Hypothalamus

The hypothalamus has already been suggested as assuming the role of a diligent 'chief executive' to the pituitary, and has been referred to in discussion of pituitary hormones. It receives a more generous blood supply than any other cerebral structure. It is mainly via this generous blood supply that stimuli promote the hypothalamus to secrete specific releasing agents to the pituitary, which in turn secretes an appropriate hormone from those listed above. It also manufactures the two hormones stored in the neurohypophysis and has a regulatory function in temperature control, thirst, hunger, sexual and emotional behaviour. It also exerts neuro endocrine control of the catecholamines in response to emotional stimuli via impulses coming down from the cerebrum.

Thyroid gland

The thyroid gland secretes three hormones: thyroxine, triiodothyronine and calcitonin. The main hormone is thyroxine, although triiodothyronine is relatively more active. The function of these two hormones is similar and it has become conventional to base discussion on thyroxine.

Thyroxine performs several functions in the body:

- it is essential to normal metabolism, and the increased metabolic rate brought about by thyroxine increases oxygen consumption and heat production (calorigenesis). Thyroxine also increases dissociation of oxygen from haemoglobin
- it is essential to the normal function of the central nervous system, but does not increase oxidative metabolism within this system
- it is essential to normal growth and development of the body when growth hormone is secreted by the adenohypophysis. Growth hormone can only work at maximum efficiency in the presence of thyroxine. Moreover, thyroxine is vital to differentiation and maturation of certain tissues such as the epiphyses in ossification
- the absorption of carbohydrate through the intestine reflects the level of thyroxine activity.
  High activity increases absorption and utilisation of glycogen by the tissues and increases glycogenolysis in the liver, muscle and heart, as well as increasing gluconeogenesis and insulin breakdown.
- it is involved in the regulation of lipid metabolism and is known to reduce cholesterol in the blood by encouraging its metabolism by the liver and by increasing the quantity excreted in bile
- excessive thyroxine causes excessive protein breakdown
- heart rate, blood pressure and cutaneous circulation may increase with an increase in thyroxine secretion
- the gonads (sexual organs) function normally only when thyroxine secretion is normal. Thyroxine levels are important factors in lactation
- the equilibrium of thyroxine secretion is also critical to normal function of the digestive tract
- hormone secretion increases with increasing exercise.

Calcitonin (thyrocalcitonin): inhibits the process of resorption of bone, and consequently calcitonin is secreted in response to increased concentration of calcium in the blood. Calcitonin should be considered as one of the three main guardians of calcium equilibrium in the body. The others are parathyroid hormone and vitamin D. Magnesium and phosphate are also linked with the body's calcium profile.

Parathyroid glands

The parathyroid glands secrete a hormone which promotes calcium resorption in the body.

Parathyroid hormone: secreted when there is a decrease in calcium concentration in the blood. When magnesium concentration is high, there is a decrease in parathyroid hormone secretion. Although phosphate concentration does not directly affect secretion, it is possible that it does so indirectly when, for example, high phosphate leads to lowered blood calcium levels. Parathyroid hormone acts directly on bone and kidney and it would appear that it also may have a direct effect on the intestine.

   Vitamin D is essential to the direct actions on bone and probably on intestine. This vitamin also increases calcium and phosphate absorption from the intestine. Secretion increases with long-term exercise.

Adrenal glands

The adrenal glands each lie above one kidney, hence their other title – the suprarenal glands. These glands comprise an inner medulla and an outer cortex, which are, in fact, two distinct organs.

The adrenal cortex

The adrenal cortex is involved in the stress response and regulates carbohydrate, fat and protein metabolism, and also saltwater balance.

   The hormones secreted by the adrenal cortex fall into three main categories, but two smaller groups of progesterone and oestradiol should also be considered (not known to have any significant feminising activity). The main groups are as follows.

The glucocorticoids *cortisol* (hydrocortisone) and *corticosterone*: promote glucose formation, hence their name. Corticosterone has little importance in man and comprises roughly a third of the glucocorticoids in blood. Consequently it is reasonable to follow convention by discussing only cortisol here. Cortisol has several functions to fulfil:

- it is essential to normal carbohydrate metabolism
- it promotes gluconeogenesis in the liver
- it is essential to breakdown of glycogen to glucose, by adrenaline or glucagon
- it promotes catabolism of proteins
- it brings about redistribution of fats via lipolysis and lipogenesis
- in excess, it reduces the response of tissue to bacterial infection
- it mimics, but is less effective, than aldosterone in saltwater balance and also plays an important role in maintaining blood pressure
- it increases the blood platelet count and shortens blood clotting time

- in excess, cortisol raises blood lipid and cholesterol levels
- it increases acidity in the stomach and when combined with a slight increase in release of pepsin (an enzyme involved in protein digestion) it is possible that peptic ulcer formation may result
- it promotes absorption from the intestine of fats which are insoluble in water
- in excess it interferes with cartilage development and the reduction of epiphysial plates. This may lead to interrupted growth in children. Also in this connection, it decreases calcium absorption from the intestine and increases calcium loss in the urine
- increased secretion in heavy prolonged exercise only.

Finally, it is well known that cortisol is used in the treatment of certain injuries. The injury site is infiltrated with a quantity of cortisol in excess of the normal physiological level. The cortisol protects the site from damage and prevents the normal response to tissue trauma, such as histamine release, or migration and infiltration of leucocytes at the injury site. Cortisol does not actively heal the injury, but creates a favourable environment for healing. However it will be appreciated, from what has been said above, that cortisol infiltration is not without considerable risk and it is hardly surprising that sport authorities in medicine are extremely cautious in suggesting its use. For example, it has a weakening effect on collagen, as in tendons, rendering them brittle over time.

The mineralocorticoids *aldosterone* and *11-deoxycorticosterone* (cortexolone): cause retention of sodium and increased excretion of potassium in the urine. Consequently they are key agents in saltwater balance. Aldosterone is approximately 30 times as powerful as 11-deoxycorticosterone in terms of sodium retention, but it is less efficient as an agent in potassium excretion. Secretion increases with increasing exercise.

Androgen secreted by the adrenal cortex has a less masculinising effect than testosterone. It is necessary for the growth of body hair in women. The principal adrenal androgen is dehydro-epi-androsterone. As stated, the hormones of the adrenal cortex follow a circadian rhythm, but their secretion is increased by stressful stimuli. The various compounds involved are all steroids and derived from cholesterol (fig. 52). It will be clear that several results of excess secretion of these corticosteroids are not compatible with good health and, consequently, persistent exposure to cumulative stressors which exhaust adaptive response should be avoided. In this respect, sport and physical recreation may be considered therapeutic.

The adrenal medulla

The adrenal medulla secretes the catecholamines adrenaline and noradrenaline. The actions of adrenaline (epinephrine) and noradrenaline (norepinephrine) are very similar, but the latter is more efficient in raising blood pressure and less

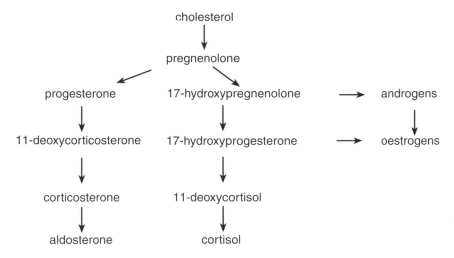

FIG. 52 Possible pathways in the synthesis of steroid hormones from cholesterol (from Samson Wright, 1973)

efficient in metabolic actions and in relaxing smooth muscle. Their secretion is stimulated by: physical and emotional stressors, cold exposure, decreased blood pressure, low blood glycogen, certain drugs (e.g. anaesthetics), afferent nerve stimulation, and increasing exercise.

Involvement of the catecholamines and the sympathetic nervous system in the 'flight and fright mechanism' is well known. These two independent systems provide a most efficient means of meeting emergency situations. Such means might be summarised as:

- increase in heart rate and cardiac output, and rise in blood pressure
- mobilisation of muscle and liver glycogen, leading to increased blood sugar
- increase in metabolic rate
- skeletal muscle fatigues less readily
- relaxation of smooth muscle in the wall of the bronchioles, which leads to a better supply of air to alveoli
- respiration rate is raised
- dilation of coronary blood vessels and those of skeletal muscle, thus providing increased blood supply to those organs urgently requiring it
- constriction of blood vessels of abdomen; contraction of sphincters of digestive tract, ureters and sphincters of urinary bladder; inhibition of digestive tract movement and wall of urinary bladder ('butterflies' and increased micturition in precompetition)
- dilation of pupils of eye
- constriction of smooth muscle of skin and cutaneous blood vessels ('goose flesh' and pallor)
- increased ability of blood to coagulate

- affect on reticular formation of brain to increase memory recall, and to increase attention and concentration.

While the value of catecholamines is clearly of advantage in the flight and fright mechanism, the value is much less clear in the face of psychological and emotional stress. In fact, Carruthers (1971) sees such secretion as part of a most undesirable chain of events (fig. 29, p. 90). They are secreted for a purpose. If not used for that purpose, they must be 'burned off' – for example, via light aerobic exercise. Adrenaline secretion increases in heavy exercise; noradrenaline increases with increasing exercise.

The pancreas

The pancreas, in addition to its exocrine function of secreting pancreatic juice, also has an endocrine function which it fulfils via the *islets of langerhans*. There are two types of cell involved in its endocrine function:

(1) cells secrete *glucagon* which increases blood glucose by glucogenolysis and gluconeogenesis
(2) cells secrete *insulin* (table 18) which decreases blood glucose by stimulating reabsorption of glucose in the kidneys, reducing liver glycolysis and increasing glycogen formation from glucose in muscle.

stimulation	inhibition
Monosaccharides	Adrenaline
Amino acids	Noradrenaline
*Ketones	Insulin
Glucogen	Fasting
Growth hormone	
* product of liver metabolism of FFA	

TABLE 18 Factors influencing insulin secretion via blood

The thymus

The thymus increases in size from childhood until adolescence, and thereafter progressively atrophies. This gland is responsible for the 'education' of the T-lymphocyte immune cells so that they do not attack the body's proteins. This process of clonal selection by deletion occurs through apoptosis, or induced cell suicide.

The testes

The testes have an exocrine function in the manufacture of sperm and an endocrine function in the secretion of testosterone. Testosterone, in addition to its initial role in the foetus of forming the male genitalia, is also responsible for development of the secondary male characteristics at puberty, the maintenance of some of these throughout adult life, and the male emotional profile.

Testosterone causes nitrogen retention in the body and increased synthesis and deposition of protein, especially in skeletal muscle. By this process, there can be little doubt that testosterone derivatives increase strength, given that dietary factors and training regimens are appropriate. In addition, testosterone and its derivatives promote retention of water, sodium, potassium, phosphorus, sulphate and calcium. It is mainly the retention of water which causes the considerable weight gains which are recorded in studies of the effect of testosterone ingestion.

For several years, some athletes have been known to illegaly take testosterone derivatives for their anabolic effect. Anabolism is the formation of energy rich phosphate compounds, proteins, fats and complex sugars by processes which take up rather than release energy. (Catabolism = releasing energy, and metabolism = energy transformations in the body.) It would appear that the taking of such substances increases strength, promotes formation of erythropoetin, and so on. However, to do so, with or without medical advice, in pursuit of competitive advantage, is, apart from being illegal in the world of sport, also highly irresponsible. By disrupting one part of the endocrine system in this way the equilibrium of the total system is compromised. For example, the following have been advanced as possible, and in some cases are probable, additional effects of taking testosterone derivatives:

- initial enlargement of the testes is followed by shrinkage because the high level of testosterone causes a negative feedback in the system resulting in no luteinising hormone being sent to the testes
- the long bones mature too rapidly
- an increase in sexual desire is followed by a decrease
- the salt/water imbalance due to fluid and electrolyte retention may lead to kidney, circulatory and coronary disorders
- the probability of prostate gland cancer would appear to be increased
- there is a higher incidence of jaundice in those taking these substances
- liver disorders are associated with testosterone ingestion.

Several of these effects may be irreversible. Secretion increases with exercise.

The ovaries

The ovaries, in addition to discharging ova, secrete two hormones: an oestrogen known as oestradiol, and a progestin known as progesterone. These hormones are responsible for the development of female primary and secondary sexual characteristics, the growth and development of the female sex organs at puberty (e.g. enlargement of uterus), the menstrual cycle, the physiological and anatomical changes associated with pregnancy, and changes in the mammary glands (e.g. conversion of pelvic outlet, broadening of hips).

Oestradiol: the involvement of oestradiol is very slight until puberty when the hypothalamus stimulates the adenohypophysis to secrete gonatrophins, which stimulate the ovary to discharge ova and secrete oestradiol and progesterone. Consequently, athletes may find performance fluctuation due to such changes as strength-weight ratio, alignment of femur relative to tibia, and basic metabolism undergoing gross adjustment. Fig. 53 outlines possible weight variations in the course of the cycle. It has been suggested that the cycle should be adjusted to make 'optimum competition weight' days coincide with major competitions. Indeed, this has been achieved by administration of certain drugs. However, it is not clear what long-term effect such adjustment of this most basic rhythm will have on other rhythms. Oestradiol, in addition to its key role in the menstrual cycle and those functions listed above, also effects:

- deposition of fatty tissue on thighs and hips
- growth rate of bones after puberty. It has a 'burning out' effect leading to an early growth spurt but also an early cessation. Looking at it another way, the male child grows longer, longer!

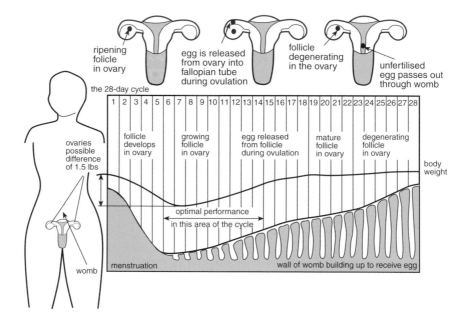

FIG. 53 Menstruation. The cycle of changes which take place in the tissue lining a woman's womb culminate about every 28 days when the blood-enriched lining comes away as the menstrual flow. The changes in the womb occur in parallel to the developments in an ovary, where an egg ripens and is released at ovulation, about halfway through the cycle. The egg travels along a fallopian tube towards the womb. It is fertilised, becomes implanted in the lining of the womb, and menstruation ceases for the duration of pregnancy (adapted from Family Health Guide, Reader's Digest, 1972).

- blood cholesterol levels are reduced by oestradiol and possibly this helps in the prevention of development of coronary heart disease
- while testosterone increases sebaceous gland secretion and the possibility of acne, oestradiol increases water content of the skin and decreases sebaceous gland secretion.

Progesterone: increases body temperature and it is thought that its secretion at ovulation is the reason for increased body temperature at that time. Combinations of these female steroids have been marketed as oral progestogens (female oral contraceptives). These oral progestogens have been used by some athletes in order to effect control of the menstrual cycle but, again, the general equilibrium of the endocrine system is exposed to the possibility of certain compromises such as weight increase, increase in emotional irritability and feelings of depression, decreased status of vitamin B6, vitamin B2, folic acid, vitamin C, vitamin B12, and of trace elements such as zinc. The depression is manageable on trying different types of 'pill', possibly with folic acid supplementation. Depending on menstrual phase, exercise increases secretion.

THE IMMUNE SYSTEM

The immune system consists of a complex, well-regulated interdependence in the grouping of hormones, cells (e.g. white blood cells, see chapter 5), and interactive adaptive mechanisms which defend the body when attacked by outside microbes – viral, bacterial and fungal; foreign macromolecules; and abnormal malignant cell growth. When infection occurs, the immune system works to reduce the severity of the condition and to accelerate repair and recovery.

Exercise, stress (emotional, physical or mental) and ill health constitute interactive factors, each impacting on the body's immune system. Each factor can independently affect immune status, immune function and, consequently, resistance to infection and disease. In the absence of adequate in-built regeneration, the collective cumulative effect of these factors expose a person to the danger of serious fitness and/or health breakdown.

Conditions from so-called 'overtraining' through to Chronic Fatigue Syndrome are all, quite simply, cumulative stress related. The body struggles to adapt to a growing aggregate of stressors, the immune system cannot cope, and the body cannot regenerate sufficiently to regain control. It is as if the body cannot get above the base line (0) following loading and tiring (fig. 89, see p. 323).

Light moderate physical activity provides some protection against upper respiratory tract infections, compared to a sedentary lifestyle, and does not seem to increase the severity of the condition. On the other hand, intense physical activity (e.g. heavy training to exhaustion) creates a period of between three and 72 hours where resistance to bacterial and viral attack is decreased. This renders the athlete easy prey to respiratory infection, which makes its presence felt within 7–11 days.

SUMMARY

The hormones are the supreme guardians of homeostasis. They regulate organic functions through their individual and combined roles. A knowledge of hormone function is essential to a comprehensive understanding of an athlete's status, not only his level of athletic fitness but also his general health. It is possible that an athlete will receive medication in the form of ingested hormone preparations (such as oral progestogens to regulate the menstrual cycle; creams for the skin such as cortisol creams for treatment of eczema; injections such as insulin for diabetes mellitus). Consequently, it is important to understand why and how the use of these preparations will affect the integrity of the endocrine system. Medical advice must be sought to establish the implication of exposing the athlete to certain training stressors. In recent years it has been tempting to see the hormones not only as regulators of total body function, but also as possible instruments to advance athletic performance. Indeed, it is not uncommon for hormone preparations to be discussed along with the athlete's nutrition. However, the equilibrium which exists within the body is very delicate and, as yet, not completely understood. Conservation is as necessary to our internal environment as it is to the external environment and, with or without medical supervision, the pursuit of 'hormonal advantage' in sport is as unwise as it is unethical. It is clear that cumulative stress threatens the immune system. In designing the personal preparation plans of athletes, a review of the total stressor profile of the athlete's lifestyle is essential.

9 PHYSIOLOGICAL DIFFERENCES IN THE GROWING CHILD

It is very easy to see training as the only stressor to which the young athlete's organism is exposed. However, this is most certainly not the case. Training is only one stressor in a complex assault on the organism which must adapt to the demands of growth and maturing function.

EFFECTS OF STRESS

As a result of multi-stressor situations, metabolic functions take place at a higher rate and the stress characteristics of circulation and respiration are quite apparent. One may rightly assume that the resistance or elasticity of the blood vessels contribute to the type of circulo-respiratory adjustments seen in youngsters in training. However, the main focus of attention should be on the heart itself and its ability to pump out blood. The measurements we are looking for, then, are *stroke volume*, *heart rate* and *blood pressure*. Consequently, considerable attention is also given to cardiac output, which is 4–5 litres at rest and over 20 litres in exercise. The increase can be affected by increasing heart rate and stroke volume. Obviously, the more blood the heart can pump out per unit of time the better it is for the athlete, so endurance training is geared in the first instance to improving cardiac output. Due to the small size of the untrained child's heart, cardiac output increase is brought about almost entirely by increased heart rate. This frequency regulation, in contrast with the volume regulation of adults and trained youths, is a particular feature of the circulation of untrained youngsters.

Research in the former German Democratic Republic (GDR) and Sweden shows a linear relationship between the heart volume and maximum oxygen uptake (VO2 maximum) with age, from 8–18 years. However, examination of heart size on its own does not give any real indication of the performance capacity of young athletes since the normal size range is very large. The relative size of the heart compared with other morphological and functional values would, however, give some indication of performance (table 19).

According to Hollmann, the greatest increase in heart volume occurs at approximately 11 years of age for girls, and approximately 14 years of age for boys. The heart weight is greatest 2–3 years later. Furthermore, as young people mature, heart rate decreases while blood pressure and the range between systole and diastole increases. Training adds to these natural growth phenomena, giving greater heart volume, range of blood pressure and maximum heart rate. This provides lower functional values at rest and higher functional values under stress, i.e. an increased range of functional ability.

age	untrained		trained		
	boys	girls	boys	girls	
11	376	349	417	392	
12	440	366	461	448	
13	483	452	508	496	
14–15	549	501	584	539	
*14–15	555.1	469.9	660.6	443.7	sprints
			620.2	498.8	middle distance
			650.9		football

TABLE 19 Heart volumes in ml of untrained and trained 11–15-year-olds (from Harre, 1986).

Muscle biochemistry in pre-puberty does not favour lactic anaerobic activity. There are significantly lower levels of the glycolytic enzyme phosphofructokinase in children compared with adults. This would suggest that 'early teens' success in sprints or endurance events may be due to aerobic and/or alactic anaerobic efficiency, or an early maturity. Attempting to 'force' anaerobesis on the pre-pubertal child is as pointless as it is unwise.

Up to 12 years of age, oxygen intake is approximately equal for boys and girls. Thereafter, girls accelerate to their maximum between 13 and 16 years of age, and boys increase their oxygen intake rather more slowly to reach their maximum at 18–19 years of age. Although it was suggested earlier that cardiac output increase is almost entirely due to heart rate increase in the child, sports physiologists now suggest that a regulation of stroke volume can be seen in trained children and youths. This manifests itself in a greater increase in systolic blood pressure, or in blood pressure range, accompanied by only a slight increase in heart rate. This is illustrated in figure 54 by comparison of trained and untrained boys and girls. It can be seen that heart rate for trained children is lower than for untrained. In recovery, the total time for trained children is shorter (fig. 55).

The peak of biological adaptability in children occurs between 10 and 15 years of age, at a period when physical capacity has by no means reached its maximum. As far as developing physical ability is concerned, youth is the best time for the athlete, bearing in mind that the growing organism is required to expend considerable energy in growing and maturing. Heavy strength work and anaerobic (lactic) work are not to be emphasised in early youth, but mobility, which will almost certainly be on the decline after 8–9 years of age, must be consciously worked for where appropriate. While aerobic endurance training and general training can often be found in simple endurance sports (e.g. orienteering, paarlauf) and field games, care must, nevertheless, be taken to ensure adequate rest periods, especially where endurance training is taken to the 'controlled'

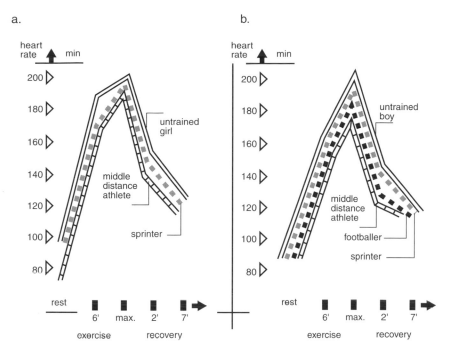

FIG 54 (a) Average heart rate at rest and in exercise for 12–14 yrs. Trained and untrained girls with standardised exercise loading (Harre, 1973); (b) average heart rate at rest and in exercise for 12–14 yrs. Trained and untrained boys with a standardised exercise loading (Harre, 1986).

environment of the track or pool. Harre has noted (1973) that 'when there has been a logical choice of training methods and due observation of the basic principles of training, functional disturbances are, as a rule, not the result of loading in training. Much more to blame here are the total stressors put upon the young athlete, and performance-diminishing features such as immoderate amount of stimuli (e.g. excessive TV watching, inadequate sleep, unsuitable diet, etc.).' On top of this, in the years 13–18, the emotional stressors of culture and the human environment with its ebb and flow of behaviour, attitudes and relationships, plus rigorous academic demands can be extremely exacting.

Fatigue is a physiological occurrence that affects every form of living substance: due to training it is an important condition for the adaptation of the organism to increasing demands. Muscles, ligaments, joints, nerve cells, bones, etc., are all subject to the process of fatigue, which is a temporary, reversible reduction of function, linked with the disinclination for further loading. The recovery period required to restore normal function following fatigue depends on the size and nature of the preceding stressor. The ability to recover improves as the young athlete grows and as his training load is systematically increased. However, long interruptions to training result in a deterioration of this ability. A regular medical check-up, accompanied by a physiotherapy check-up, will help avoid any functional problems which can arise

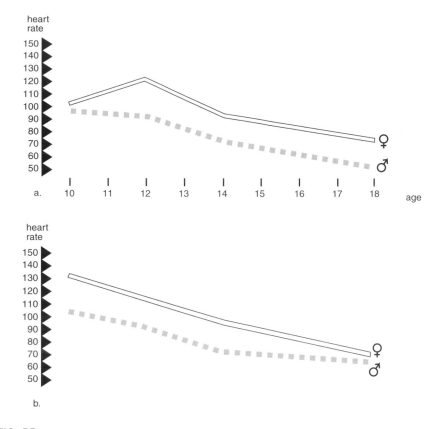

FIG. 55 (a) Heart rate in the third minute of recovery for 65 10–14-year-old athletes in preliminary training for speed sports (Harre, 1986); (b) heart rate in the third minute of recovery for 43 10–18-year-old athletes in preliminary training for endurance sport (Harre, 1986).

due to excessive stressor bombardment. This done, training will always, if accompanied by careful thought, be to the athlete's benefit.

Due to the existence of natural androgenic hormone to an extent never matched elsewhere in their life, girls should be exposed to regular moderate strength training as soon as they finish their adolescent growth spurt, but before sexual maturity. Menstruation is occurring earlier now (13 years 2 months – 13 years 4 months) than in 1890 when 15 years was the age of menarche (it may be earlier or later). The combined stressors of the relatively 'new' phenomenon of menstruation, plus growing itself, suggest avoidance of training loads which produce excessive fatigue in the early teenage athlete.

Finally, although the importance has been stressed of regarding the child as a child and not a mini-adult (because of basic dimensional differences), many measurements and values are, in fact, proportionate to, or 'scaled down versions' of, the adult's. For example, blood volume in terms of ml/kg of body weight is 75 for men, 65 for women and 60 for children (fig. 57).

FIG 56 Schematic illustration of the influence of dimensions on some static and dynamic functions in geometrically similar individuals. A and B represent two persons with body height 120 and 180 cm respectively (partly modified from Asmussen and Christensen, 1967) (from Astrand and Rodahl, 1986).

SUMMARY

The process of growing reaches beyond the readily observed anatomical indications. Within the athlete there are proceeding structural and functional changes which are part of the growing process. While these changes in the athlete's physiology are preparation for adult life and the possibility of a progressive intensity and extent of loading consistent with the advanced athlete's training, they also represent high-energy expenditure. Moderate exercise reflecting a varied intensity and extent of loading is essential to normal growth. Organised training for boys and girls should be introduced around 10–12 years of age. However, the coach must see the growing athlete's training as characterised by a sound programme of all-round development which does not produce exhaustion of already reduced energy reserves.

SUMMARY OF PART 2

Training might be thought of as the practical means of adapting the organism to certain specific demands of a sport. The systems which have been reviewed in these chapters are all involved in the adaptation process, or permit adaptation to take place. Some specific effects of training, which illustrate adaptation by the increase or decrease of certain functional capacities, are listed in table 20. It should be said here, however, that no single form of training will affect all of these adaptations.

increase	*decrease*	
Strength of bone	Heart rate at rest	
Strength of ligaments	Heart rate at submaximal workloads	
Thickness of articular cartilage	Oxygen uptake	for
Cross-section area of muscle	Blood lactate	given
Muscle strength and power	Pulmonary ventilation	workload
Creatine phosphate and ATP in muscle	Triglycerides in blood	
Myoglobin	Arterial blood pressure	
Capillarisation of muscle (including heart)	Glycogen utilisation	
Heart volume	Blood cholesterol	
Heart weight	Risk of myocardial infarction	
Myocardial contractility	Obesity-adiposity	
Blood volume	Platelet stickiness	
Total haemoglobin	Stress associated with physical/ psychological stressors e.g. humidity, altitude, emotion, etc.	
2,3 diphosphoglycerates		
Fibrolytic activity		
Maximum heart rate		
Stroke volume		
a-v02 difference at maximal workload		
Blood lactate at maximal workload		

TABLE 20 Summary of cumulative effects of sub-maximal and maximal exercise

increase	decrease
Pulmonary ventilation at maximal workload	
Respiratory rate at maximal workload	
Diffusing capacity of lung at maximal workload	
Lean body mass	
Glycogen content of muscle	
Size and number of muscle mitochondria	
Mitochondrial activity (succinic dehydrogenase, phosphofructokinase)	
Range of joint action	
Speed of limb movement	
Tolerance to stress	

TABLE 20 Continued

The athlete trains to compete or participate in physical activity. The demands of each sport, and the specific environment of any contest, are unique to the individual athlete concerned. Thus, when training for a given sport, the specific adaptation of that athlete's organism to meet the demands of that sport is also unique. Adaptation will also vary according to whether it is a final or a friendly competition, or at altitude or in high humidity, in pursuit or defence of a title, the location in a circadian or monthly cycle, at home or following lengthy travel, and so on.

Not every problem relating to specific adaptation will be resolved by a study of the human organism, but at least these problems can be more clearly defined and identified, even within the limits of our understanding of organic function.

REFERENCES FOR PART 2

Astrand, P. O. (1967) *Federation Proceedings 26*, 1772

Astrand, P. O. & Christensen, E. H. (1964) Aerobic work capacity. In *Oxygen in the Animal Organism* by Dickens, F., Neill, E. & Wicklas, W. F. (eds). Pergamon Press, New York

Astrand, P. O. & Rodahl, K. (1986 and 2003) *Textbook of Work Physiology*. 3rd and 4th Edns. McGrawHill

BadewitzDodd, L. (1991) *Drugs and Sport*. Media Medica

Bloomfield, J., Fricker, P. A and Fitch, K. D. (1992) *Textbook of Science and Medicine in Sport*. Blackwell Scientific Publications, Melbourne

Brooks, G. A. and Fahey, T. D. (1984) *Exercise Physiology: Human Bioenergetics and its applications.* John Wiley and Sons, New York

Buskirk, E. R. & Bass, D. E. (1974) *Climate and Exercise in Science and Medicine of Exercise and Sports.* Johnson, W. R. & Buskirk, E. R. (eds). Harper and Row, London

Carlile, F. & Carlile, U. (1960) T-wave changes in strenuous exercise. *Track Technique, No. 2.* (From paper to New South Wales, Australia, Sports Medicine Association, 1959)

Carruthers, M. E. (1971) *Biomechanical Effects of Psychological Factors on Physical Performance.* Paper to British Association of Sports Medicine and Scottish Amateur Athletic Joint Coaching Committee Conference on Bioprofiling, Glenrothes

Dahl, H. A. & Ribvik, E. (1999). *Menneskets Funksjonelle Anatom.* J.W. Cappelems Forlag, Oslo, Norway

Durnin, J. V. G. A. (1975) *Protein Requirements of Physical Activity.* VIth Coaches' Convention Report Ekblom, B., Goldbarg, A. N. & Gullbring, B. (1972) Response to exercise after blood loss and reinfusion. *Journal of Applied Physiology, Vol 32,* No. 2 (from Harre, 1986)

*Entrants to Deutsche Hochschule fur Korperkultur (DHfK), Leipzig, GDR.

Giampietro, M., Bellotto, P. & Cardavone, G. (1998) *Nutritional Supplements.* NSA 13:2; pp 31–33

Golnick, P. D., Armstrong, R. B., Saltin, B., Saubert, C. W., Sembrowich, W. K. & Shephard, R. E. (1973) Effect of training on enzyme activities and fibre composition of human skeletal muscle. *Journal of Applied Physiology,* No. 34, pp 107–111

Grisogono, V. (1991) *Children and Sport: fitness, injuries, diet.* John Murray

Guyton, A. C. (1990) *Physiology of the Human Body.* Holt Saunders, Philadelphia

Harre, D. (1986) *Principles of Sports Training.* Sportverlag, Berlin

Harries, M. (1994) *The Oxford Textbook of Sports Medicine.* Oxford University Press

Harris, R.C., Sodeland, K. & Hultman, E. (1992) Elevation of creative in resting and exercised muscle of normal subjects by creative supplementation. *Clinical Science* 83, 367–374

Huxley, H. E. (1958) The contraction of muscle. *Scientific American* 19.3

International Athletic Foundation. (1989) *Too Thin to Win.* IAAF

Jäger, K. & Oelschlägel, G. (1974) *Kleine Trainingslehre.* 2nd Edn. Sportverlag, Berlin

Jones, D. A. and Round, J. (1990) *Skeleta. Muscle in Health and Disease.* Manchester University Press

Keele, C. A. & Neil, E. (1973) *Samson Wright's Applied Physiology.* 12th Edn. Oxford University Press, London

King, J. B. *Sports Medicine.* British Medical Bulletin Publication. Churchill Livingstone, Edinburgh

Komi, P. V. (1992) *Strength and Power in Sport.* Blackwell Scientific Publications, Oxford

Lee, M. (1993) *Coaching Children in Sport: principles and practice.* E & F N Spon

MacKenna, B. R. and Callender, R. (1998) *Illustrated Physiology.* 5th Edn. Churchill Livingstone, Edinburgh

Macleod, D. A. D., Maughan, R. J., Nimmo, M., Reilly, T. and Williams, C. (1991) *Exercise: benefits, limitations and adaptations.* E & F N Spon, London

Macleod, D. A. D., Maughan, R. J., Williams, C., Madeley, C. R., Sharp, J. C. M. and Nutton, R. W. (1993) *Intermittent High Intensity Exercise.* E & F N Spon, London

Maffulif, N. (1993) *Color Atlas and Text of Sports Medicine in Childhood and Adolescence.* MosbyWolfe

McArdle, W. O., Katch, F. I. and Katch, V. L. (2000) *Essentials of Exercise Physiology.* Lippihcott, Williams & Wilkins, Baltimore, Maryland, USA

McArdle, W., Katch, F. F. and Katch, V. L. (1994) *Essentials of Exercise Physiology.* Lea and Febiger, Philadelphia

McNaught, A. B. & Callender, R. (1963) *Illustrated Physiology.* Churchill Livingstone, Edinburgh

McNeill, Alexander, R. (1992) *The Human Machine.* Natural History Museum Publications, London

Maffetone, Phillip (2002) *In Fitness and In Health.* David Barmore Productions, Stamford, NY

Newsholme, E. A., Leech, T. and Duester, G. (1994) *Keep on Running: The science of training and performance.* John Wiley and Sons, Chichester

Noakes, T. *Lore of Running: Discover the Science and Spirit of Running.* Leisure Press, Champaign, IL.

Pappenheimer, J. R. (1950) Standardisation of definitions and symbols in respiratory physiology. *Fed. Proc.* 9, 602

Pyke, M. (1975) *Success in Nutrition.* John Murray Ltd, London

Robergs, R. A. & Roberts, S. O. (1997) *Exercise Physiology.* Mosby Year Book inc., St Louis, Missouri, USA

Saltin, B. & Hermansen, L. (1967) *Glycogen Stores and Prolonged Severe Exercise, Nutrition and Physical Activity.* Almqvist & Wiksell, Uppsala

Schreiner, K. E. & Schreiner, A. (1964) *Menneskeorganismen.* 6th Edn. J. Jansen (ed.). Universitetets Anatomiske Inst., Oslo

Sergeant, A. J. and Kernell, D. (1993) *Neuromuscular Fatigue.* NorthHolland, Amsterdam

Sharp, N. C. C. (1995) The Health of the Next Generation: Health through fitness and sport. *J. Royal Soc. Health,* 116, No 1, 48–55

Shepherd, R. J. and Astrand, P. O. (1992) *Endurance in Sport.* Blackwell Scientific Publications, Oxford

Stanton, R. (1988) *Eating for Peak Performance.* Unwin Hyam

Sufte, N. K., Gushiken, T. T. and Zarins, B. (1986) *The Elite Athlete.* SP Medical and Scientific Books, New York

Suslov, F. (1972) Views on middle and long distance training. *Modern Athlete and Coach,* 10, No. 1

Vander, A. J., Sherman, J. H. & Luciano, D. S. (1970) *Human Physiology, The Mechanism of Body Function.* McGrawHill, New York

Wells, C. L. (1985) *Women, Sport and Performance: A physiological perspective.* Human Kinetics, Champaign, IL

Williams, C. (1974) *Special Forms and Effects of Endurance Training.* Vth Coaches' Convention Report

Williams, C. (1975) *Adaptation to Stressors of a Changing Environment.* VIth Coaches' Convention Report

Williams, C., Kelman, G. R., Couper, D. C. & Harris, C. G. (1975) Changes in plasma FFA concentrations before and after reduction in high intensity exercise. *Journal of Sports Medicine and Physical Fitness, Vol 15,* 2–12

Wilmore, J. H. and Costill, D. L. (1994) *Physiology of Sport and Exercise.* Human Kinetics, Champaign, IL

Woofton, S. (1988) *Nutrition for Sport.* Simon and Schuster

Yakovlev, N. N. (1961) Nutrition of the athlete. *Track Technique,* Nos 20-26, June 1965

BIBLIOGRAPHY

Browns, F. (1993) *Nutritional Needs of Athletes.* Wiley, Chichester, UK

Cohn, E. E. & Stumpf, P. K. (1972) *Outlines of Biochemistry.* 3rd Edn. John Wiley & Sons, New York

De Vries, H. A. & Housh, T. J. (1994) *Physiology of Exercise.* 6th Edn. Brown and Benchmark, Madison Wisconsin

Donath, R. & Schüler, K. P. (1972) *Enharung Der Sportler.* Sportverlag, Berlin

Folk, G. E. (1974) *Textbook of Environmental Physiology (2).* Lea & Febiger, Philadelphia

Ganong, W. F. (1973) *Review of Medical Physiology.* 6th Edn. Lange Medical Publications, California

Hill, A. V. (1945) *Living Machinery.* G. Bell & Sons Ltd, London

Holmer, I. (1974) Physiology of swimming man. *Acta Physiologica Scandanavica,* Supp 407

Howard, H. & Poortmans, J. R. (1975) *Metabolic Adaptation to Prolonged Physical Exercise.* Birkhauser Verlag, Basel

Jeffries, M. (1976) *Know Your Body.* BBC Publications, London

Karlsson, J. (1971) Lactate and Phosphagen concentrations in the working muscle of man. *Acta Physiologica Scandanavica,* Supp 358

Kelman, G. R., Maughan, R. J. & Williams, C. (1975) The effects of dietary modifications on blood lactate during exercise. *Journal of Physiology,* 251, pp 34–35

Luce, G. G. (1972) *Body Time.* Temple Smith, London

Margaria, R. (1976) *Biomechanics and Energetics of Muscular Exercise.* Clarendon Press, Oxford

Martin, G. E. (1997) Influence of elevated climatic heat stress on competition in Atlanta 1996. HSA 12:4; 65–78

McLintic, J. R. (1975) *Basic Anatomy and Physiology of the Human Body.* John Wiley & Sons, New York

Morehouse, L. E. & Miller, A. T. (1967) *Physiology of Exercise.* 5th Edn. C. V. Mosby, St Louis

Pernow, B. & Saltin B. (1971) *Muscle Metabolism During Exercise.* Plenum Press, New York

Richardson, R. G. (1974) Proceedings of the Joint Conference with the British Olympic Committee on Altitude Training. *BASM, Vol 8,* No 1

Robson, H. E. (1973) Proceedings of the XVIIIth World Congress of Sports Medicine (1970). Special issue of *The British Journal of Sports Medicine, BASM, Vol 7,* Nos 1 & 2

Scheuer, J. & Tipton, C. N. (1977) Cardiovascular adaptation to physical training. *Annual Review of Physiology,* 39, pp 221–251

Sperryn, P. (1975) Proceedings of the International Symposium on Anabolic Steroids in Sport. *BASM, Vol 9,* No 2

Tanner, J. M. & Taylor, G. R. (1975) *Growth.* 5th Edn. TimeLife International, Amsterdam.

Videonova, S. (1999) *Sports, Stress, Adaptation:* 1st International Scientific Congress, Sofia, Bulgaria

PART 3

MISSION CONTROL

It has been suggested that coaching is 'more of an art than a science'. Perhaps this idea evolved to explain the existence of several outstanding coaches who have had little, or no, formal scientific education. They may not have studied biomechanics, physiology, anatomy, and so on, but they will almost certainly claim to be students of human behaviour; students, moreover, who derive their knowledge from practical experience of working with athletes, rather than from textbooks. This knowledge might include an understanding of teaching methods, individual motivation, and the relationships between athletes in a team or squad. In his own way, such a coach is using a scientific approach, for the study of behaviour is the science of psychology. The 'art' of coaching is the ability to relate several sciences to assist an athlete in his pursuit of excellence. Not only is psychology one of these sciences, it is central to equip the coach in relating them to athlete and sport. This is the framework within which the 'people business' of coaching operates effectively. The art is also, then, the ability to make those judgement calls which redirect behaviour and ensure delivery of intended performance excellence. The most relevant aspects of psychology for coach and athlete are discussed in this section. Chapter 10 has been prepared by Dr Pamela F. Murray who has also revised chapters 11 and 12.

10 VICTOR IN MENTE, VICTOR IN CORPORE
(A mind to conquer, a body to conquer)

The education of the athlete by the coach and supporting team of specialists, and the athlete's self-education thereafter, is an under-optimised, if not underestimated, aspect of training.

Critical reflection is a coaching skill concerned with both the aims and consequences of technical efficiency, accompanied by open enquiry guided by 'attitudes of open mindedness, responsibility, and wholeheartedness' (Pollard, 1988). It reminds us that coaching does not take place in a social vacuum. Yet, on a practical level, the coach receives more technical guidance than assistance in comprehending human interactions. As coaching has developed in scientific literacy, its fundamental humanistic, social nature remains less understood. Less time is invested in what we are less familiar with, and, consequently, the technical preparation of the performer is a stronger element than the preparation of the less visible, intangible aspects of performance. Technical literacy has appeared as a baseline coaching skill where coach-differentiating variables such as imagination, vision and risk-taking are rare (Murray, 1999). While the science of sport psychology has physical indicators, such as biofeedback training, part of its attraction and inherent challenge is the non-quantifiable, synergistic impact when intuitive and creative variables are optimised, resulting in the realisation of true athletic potential.

The coach has two main responsibilities: to prepare the athlete physically and technically *for* the sport, and to develop the athlete socially and ethically *through* the sport. This begins with sensitising the athlete via self-awareness.

INTELLECTUAL PREPARATION OF THE ATHLETE

As with physical preparation, where adaptation is central to training development, psychological adaptation must also occur, carefully extending existing cognitive and emotional thresholds. Before the performer can learn about self-regulation under competitive conditions, self-awareness must exist. Martens (1987) stated that sport psychology's motto is 'know thyself'. If the optimisation of sports performance can be described as a journey, then it begins with self-awareness. This takes two formats: the management of the psychological preparation, and the management of the psychological performance.

To develop a full understanding of the self may require many years of exposure to varied intensities of experience, useful guidance, and access to constructive feedback. Yet often the performer cannot wait so long. In order to address this possible imbalance, a proactive educational stance is necessary through which both coach and athlete benefit. One option available is to gradually and systematically expose the athlete to varied learning inputs and experiences using compatible styles of coaching (Murray & Krastev, 1992). The association of certain behaviours with an identifiable style of coaching implies the notion of a behavioural continuum. A style is a preferred way of thinking. It is not ability, but rather the way we choose to use our abilities. The style of coaching can support the maturing of an independent, competent performer.

Additionally, it is accepted that a higher calibre of performer results from a background system of training (Nolan, 1997; Tellez, 1991). Coaches benefit from the application of systematisation to their activities leading to a greater understanding of the coaching process (Côté, et. al, 1995). Within a recognisable system, a special personality with accompanying style is also necessary for the successful coach (Massimo, 1980). Don Schula, Miami Dolphin NFL coach stated, 'I don't know any other way to lead but by example' (Blanchard & Schula, 1995). There exists a strong association between coaching behaviours and team motivational climate (Amrose & Horn, 1997). This highlights both the existence and the centrality of styles of coaching. Despite the pressure brought to bear upon the coach, the style should be compatible with the needs of the performer. A coaching style, comprising three elements – commitment, contact, and development – is necessary to operationalise coaching functions rationally.

Generally, individuals acquire their styles through a process of socialisation. We might perceive that certain styles receive greater reward in any given environment, and so emulate these. If an inclination to any specific style orientation is evident, it is worth noting that the athlete will assimilate aspects of the demonstrated style (see p. 160, role modelling). The style is related to the function performed. Due to situational differences, distinct developmental stages and individual personality divergence, the coach operating along a spectrum can gain from the increased range of options that a diverse style profile offers. It is also advantageous for the athlete more adept in managing mobile styles of coaching, increasing individual versatility and discouraging dependency. Dick's (1992) coaching continuum is one such approach. It consists of four styles of coaching that trace the developmental needs of the athlete: directing, coaching, supporting and counselling. This type of conceptual framework has antecedents in business with situational management (Blanchard & Johnson, 1983), and has received further application in sport (Kinlaw, 1993).

As a performance agreement shifts from control to release management (Covey, 1992), the utility of a versatile application of coaching approach is evident. Intuitive notions about the operationalisation of such styles tracing chronological performance development are unfounded, although certain aspects of athletic progression do lend themselves to a pre-selected style of coaching (Murray, 1999). The influence of the nature of the sport over style selection has been underplayed, and the weighting given to style selection by the performance level over-emphasised. Yet this has something to offer coaching. The behaviour of the coach has been determined influential in performance status, although a cause-effect relationship between style and result is refuted.

While a general relationship between authoritarian or instrumental behaviours and coaching effectiveness is not proven, there are coaching scenarios that benefit from such an approach. For example, lower level performers, novices learning new techniques, set play practices, safety issues or working with large groups or squads are well served by a *directive* style. There is little negotiation between coach and athlete given the lack of experience and knowledge on the part of the athlete, or requirement for firmness in safety issues, or clear communication with numbers. While single style application can be appropriate, styles are not mutually exclusive. Directing, combined with a more applied approach, is useful for coaching late-starters and immature athletes, working with development squads, transition from junior to senior competition, technical skills training and throughout the progression from club to regional level competition.

With more time in the training environment, a more hands-on approach is applied. The *coaching* style allows the athlete to begin to contribute to the session makeup, perhaps by participating in decision-making about session format, or by conducting his own warm-up routine. This style is more interactive and a catalyst for the expansion of athlete initiative. Developing the psychological awareness of the performer can shadow this approach, as the athlete is encouraged to consider why goals are set. Within the directive style there is no place for reflection. Outsiders to the coach-athlete relationship, such as specialists dealing with aspects of sport science support, or skilled performers, may offer input. The athlete gains early experience in dealing with such external inputs. The coach is encouraging the athlete to remain proactive, not allowing a gradual slip into mere receive mode: 'What are we doing today, coach?'. That alternative creates dependency, the key to a non-fulfilling athletic career.

It is unusual to see a standalone application of the coaching style, as it combines well with supporting and counselling styles when dealing with natural talents, one-to-one situations, individual development, tactics, guidance, athlete education, mental training and the training of coaches.

With the notion of a shared approach, the subsequent style along the continuum is that of *supporting*. With increasing performance level, the style of coaching becomes more athlete-orientated. The athlete accepts and shares responsibilities, by, for instance, contributing to training programme design and the planning of competitive activity. Supporting activity is valuable in conflict management and its resolution. Behaviours characterised by this style under such circumstances include listening, arbitration, patience, cooperation, negotiation, firmness with flexibility, one-to-one inputs, accepting advice, and consulting others. Supporting forms a favourable partnership with the counselling style for technical skill refinement, event specialisation, coaching more mature and experienced athletes, lifestyle management issues, planning and goal-setting.

The *counselling* style is used with an accomplished athlete able to arrange a lifestyle compatible with training and performance demands. Sufficient input has enabled the athlete to combine personal experience with systematic support. The mature individual, following a progressive journey of style-related development, is now in a position to exercise self-determination. In its solo form it has been used when coaching mavericks, treating team members as individuals, and for use in competition modelling. Athletic maturity is not possible under conditions of athlete control. Many forms of relinquishing direction exist, forming part of the performer's education as he learns about the accompanying accountability. Additionally, this democratic approach has led to players engaging in higher levels of social support, training instruction, and positive feedback (Westre & Weiss, 1991).

While described as a progression, an athlete may well respond best to one style when concentrating on technical form, but prefer another when handling another aspect of training or performance regulation. The coach should be able to give the athlete two gifts – the roots to grow and the wings to fly (Bolton, 1992). A style-shifting ability is inestimable. Notwithstanding specific coaching function, leadership is required (Katzenbach, 1995). Although it is not possible to identify predominant behaviour or leadership style engaged in by winning coaches (those having a win/loss record of greater than 50 per cent) (Iso-Ahola & Hatfield, 1986), an assured athlete with maturity and emotional stability is required for athletic success (Counsilman, 1977). Non-successful coaches tend not to distinguish themselves in terms of certain styles of leader behaviour. Linked with such effectiveness is coach-athlete compatibility (Horne & Carron, 1985). The quality of the relationship between athlete and coach is an important determinant of team success and satisfaction (Cox, 1998).

The intellectual preparation of the athlete is designed to develop the ability to accumulate a relevant reservoir of knowledge necessary for successful participation in sport. Decision-making ability and cognitive creativity in part determine how efficiently the athlete will compete. The athlete must be independent, not vulnerable to manipulation by the coach nor any other person within the sport, and be able to control himself in the chosen competitive arena. Such development of thought capacity requires a patient coach who strategically plans the individual's preparation through integrated inputs. Sport science support is necessary to give an objective foundation to the development of athlete cognition.

An all-encompassing preparation is now a basic requirement for the athlete competing against organised coaching systems operating in other countries, which emphasise overall development. The terminology should not put coaches off making use of specialist input; it is simply that a cognitive strategy is needed for a thinking competitor. Given that competition implies adaptation to changing variables, the athlete should not be limited through lack of intellectual preparation.

This also applies to the coach whose education is a continuous engagement. While research has indicated that athletes categorise their coaches by behaviour (Cox, 1998), the impact of the behaviour of the coach has perhaps been disregarded. Anecdotal evidence suggests that coaching 'tyrants', for example, were renowned for inconsistent behaviour. As coaching behaviour has been shown to impact both positively and negatively on the performer, it would appear a valuable avenue for further research. Formal recognition of this situation is notable by its omission from coach education programmes. There is investigative activity examining the relationship between coaching behaviours and other constructs, but this area remains lacking.

Role modelling

Performers observe role models and can often internalise many of the observed attributes over time. An athlete observing authoritarian role models may be susceptible to becoming authoritarian (Sternberg, 1999). The coach can proactively promote ethical role models within the training and competitive environments. In addition to the coach, other sources for role modelling exist, such as the immediate peer group, the behaviour of professionals in sport and their portrayal by the media. Sources are deemed positive if they encourage and reinforce behaviour that reflects the values associated with sportsmanship and etiquette.

Occasionally, top-level sport offers invaluable role models who can influence many coaches and athletes. At the 1994 European Athletics Championships in Helsinki, the reigning champion at 3000 m steeplechase, Panetta (Italy), was, on paper, worth fourth place as he neared the end of his career. Another Italian, Lambruschini, was favourite for gold. If anything happened to Lambruschini, Panetta could win a bronze medal. Lambruschini's misfortune could be Panetta's good fortune, but Italy would have a bronze medal not gold. Lambruschini crashed to the ground after misjudging a hurdle. Panetta, less than two seconds behind him, pulled him up from the trackside, led him back into the race, then set the pace to favour his team-mate and rival. Lambruschini went on to win; Panetta finished in eighth place. What an athlete does to achieve status as a champion does not establish him as a role model. It is how he behaves in the arena and outside it. While generous gestures within a competitive environment are rare, the coach can support more socially aware and responsible behaviour.

Modelling using Sensory Motor Training (SMT)

Training the senses is the most highly developed form of preparation for those stressful, competitive conditions to which the athlete is exposed. Sensory Motor Training (SMT), if handled well, will give the athlete the opportunity to enhance event-specific sensory perception. As a leading sense from the sensory complex will inform the athlete of actual happenings during performance, the coach can rehearse competitive conditions with the aim of developing sensory reception and the ability to read a situation and respond. Modelling is a form of SMT that seeks to reproduce aspects of competitive performance, using competition as a vehicle for specific sensory motor training. It must be said that some competitive characteristics cannot be reproduced, such as the atmosphere. The use of noise or music will not elicit the same response in the athlete as on the day of the event, as was previously thought possible, and the coach is better advised to replicate environmental conditions such as altitude, humidity, time and temperature.

That said, role playing has proved to be a most effective technique within modelling, where the role of the opposition can be taken on by some of the potential competitors. Prior to a major championship, the Czechoslovakian artistic gymnastic team were divided into two groups: one group played the role of the then Soviet team, and the other group retained home nation identity. So realistic were the accompanying conditions, with the roles of dressed officials also being played, that a strong emotional element was created within the model competition. Coaches and gymnasts were effectively guided in the refinement of individual preparation strategies as a result of the emotional accuracy of the rehearsal. It is important for the coach to consider factors that directly affect the performer within competitively induced situations when creating a situational model. While there are limitations to this kind of approach, it can benefit the performer. There can be no better rehearsal for the Olympics than the Olympics, but it is possible to practise compatible skills by becoming more familiar with our responses under related conditions.

The opposition cannot be controlled, but self-regulation is possible, preceded by practice under a comprehensive range of potential circumstances. To turn on a switch requires a predetermined route for the expected current to pass through. Likewise a coping strategy is optimised if established prior to required use. Effective coping strategies can be a differentiating factor in creating performance consistency. Team sports, similarly, can make use of tactical advantages and disadvantages during rehearsal activity, such as playing with the restricted use of a particular shot or space. Normal parameters must be adhered to, as if in match play or competition, so disallowing an easy 'get-out'. If the performer reacts with: 'It's okay, it's not the real thing!' no benefit will be experienced. Effective models have been created in soccer for goal practice for striker and keeper using an overcrowded goal area, reducing decision-making time and thereby imitating real-game characteristics. Decisions to be taken by striker and keeper are left open to continually rehearse spontaneous situational coping. Such practices without the inclusion of real-game conditions are not maximised in terms of SMT.

The coach can produce innovative practices, taxing the player through the combination of technical and tactical demands. Very occasionally, the coach may suddenly change a previously agreed session, thereby surprising the athlete. For example, if a track athlete is coming to the end of a 300 m run and the coach shouts instructions to carry on for a further 150 m, the athlete will be forced to mobilise his reserves. While immediately unpopular, the coach has in fact used a technique which will help the athlete when moving into stressful conditions. This cannot be used on a regular basis. The sensory motor training involved will teach the athlete how to make appropriate adjustments conducive to success-related activity under varying conditions. The design of models is a result of coaching experience, careful observation (perhaps using technological means), and subjective measurement using esteem and self-esteem scales.

Image and self-image of the athlete

'Image' is the product of the commercial sphere. The media creates and develops an image compatible with product advertising. A positive image is not the same as a positive self-image; self-image is more important for dealing with success and coping with failure. A winner must know himself and be comfortable pursuing his aims. This is in marked contrast to self-image. Self-image is the result of self-reflection. The starting point comes with dealing with adversity – 'Why did I not succeed?'. The point of failure is analysed, giving the athlete the opportunity to compensate for practical aspects revealed in the analysis. If the self-image of the athlete is a positive one, where the athlete feels good about himself, he will comfortably identify with the goal and related activities in a confident manner. The athlete must accept himself regardless of any result at a competition.

A non-achieved goal is not apparently as devastating as a failure. The coach observing the attributions selected by the athlete can evaluate the perceptions of cause and effect displayed. It makes sense for the athlete to attribute failure to an unstable cause, such as luck, conditions, or commitment as this implies that the result may not be repeated. If, on the other hand, the athlete attributes the failure to a stable cause, such as lack of necessary skill, then this is in part predicting future failure (Weiner, 1985). The coach can encourage the athlete to attribute failure to a variable that the performer can exert control over at a future time. The converse of this relationship advises the athlete to attribute success to an internal, stable cause, such as ability, tactical awareness or skill, resulting in increased confidence. This approach does not imply that the responsibility for a poor performance is reneged, but attempts to reinforce reasoning that does not detract from the player's perceived efficacy.

Self-efficacy

If belief in one's ability describes self-confidence, a self-efficacious individual believes that he is competent and consequently can succeed in a given task. Self-efficacy is needed by every athlete hoping to translate the time, energy and commitment involved in training into performance advantage. As with confidence, self-efficacy links self-belief with perceived ability, potentially impacting upon performance. Compared with individuals who doubt their capabilities, those demonstrating high self-efficacy display greater task persistence, work harder, and achieve at higher level (Cox, 1998). A collective effect within a training squad is also possible.

By understanding the performer, the coach is in a better position to support efficacy in his athletes. By using an esteem scale to capture the athletes' response, reactions and feelings on certain matters, or to establish the coach's perspective, a framework for supporting self-efficacy is provided.

Self-esteem scales and esteem scales

A self-esteem scale is a form of self-evaluation conducted by the athlete, establishing a clear picture of the individual's perceived responses to included items. The esteem scale is used by the coach to assess the athlete's response to a range of variables within the training or competitive environment. Both are examples of psychodiagnostic tools at the disposal of the coach. The coach can compare information revealed through other observational techniques, such as video performance, training diary and observations.

The rating scales can be designed to provide, for example, feedback on training organisation and preparation planning (fig. 57). Flexible designs that alter according to the information required give both coach and athlete the opportunity to reflect on aspects related to training and competing, found to assist efforts or detract from optimum conditions (fig. 58). Overuse is not encouraged, but their use pre, mid and postseason is certainly beneficial, with occasional use when the coach wishes to identify specific predetermined characteristics, whether positive for reinforcement, or negative for eradication. The layout shown (fig. 57) helps

> Please comment on the following aspects of your training management using the scale where 1 = not good, 5 = excellent. Using the second scale, indicate to what extent you feel that rated item detracts from or helps your efforts: -3 = detrimental; +3 = very helpful

training	rating	perception
Training organisation		
Session organisation	1 2 3 4 5	-3 -2 -1 0 1 2 3
Enthusiasm while training	1 2 3 4 5	-3 -2 -1 0 1 2 3
Ability to give maximum effort	1 2 3 4 5	-3 -2 -1 0 1 2 3
Communication with coach	1 2 3 4 5	-3 -2 -1 0 1 2 3
Commitment to programme	1 2 3 4 5	-3 -2 -1 0 1 2 3
Technical support		
Technical expertise of coach	1 2 3 4 5	-3 -2 -1 0 1 2 3
Technical understanding of event	1 2 3 4 5	-3 -2 -1 0 1 2 3
Sport science support	1 2 3 4 5	-3 -2 -1 0 1 2 3
Input to technical programme	1 2 3 4 5	-3 -2 -1 0 1 2 3
Support of other coaches/athletes	1 2 3 4 5	-3 -2 -1 0 1 2 3
Recovery		
Recovery between sessions	1 2 3 4 5	-3 -2 -1 0 1 2 3
Effectiveness of active regeneration	1 2 3 4 5	-3 -2 -1 0 1 2 3
Nutritional care	1 2 3 4 5	-3 -2 -1 0 1 2 3
Sleep pattern	1 2 3 4 5	-3 -2 -1 0 1 2 3
Out of training worries	1 2 3 4 5	-3 -2 -1 0 1 2 3

FIG. 57 Self-esteem scale

the athlete to evaluate his training management. If the athlete is seen to be constantly distracted, the design will allow for the consideration of lifestyle management, giving an insight into the broader aspects of the athlete's activities. The athlete uses a self-rating style in this example.

Athlete gives maximum effort	-3 -2 -1 0 1 2 3
Responds well to informative feedback	-3 -2 -1 0 1 2 3
Communicates feelings	-3 -2 -1 0 1 2 3
Follows the agreed programme	-3 -2 -1 0 1 2 3

Loses motivation when tired	never	sometimes	frequently
Loses concentration easily	never	sometimes	frequently
Can mobilise reserves	never	sometimes	frequently
Is prone to negative feelings	never	sometimes	frequently

```
☺                                          ☺
☺  ☺                                       ☺  ☺
☺  ☺  ☺        Pre-game prep               ☺  ☺  ☺        Confidence
☺  ☺  ☺  ☺                                 ☺  ☺  ☺  ☺
☺  ☺  ☺  ☺  ☺                              ☺  ☺  ☺  ☺  ☺
```

Ability to focus	poor	fair	good
Easily distracted	poor	fair	good
Relaxes following goal score	poor	fair	good
Ability to recover from loss of focus	poor	fair	good
Narrow attention under pressure	poor	fair	good

FIG. 58 Esteem scale formats

Motivation

A highly researched area with many schools of thought, motivation continues to elude coaches and researchers alike, given that there is no finite or precise list of motives, and also due to the fact that motives cannot be identified through experiment. Many current theories are based on the concept of perceived competence, such as attributions, goal orientations and intrinsic motivation (Biddle, 1995). We accept some operational theories which fit the competitive basis of sport. In this case we refer to motivation as considered by the McClelland-Atkinson model (McClelland, Atkinson, Clark & Lowell, 1953; Arkes & Garske, 1982), where two factors determine whether an athlete will engage in competition: the motive to achieve success and the motive to avoid failure. Often referred to as 'competitiveness', achievement motivation has been considered by sport psychologists as a personality factor, where personality traits influence the athlete's need for achievement. An interactional view accounts for more changeable goals, identifying how these affect the situation and the influence the goals themselves exert over the situation.

A motive is the basis for energy and direction of behaviour where the athlete requires both movement and mental skill to reach a goal. The motive to achieve success, regarded as the athlete's self-confidence or efficacy, is believed to represent an athlete's intrinsic motivation when approaching a competitive situation. The motive to avoid failure is represented by the individual's personality disposition for anxiety.

Motivation consists of a cluster of motives which are inner needs (urges or tendencies), plus external stimulus; motivation = motive + external stimulus (actual or signal). Inner and external stimuli create the motive. However, the final behaviour will depend on the mental capacity of the athlete. Singer (1968) proposed that performance (p) is a function of motivation (m) and skill (s): $p = f(m+s)$. The specific cluster of motives is important given that some combinations may be incompatible: 'do not like training' (negative), with 'have to compete' (negative); 'want to go out with friends' (negative), with 'look forward to training' (positive); 'want to win' (positive), with 'want to train' (positive).

Achievement motivation can be described as the predisposition of the athlete to win. Athlete's motives are not static. Emotions such as fear, joy or anger are also regarded as motives. The athlete will respond at every moment to the dominant motive according to his intellectual capacity. Intrinsic and extrinsic motivation should be combined to establish an optimum motivatory effect. While a balance exists, intrinsic motivation should prevail as the goal-centred athlete has greater motivation. If we take the example of the professional footballer anticipating payment, he must first win, and so attend to the actual performance goal before considering the financial bonus following success. Risk-taking behaviour describes a situation where the athlete seeks challenging achievement situations where there is a 50 per cent probability of failure. A situation with a low or very high chance of failure would depict an athlete low in the motive to achieve success, as the athlete will either win easily, or be excused for losing against such tough opposition. In this way his self-esteem is not threatened.

Motivation and goal-setting

Dealing with success and coping with failure directly impact upon the individual's motivation. Motivation does not operate in isolation. Coupled with cognition, it is thought to form the motivation for the next goal. Goals permit the opportunity to devote sufficient attention to implementing intentions, while enhancing confidence, so that no ambiguity about what needs to be done exists. With this increased clarity, decision-making is less time-intensive because an overriding aim and focus exist. The effect of goal-setting is not, in itself, unlike competition, as challenging goals can be perceived as stressors (Huber, 1985). Proximity, difficulty and specificity have been shown to be crucial goal-setting characteristics.

Proximal goals in training, those closer to the athlete rather than distant future goals, are reported to increase the athlete's confidence, strength, stamina and skill, reducing the likelihood of the athlete being adversely affected by competitive stress (Beggs, 1993). Short-term goals should be used as a means to achieve long-term goals (Bar Eli, et al, 1994). It has been suggested that moderately difficult goals are preferable to difficult goals (Kyllo & Landers, 1995). *Scram* denotes the properties of effective goals: Specific, Challenging, Realistic, and Measurable (Fuoss & Troppman, 1981).

Optimal goals are not just verbalised but assimilated by the performer to the extent that he can visualise himself carrying out what is required for goal accomplishment (Hill, 2001). Goals are coupled with feedback, identifying any discrepancies as they occur. More is gained from goal review if mid and long-term perspectives are considered. The athlete who performs poorly at a minor or low priority competition should examine the performance in terms of major game preparation – what can be maintained, adjusted, abandoned, reinforced or added. This would be impossible to do without first, the motivation, and second, the cognition reinforcing the relationship between the actual state and expected state (Vanek, Hosek & Man, 1982). The cognition ensures that the process of goal-setting and its subsequent treatment, attainment or non-attainment, provide learning opportunities.

Appropriate values for identified goals should be assigned in light of the competitive experience. Performance goals, referring to the application of strategies and techniques that help the athlete attain skill mastery, are superior to outcome goals (Zimmerman & Kitsantus, 1996). A personal goal does not clash with a team goal but ensures a source of individual learning regardless of the outcome.

Emotions and arousal effect

Emotions are inborn, generated automatically in the most primitive portion of the brain. There exists a biology to basic emotions in which certain points in the brain house emotions such as fear, aggression and pleasure. One point of stimulation can be continually aroused, as with the drug abuser becoming addicted, and the individual will behave in a certain way to bring about that specific emotion. Sport is one such stimulus, a need to be fulfilled by the athlete. Participation in competitive sport is related to pleasure, whether through the actual movement itself, or through commercial consequence of achievement, glory, or the physical effort accompanying training. By understanding such emotions – expressing them productively, listening to others and empathising – the individual may access the best of what he has to offer. This is fundamental in achieving performance literacy, our ability to identify and understand competition-related emotions, and their subsequent acceptance, or regulation. Without an awareness of what emotions we feel, a lack of empathetic and interactive skills exists (Steiner, 1999).

New emotions and needs come from the external environment, and so the athlete will internalise emotions related to the fulfilment of those needs. The level of the athlete's needs is then raised. Role modelling in accordance with ethical values will help stabilise the athlete throughout periods of extreme external pressure, for example when faced with the dilemma of additional lucrative competition versus much needed regeneration, or the selection of behavioural response to a badly behaving opponent. An established behavioural code can be likened to motor learning, where dominant movement patterns, such as jumping or landing, influence our patterns of physical movement thereafter. In this sense, the more secure the athlete feels in terms of the expression of values and emotions, the greater the ability to cope, mobilise reserves and recover following upsets or unexpected overloading.

With further internalisation, the athlete will have greater influence over the external environment, and be in a position to give others new values, skills and approaches to society. This process is called externalisation. The autonomous athlete, having reached a fulfilling performance level, should not divorce himself from those values which underpinned his early career, nor the emotions and behaviours of that period. A higher complex of values now influence the athlete, and this in turn provides others with 'messages' due to the process of externalisation. It is vital that replacement emotions are guided by ethical values. Ethical behaviour does not simply arrive with the rise to elite performance level, and yet performers at this level carry a great responsibility to ensure that their behaviour is commendable. Behaviours can be changed through education, a continuing responsibility of both coach and athlete. Coaching systems should be based on the process of athlete internalisation-externalisation, ensuring the necessary progressive development.

Extreme positive or negative emotion can detract from an appropriate mental state for performance; a dramatic increase in arousal may serve to block movement coordination and mental processes such as cognition. Under such conditions, the athlete is unable to produce a normal performance. The personality of the athlete will determine how the stressors are managed. For those individuals who perform better when external pressures cause inner tension, performance in competition exceeds that of training. Such athletes have frustration tolerance, a higher level of resistance, whereas those who perform better in training than in competition have a very low frustration tolerance.

From the coaching point of view it is important to realise that mental resistance, sometimes referred to as mental toughness, is either inborn, informed by the type of education received by the athlete, or influenced by experiences under stressful conditions. It is advisable to create a system of athlete education leading to the independence of the athlete, involving complete knowledge of the self, and optimal risk-taking.

The resistance level and frustration tolerance of the athlete becomes evident when working with the athlete throughout training and competitive calendars. Competitive stress has been approached by both emotion-focused and task-centred methods: emotion-focused coping methods, such as relaxation techniques and self-talk, attempt to address anxiety and other non-facilitative emotions; task-centred coping methods, such as goal-setting, aim to remove the cause of unwanted emotions (Cohen & Lazarus, 1979).

Psychological management of the opposition, and self-management

It is important to teach the athlete how to handle the opponent psychologically, as he will not be looking out for the best interests of fellow competitors. There are many behaviour patterns of potential value to the athlete prior to the event, at the competition site, and in other areas such as the athletes' village. As with all event favourites, Danek, a Czech discus thrower and world record holder at 64.54 m, received much media attention and support prior to the 1964 Tokyo Olympic Games. His main opposition came from the American, Oerter, who also proceeded to confirm Danek as firm favourite, sure to win the competition in his absence as he was too injured to throw. On the day of the competition, Oerter turned up heavily taped up, visibly distracting Danek. Danek started with a throw of 59.73 m, improving in round four to 60.52 m. Oerter's fifth throw was 61.00 m, an Olympic record. At this moment Danek was crushed; his arousal was so high that further attempts were not completely coordinated.

Although the opposition cannot be controlled, the athlete can learn to regulate himself psychologically and so feel better positioned to manage the opponent. This is not unethical but more along the lines of self-preservation and pragmatism. Pre-performance and performance routines should cover a range of potential incidents as thorough risk-management. Every activity must feed the athlete's performance, and not detract from it in any way. To reduce pressure as event favourite, he must think of challenging for the medal rather than defending himself against challengers. If he has a high performance expectation, it is easier to achieve this goal from the position of outsider than from the limelight.

Competition strategy involves learning about self-portrayal, where the focus on goal fulfilment should be clear of distractions. Each athlete will create his own recipe establishing flexible, successful ingredients. The athlete must also exert complete self-control learning to adapt to a range of situations. A British international high jumper reported that he liked to feel 'bouncy' before competing. When asked how this was achieved, the athlete stated: 'by running round a 400 m track and springing over an occasional hurdle'. This same athlete was about to compete in an indoor arena with a 200 m track! Clearly the performance was not supported by this rigid performance plan.

Competitive experience does assist in the design of such plans, and various viable alternatives should be devised and rehearsed in light of changeable conditions. The mental plan will direct energy and effort carefully in light of familiar experience. Contingency for the unknown is not as difficult as it may sound – the athlete will have a range of mental skills at his disposal, which provide tools with which to approach adversity. Daley Thompson, double Olympic Champion and World Record holder in decathlon in the 1990s, mentally rehearsed different scenarios where he would put himself at the very edge of risk in the arena. Should any similar situation occur in reality, he felt that he had been there already. Confidence is instilled by the very fact that the performer can call upon internal resources to help deal with the unexpected. This additional option at the athlete's disposal provides added security. Central to the success of a plan is athlete control, that is self-control. No athlete can afford to wait for the opposition to impose competitive conditions. If the athlete allows this to happen, he is abdicating responsibility for the performance.

Development of the mental plan

As more successful athletes have been shown to demonstrate higher levels of energy and possess an ability to turn potentially challenging situations to their advantage (Apitzsch & Berggren, 1993), mental training can tap into such energy reserves. The extent to which an individual succumbs to competition-induced anxiety is determined by internal factors, such as previous experience, unconscious processes, but also by external variables that act systematically to modify and influence the individual's responses. Mental plans take various formats dependent on athlete preference: words to describe distinct scenarios; trigger words only depicting established preparation patterns; visual symbols such as the shape of a throwing circle or podium; associated noises such as the swirl of the rotation in shot put; or combination recipes. Tom McKean, 800 m European Champion and World Indoor Champion, followed his plan from the lower section upwards, as he visualised each step towards a successful outcome (table 21). The performer was shadowed in training and competition to establish relevant plan ingredients. A loose structure was implemented to guide the acquisition of mental training skills. Warm-up races such as club commitments and national championships were used to refine the flexible framework.

600–800 m	trigger '*squeeze*'; kick hard
600 m	get ready to kick
500 m	trigger '*stay up*'; work onto the back straight
200 m	in position, stay relaxed
Start	trigger '*get out fast*'
Pre-start	alone, ignore people around me, avoid eye contact attention on breath control, relaxation routine

TABLE 21 Race focus plan for GB international 800 m runner

KEY: when you pass the ball, you don't give away responsibility

1. Loss of concentration through mistakes

Loss of attention	missed kick . . . it's gone, park it
Use gearbox	select a gear, 1st to recover
2nd gear	up to playing speed
Concentration 1	use movement pattern (fist hit on leg)
Loss of focus	come back to here and now
5-point kick plan	visualise, successful imagery
Concentration 2	use trigger word '*precise*'
Return to game pace	change gear, 3rd for aggressive pace change
Acceleration	4th gear in control, smooth play

2. Loss of concentration through fatigue

Reinforce gearbox	keep changing gear
Positive self-talk	use triggers '*big hit*'; '*safe hands*'
Team energy	talk to team-mates, remember 'the hill'
Energise	energy-ball imagery
Be aware of roles	attack, support

3. Heads are down

4 points down	we need 5 to win
Team energy	keep recycling
Basics	keep it simple
Time	use every second

TABLE 22 Refocusing plan for Tim Stimpson (of West Hartlepool), Leicester and England, Rugby Union

Tim Stimpson established a range of plans reflecting his individual needs throughout the game. Training camp venues were used to introduce and practise mental training techniques in controlled and modified conditions. Personal reserves such as emotional and physical commitment were necessary throughout the intense training activities. The 'hill' cited in table 22 referred to a specific training session in Loughborough's Charnwood Forest: 10 × hill run. Not only was it immensely difficult for all players to make it up the hill after the halfway point, with their vast range of weights and builds, but also, additionally, the recovery walk down the hill was hugely draining on the quads. The active recovery provided no relief, just further energy expenditure. It visibly distracted some and became a source of attrition to others. An individual task became a team challenge as every member gave 100 per cent effort, shouting on their team-mates; and those who managed to finish joined in with the last efforts of their struggling team-mates, ensuring that every man completed the session. The levels of physical, psychological, and emotional effort accessed were memorable, converting a single training session to a resource to be called upon in times of pressure. Individual and collective strategies were implemented, where any player could call upon internal reserves and the accumulated willpower of the group. During match play, players recalled associated emotions, helping to elicit a similar cohesive response. Technical training sessions were used to rehearse the different techniques, where conditions reflected the real game demands more closely.

Non-league games theoretically provided the next step in plan refinement. However, due to the difference in the approach of the player to this level of game as opposed to a league game, and the difference in the level of performance arousal, it rarely provided a sequential progression. The practice did, however, serve to secure the learning of techniques. The player developed a range of creative adaptations thereafter.

Another player, who competed for the British Lions, quick on his feet but often slow off the ground following a tackle, was awarded the 'armchair award', dependent on the number of seconds it took him to engage in the game following going to the ground. This was both light-hearted and serious. Resting or injured players helped put together a series of time profiles comparing his recovery with those of less experienced players. Consequently, he learned to actively attenuate to the game play, remaining switched-on at all times. Before that, he had slipped into a habit of switching-off for a few seconds after he had 'done his bit'. Being aware of this potential weakness in his game made the difference, and other squad members learned in the process.

This detailed planning necessitates the time and proactive attention of the player. The mental plan can be reviewed through post-game analysis as soon as possible after the event. Practice is essential. Confidence in mental plans is fundamental, therefore supporting staff should be careful to refer to aspects of the player's plan so as to publicly reinforce its practical value. An inability to integrate mental training with physical preparation will diminish the potential impact.

There are also potential problems away from the competition site that the athlete can address. The athletes' village or team hotel at any major championship plays host to many potential stressors, which may have a negative impact. For instance, distractions from social activities, nearby presence of the opposition, and the constant intensity that distinguishes the site from the home environment can be energy drains. Experience reveals that it can be a testing ground for athletes wishing to 'psyche-out' opposition. The athlete must live among failures, those with great aspirations, and those with unethical values. Some athletes thrive within such an environment, using the numerous goings-on to continually keep their mind off competing.

To live in comfortable isolation may suit those wishing to conserve performance energy. Carl Lewis did not stay at any Olympic village, preferring to stay away from that type of environment and successfully minimising his exposure to other variables, which he perceived as potentially distracting. Refraining from other athletes' psychological handles can be difficult, and so the athlete can be comfortable in the knowledge that predetermined routines will look after his respective interests. Other great Olympians have also demonstrated similar distancing approaches, most notably five-times gold medallist Sir Steven Redgrave.

On the other hand, an athlete may use the village situation as a vehicle for imposing his psychological strength on the opposition. Olympic Champion, Linford Christie did so with the utmost skill.

Performance support should also be aware of the potential downfalls associated with athlete deprivation at competition sites. Athletes competing abroad may experience taste deprivation, a desire for food that satisfies their specific requirement. While competition hosts may offer excellent facilities, it is important for the athlete to operate within a comfortable zone, in touch with aspects typical of the home environment. It is worth sending a cook from home with any travelling team, as did Nestlé, who sponsored the Swiss team during the 1980 Moscow Olympics, or Bayern Munich FC, when playing away in UEFA Champions League games. The athlete should not expend too much energy adapting to constant change. This type of practice is now regarded as normal, assisting performers with established routines that contribute to their self-regulation.

Pre-performance routines within the long pre-start conditions (fig. 60) provide familiar structures and flexible, but controlled, patterns. The performance routine within the competition itself will facilitate consistency. Boutcher (1993) reported further advantages: attention control is increased, helping the athlete to concentrate more efficiently; the warm-up decrement is addressed, dealing with a loss in motor performance following a short break by giving psychological and physiological warm-ups in stop-start activities; and automatic skill execution is encouraged. Despite the use of naive, so-called, non-scientific techniques designed to harmonise body and mental states, there are occasions when the desired result is not achieved. The athlete should have an operational understanding of mental training techniques with a scientific basis, such as progressive relaxation (Jacobson, 1929), involving the systematic tensing and relaxing of muscle groups. Autogenic training is similar to progressive relaxation with an emphasis on how the body parts feel (Schultz & Luthe, 1959; Harris & Harris, 1984; Nideffer, 1985; Orlick, 1986).

Mental training can be the difference between successful and less successful athletes (Weinberg & Gould, 1985). Medal winners in the 1988 US Olympic wrestling teams used more positive self-talk, had a narrower and more immediate focus of attention, had better mental preparation for unforeseen negative circumstances and had more extensive mental practice.

Many procedures have been developed, but not all are as effective as they are claimed to be. While the athlete should learn to relax the body as a basis for intervention strategies, he must also learn reactivation, depending on the athlete and sport. Players in English first division rugby and Premier division football make effective use of a combination of pre-game relaxation followed by individually designed reactivation strategies. Individual programming is crucial for both team and individual sports where blanket strategies may even serve to distract some players and compromise a viable ideal performance state for all within the team. The relaxation-reactivation is rehearsed for competition-type, whether for home and away games, or national and international events. Competition-induced arousal is given a new direction avoiding a negative spiral effect.

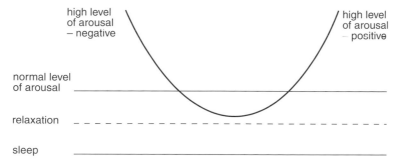

FIG. 59 Competition-induced arousal (Vanek, 1967)

Theoretically, arousal can be very low, such as sleep, or higher for normal daily activities. It is described as physiological and psychological activation (Gould & Krane, 1992). A high level of arousal results in mental activation, which can manifest itself in sweating, increased heart rate and respiration. Some individuals may experience over-arousal to the extent that they lose control over their actions. Arousal does not imply either negative or positive reactions. Anxiety, however, is a negative emotional state characterised by feelings of apprehension associated with the activation or arousal of the body. Figure 59 shows the level of arousal prior to competition (on the left), which is negatively affecting the individual. Using a mental training technique, this is reduced to a relaxed level, but not sleep. From there, reactivation occurs with the use of an appropriate follow-on technique. The arousal again increases but this time with a new direction, positively affecting the athlete (to the right of the figure). The performer has controlled pre-competition anxiety avoiding, for example, loss of energy leading to a feeling of flatness. In addition, an indirect consequence is that of increasing self-confidence. The athlete, in the knowledge that self-management techniques have been learned and rehearsed, will approach competition with self-assurance.

Many arousal models exist describing the anxiety of the athlete and subsequent behaviour; Hardy and Fazey's (1987) catastrophe model assumes that anxiety is made up of cognitive anxiety and a physiological response. Cognitive anxiety is caused by either negative expectations of success, negative self-evaluation, or diversion of attentional focus (Burton, 1990). It is characterised by worry, negative self-talk and imagery, and loss of attention. When physiological arousal is high, such as on competition day, this model predicts that a negative correlation between cognitive anxiety and performance exists, although moderately high levels of physiological arousal are necessary for peak performance. Reversal theory (Apter, 1982) asserts that a high arousal level occurring within an evaluative state will be negatively interpreted as anxiety, whereas the same level of arousal occurring when the athlete is within a non-evaluative state will be interpreted positively. The category and perception of anxiety determines the athlete's responses and learning of appropriate coping strategies. The manifestation of anxiety, whether cognitive and/or somatic, influences the selection of stress management models (Davidson & Schwartz, 1976). Somatic anxiety is the physiological or affective component related directly to autonomic arousal, which may be exhibited in a range of physiological responses including clammy hands, muscular tension and rapid heart rate.

Important for both coach and athlete when giving attention to the arousal performance relationship is a multi-dimensional perspective (Martens et al, 1990). The athlete is potentially vulnerable to differential effects on aspects of the information-processing system when under the stress of competition (Jones, 1990). The aim of mental training is to harmonise the mental and training/competing states. It may take several months to master control over arousal. Coping skills must be rehearsed and practised under simulated conditions to maximise their efficiency. These techniques should not be carried out without specialist training and objective measurement. Imagery, audio and video tapes are components of any procedure. This said, mental training is not to be overestimated, as it is only part of the overall psychological preparation.

Performance management

Athletic performance can be segmented according to the engagement of the individual leading up to the event, and subsequent disengagement from the activity. The ability to understand and manage the stages of time of competition optimises the conditions which are under the athlete's control. Each stage should be carefully analysed so that coach and athlete can manipulate existing variables. In no single stage should the athlete feel loss of self-control or uneasy about how things are going. Of particular importance is the handling of the post-competitive mental state (5) as this stage influences long pre-start conditions (3) (fig. 60). This determines the actions of the coach following defeat and success to ensure that the athlete is able to re-enter at the pre-competition stage in a comfortable mental state. Care of the athlete is personality-related, however sensitivity on the part of the coach following competition is more likely to contribute to the athlete's recovery from one competition and thereby assist his preparation for the next.

Arousal can be depicted along the stages of time of competition. A simplified approach highlights the profiles of three athletes, A, B and C (fig. 61).

Each athlete is, of course, different and will display a unique arousal pattern. It is responsible to explore the varied conditions under which the athlete will perform well, or under-perform, so that the accompanying skills and coping strategies can be learned. The day of the competition should not bring unexpected conditions, only a mixture of familiar experiences, or at least those that the athlete can relate to. Post-competitive conditions are closely associated with the finishing arousal and effort of the athlete. Reactions may include euphoria or depression, as these are part of the motivational cluster associated with the new training phase. Immediate post-game/competition input should be neutral, free of value judgements. If

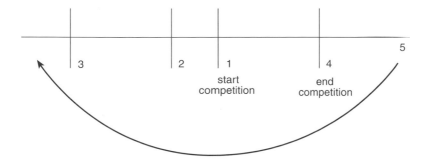

FIG. 60 The stages of time of competition
(1)   start conditions – the starting mental state of the athlete (minutes and seconds prior to the start)
(2)   short pre-start conditions – short-term pre-start mental state (minutes, hours)
(3)   long pre-start conditions – long-term pre-start mental state (weeks, days, hours)
(1–4)   competitive conditions – competitive mental state
(4–5)   post-competitive conditions – post-competitive mental state.

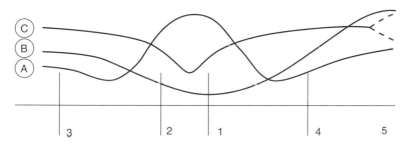

FIG. 61 Arousal A: the arousal is too high in the short pre-start conditions. Thereafter, during the competition, the arousal falls due to its premature intensity prior to competition, leaving Athlete A feeling flat and drained; Arousal B: this profile represents low arousal in training, such as when there is little effort on the part of the athlete (long pre-start conditions). It slowly rises but optimal arousal is only reached following the competition. A poor performance for Athlete B; Arousal C: falls in the short pre-start conditions, rising in competition to a facilitating level. This demonstrates the correct timing and level according to the arousal level of the finished effort for Athlete C.

performance management receives insufficient attention, all preceding training investment converts to a lottery scenario where there exists no guarantee of producing a performance that was indicated as possible in training. It is the performer's perception of the anxiety experienced that is important to clarify.

PERSONALITY OF THE ATHLETE

Given that personality is determined by an individual's characteristics, each person is unique. Hollander's (1971) notion of personality divides it into three separate but related levels: the psychological core, typical responses, and role related behaviours. The psychological core, internal and most consistent in nature, includes the individual's self-concept, central attitudes, values and motives. As the deepest component of the personality, it represents the 'real you' (Weinberg & Gould, 1995). Typical responses, represented by the way in which the individual responds to an environmental situation, will give an indication of their psychological core: 'That's just like him' implies that the behaviour reflects the core person. Role-related behaviour is engaged in to fit the individual's perception of the environment. As the environment or perception changes, so too does the behaviour. This aspect of the personality structure is most superficial and changeable. The parent-coach can often have difficulty with the coexistence of both roles.

Despite the fact that various methods have been designed to measure personality, such as rating scales, questionnaires and unstructured projective tests, it is highly unlikely that a cause-and-effect relationship exists between a personality trait and athletic performance. Examples include the Athletic Motivation Inventory (AMI), (Tutko & Richards, 1971, 1972); Cattell (16PF) Personality Factor Questionnaire, (1965); the Eysenck Personality Inventory (EPI), (1968); and the Rorschach Test (Fredenburgh, 1971). Cattell's 16PF has proven to be very useful in measurement of athlete personality.

Generally speaking, there is a difference between the athletic population and the non-athletic population. Athletes are shown to be more independent, objective and extrovert, yet less anxious than non-athletes. A process of natural selection can attract certain personality types to sport. Differences do exist between athletes of different sports, for example between co-acting and interacting sports. Team sport athletes are more dependent, anxious and extrovert than individual sport athletes (Cox, 1998). The female athlete has been shown to differ from the normative (non-athlete) female, but to share personality traits with her counterpart, the male athlete and the normative male, such as assertiveness, achievement orientation, dominance, self-sufficiency, intelligence and reservation. Fencing, ice hockey, track and field, and lacrosse demonstrated low personality variation, suggesting the viability of specific personality profiles in different sports (Williams, 1980). The coach must treat all athletes as individuals, recognising that an exceptional talent may differ from the norm.

Some researchers have turned their attention to how the situation and the environment affect the individual's behaviour (Bandura, 1977). According to the situational approach, environmental influences determine the way an individual behaves. A timid individual may play an extremely assertive game of soccer, the game situation necessitating the behavioural change. Despite the fact that the situation can certainly influence behaviour, it cannot accurately predict behaviour (Weinberg & Gould, 1995).

Contrary to the application of superficial inventories unable to penetrate the personality, former East European approaches were distinct in their inclination to use experimental methods, trying to establish and record objective data associated with the nervous activity of the subjects under observation (Vanek & Hosek, 1974). Personality measurement is most accurate if the psychological core is accessed. This can be achieved by measuring the level of typical responses using some form of questionnaire. The coach, using personal experience and time spent with the athlete, combined with paper and pencil inventories, can make a fairly accurate assessment. It is better to construct an athlete profile over a period of time using simple observation techniques to get to know the athlete in different situations. Personality measurement should not be used to discriminate against athletes in terms of the sport they choose to participate in, nor their ultimate selection or skill capability.

While it cannot predict performance, it can be used to gain further insight into behaviour in certain playing positions or competitions.

RELATIONSHIP BETWEEN ATHLETE AND COACH

Initially, the athlete must adjust to the disposition of the coach, given that the coach is stable and the athlete transitory. The coach has an approach consisting of systems and styles with which to influence the athlete directly and indirectly. Within this stabilising period, the athlete should maintain self-determination while the coach identifies with the athlete's personality. A flexible structure is used by the coach throughout his operations – adapting to the changing needs of the athlete with their development.

The science of coaching as a body of knowledge must be constantly innovative. The coach has a responsibility to continue his own learning by reading, listening, and attending workshops, clinics and courses. Only by thinking and reflecting on his work, and by integrating the supporting disciplines such as sport psychology, nutrition, physiology and biomechanics, can the coach continue to develop the discipline and his position within it. Sports science support was often independently conducted, the physiologist with coach and athlete, or the nutritionist with coach and athlete, sometimes leading to confusing or conflicting overall advice. The synthesis of sport science has since produced a shift from multidisciplinary to interdisciplinary activity (Murray, 1995). Specialists can provide a supporting network, informing, reinforcing and enhancing the operations of the coach-athlete partnership, reducing the possibilities of contradictory information. Coaching methodology is, as a consequence, extended, broadening the scope for decision-making. The coach should learn to lead and coordinate the work of the support team, optimising individual input within a context specific to the athlete's needs (Dick 1992). Within professional sport, such support should not be financed in accordance with session input, but should reinforce the partnership with specialist and coach by linking payment with performance outcome. Martina Navratilova maintained such a support team of eight or nine specialists, including two sport psychologists, one handling training motivation, and the other tournament motivation, given that she felt it difficult to be constantly motivated.

Communication between coach, athlete and specialist is fundamental to performance support. The coach should be informed of discussions, for example between psychologist and athlete, where the psychologist is respectful of confidential information. Unethical activities on the part of the sport psychologist include betrayal of trust and over-estimation of abilities as a psychologist. The sport psychologist will work in different ways, observing, assessing, and testing players where results inform coaching activity and performance preparation, or again, as a consultant with both coach and athlete, giving guidance. The number of people operating around the coach can either contribute to coaching aims or detract from them. Over-involvement can be avoided by strategically planning support and clearly identifying roles.

The art of coaching is the experimental learning from informed determination on a trial-and-error basis. The coach records daily input so that decisions can be reflected upon in terms of the related outcomes. Emotionally sensitive individuals are more able to accumulate progressively and develop the art of coaching. The centrality of the people business cannot be substituted by any other factor such as supporting technology. Technology should not detract from the creativity of the coach; it should play a facilitative role rather than replace intuitive-orientated judgement. At the disposal of the coach is a complex system of metacommunication, where the tone of the voice, a certain look or small signal can provide the athlete with very clear information. The coach does not need to use too many words, but should also find a variety of metacommunicative methods. Short instructions are best used prior to and during events. Following defeat there should only be instruction on immediate activities, such as showering or refreshments. The coach may be in an emotional state and should not risk saying anything which might damage the coach/athlete relationship. Although post-match/event review should be pursued soon after the match, an emotional coach may not be the best person to conduct the review process, which must be seen as the opportunity to learn, and not to judge.

Full team/squad meetings should be democratically executed – a formal and open route which the athlete can use without fear of recriminations. The athlete should be an active participant in the planning of his own destiny and be able to accept responsibility for under-achievement or other problems because he has continuing personal involvement. End-of-season team meetings provide the opportunity to evaluate results fully with the benefit of hindsight, where responsibility for shortfalls can be attributed, providing useful information for the planning of postseason screening and guiding the preseason training structure. Weekly, six-weekly and quarterly meetings occur in light of flexible adjustments to the coaching or performance programme and should follow a similar pattern. Consistency on the part of the coach creates a force on which the athletes can rely. Meeting procedures will allow the attending parties to focus on the relevant issues rather than be distracted by the order of the day. Language should also be grammatically uniform: for example, it is not acceptable to use 'we' when the team wins, and 'you' when the team loses! Players subjected to coach inconsistency will begin to doubt the sincerity of the coach, before losing trust completely.

Notion of team

In order to understand fully the issues pertaining to team climate, it is important to appreciate how and why people communicate (Pope, 1998). A team approach has been shown to benefit performance in both co-acting and interacting sports. A sociological perspective identifies a group as more than a collection of individuals. Individuals working together towards a common goal are much more effective than if they were to work independently of one another. The team unit receives much coverage in literature, which is generally uncompromising in its discerning views of the team unit versus the less effective counterpart, the group (Donnellon, 1996; Frankel, 1997; Slepicka, 1981), although the development of the group can be an essential part of team development. Synergistic properties are associated with cohesive teams. Although performance success has been reported in the absence of team cohesion (Landers & Leuschen, 1974; Lenk, 1969), the majority of research indicates that greater levels of cohesion lead to success (Carron, 1982; Carron & Ball, 1977).

Cohesion has been linked with certain factors fundamental to development, such as increased communication, productivity, satisfaction, behavioural change, persistence, conformity and attendance (Carron, Widmeyer & Brawley, 1985). Within this context, cohesion is seen to contribute to the development of the team, its maintenance, and to the accomplishment of group goals. Certainly there exists a potential team synergy which is found to raise performance. Cohesion acts as a uniting force influenced by both external and internal factors. Where pressure exists from other teams, the unit will be more resistant, although excessive pressure can break its spirit. In times of intense emotion associated with failure, individuals may seek to look after themselves. Low external pressure will not serve to increase team cohesion.

Inter- and intra-team conflict need not relate to a negative scenario. As the sport environment evolves, so too does the range of potential differences, such as between team member and opponent, player and manager, athlete and coach, or coach and agent. Inter- and intra-team differences can be used to resolve conflict if the method used follows a pattern of integration; to bring together the various points of view without diluting respective principles or merely achieving a short-term compromise. A satisfactory conclusion for those involved is more demanding intellectually than simply adhering to a decision made unilaterally. This type of approach will maintain consistent variables crucial to a team's operating efficiency.

Some members of the team may be more interested in the task at hand and therefore integrate well together during a set practice or a game. Others may be attracted to the group for social reasons and find that they integrate better if allowed social opportunities with other team members. Each cohesiveness construct is assumed to be related through the interaction of task and social orientations as perceived by the group. The coach can obtain a measure of the cohesion level within a team or squad setting, indicating the orientation of the team players. A range of instruments has been designed to measure cohesion, as follows:

> Group Environment Questionnaire (GEQ) – Carron, Widmeyer & Brawley (1985)
> Sports Cohesiveness Questionnaire (SCQ) – Martens & Peterson (1971)
> Team Cohesiveness Questionnaire (TCQ) – Gruber & Gray (1981, 1982)
> Sport Cohesion Instrument (SCI) – Yukelson, Weinberg & Jackson (1983, 1984)
> Team Psychology Questionnaire – Partington & Shangi (1992)

The information provided will help the coach rate the importance of activities associated with the training environment in terms of the wellbeing of the group. Player requirements may point to higher involvement of injured players in the coaching setup, more regular meetings or opportunities to socialise.

The team-cohesion instrument should reflect the interests of both coach and athlete, and therefore the selection should be made carefully and in consultation with a sports psychologist. Coaches of individual sports can also benefit from an understanding of the cohesion profile of individual athletes, given that there are many aspects to training. A training component, for example a speed or plyometric session, may be optimised in terms of training with a partner, within a squad or in the presence of the coach. Each athlete will train best in relation to a facilitating cohesive element that supports their personal motivations. For the coach to be comfortable in the knowledge that a custom-designed programme fully serves the needs of the athlete, he should appreciate the conditions under which the athlete operates best.

Age and gender differences

The coach often has to respond to both individual differences and group patterns characterised by age and gender. Former East European approaches differentiated between individuals according to maturation rates: prior to puberty, girls and boys were differentiated with the aim of instilling confidence. A mother figure among pre-school age children was thought to provide an input compatible with the child's level of development. Accordingly, the coach could demand more from the school age group. This was not limited to support and encouragement, but also involved the introduction of a father figure into the family. Following puberty, a more sensitive, warmer approach was used, with girls perceived to be more sensitive at this time. It was suggested that junior boys reacted more positively to a stronger handling. While of guiding value, personality differences, rather than age and gender differences, influence coaching approaches. The promotion of self-efficacy is inherent within all coaching activity regardless of the age or gender of the athlete.

Performance attribution does exhibit gender-based variation, although generalisations should not dictate specific coaching responses (Hendy & Boyer, 1993). A consistent difference between the causal attributions of men and women is not proven but evidence suggests that males are more likely to attribute their successes internally than females (Ickes & Layden, 1978). The coach to the female athlete should encourage the athlete to consider poor performance in terms of unstable characteristics such as effort and luck. Olympic volleyball player Peppler (1977) commented on the fact that male players participating in her volleyball clinics could be repeatedly beaten but were ready to try again, showing complete confidence. External attribution of failure should be encouraged so that it is viewed as a passing result not adversely affecting self-confidence or self-esteem. The athlete does not always attribute performance outcome in a logical manner, such as when using an ego-enhancing strategy, attributing all successes to internal causes, or when using an ego-protecting strategy, attributing all failures to external causes. If another party is constantly blamed for failure, a sense of ownership will not be developed. The coach has to maintain a balance between enhancing the athlete's self-esteem, ensuring protection at vulnerable times such as following a defeat, and maintaining a realistic perspective on the actual performance.

Extending competitive opportunities

Talent scouts can ensure that no child misses the chance to develop a natural talent. An athletic youngster may be identified through deliberate and moderate exposure to a competitive structure such as class v class and school v school. The elevation of competition level is gradual, progressing from regional representation to national and international competition. Consequently, young gifted talent may be identified. Where the child can enter a sport (depending on the accepted system operating in the country), his subsequent participation remains his decision and that of his parents. The UK has traditionally tolerated a club-driven system and regards specialist training schools as rather extreme. Yet it makes a lot of sense to observe young athletes and this provides useful information to help with their sport selection. Taking into account somatotype, displayed behavioural tendencies, tolerances, and dominant movement patterns can reduce the chance of disappointments at a later stage or provide the opportunity to move on to another sport which shares a similar core training preparation. The youngster finishing with artistic gymnastics could make a very useful transition to athletics, particularly with the addition of more jumping events for women. A highly anxious individual may be better suited to individual performance, alleviating the perceived pressure of letting others down. Conversely, a team sport offers the athlete the chance to share responsibility which might suit him better.

It is up to the coach to provide the orientation for the young athlete. An integrated coaching network where core skills are imparted would ensure that every child has a basic preparation appropriate for a variety of sports, increasing the young athlete's choice and access to sport in general. Non-residential or residential academies of sport can provide an ideal base for a balanced approach to the preparation and care of the young athlete. One sport's loss should simply be another sport's gain. This situation is preferable to losing the child to sport altogether. Evolving national institutes of sport, backed by Government, by lottery, and/or sponsorship, and/or public funding may serve as a catalyst for a considerable change for the better in managing and coordinating the development of young talent.

SUMMARY

There are no fixed ingredients for success, but the coach can teach the athlete to be aware of every possible ethical performance indicator and facilitator. Despite the belief on the part of some sport psychologists that the most influential parameter in a team's success is the player (Fouss & Troppman, 1981), mirrored by coaches advocating that a good athlete makes a good coach (Walton, 1992), coaches can be differentiated according to their skinl base (Brown & Miller, 1994; Bull, 1995; Rushall, 1995; Tinning, 1982). Skills specifically relating to training theory are regarded as the base line for all coaches (Ozolin, 1995; Voelz, 1982). Ultimately the performance of the athlete is used as a yardstick for coaching competence, which is surprising as more than technical mastery is associated with the successful coach (Loehr, 1982).

The difficulty in surmising any difference between coaches more concerned with the care and development of the person than their performance achievement is the lack of measurement parameter. The nature of the skilful coach has been captured by phrases like 'intuitive' (Loehr, 1982), 'experiential knowledge' (Klausner, 1977), 'introspection' (Terry, 1995), 'attitude' (Horung, 1982), and 'personal development' (Martens, 1980). People-centred skills are considered essential to team development (Carron & Spink, 1993; Nolan, 1990; Syer & Connelly, 1984). Such coaches invest their time, knowledge and experience in the development firstly of the person, and secondly, the performer.

Good organisation of each preparatory step, from the management of coaching staff and integration with the sport science support team, to the actual movement of the athlete on the day of the competition, is vital. Accompanying administrators should also be carefully selected, performance goal-orientated and trained for the event conditions. Every step towards competition preparation is a step towards achieving the goals of athlete or team.

11 PERCEPTUAL-MOTOR LEARNING

In most Western countries, knowledge about the acquisition of skill is frequently neglected. This may be due to the nature versus nurture emphasis of recent years, with controversial statements such as 'winners are born not made!', or to the fact that new information on the perceptual and decision-making aspects of sport has not been effectively disseminated through coach education programmes.

Regardless of the reasons for this oversight, every individual has a need of movement, whether this is the fundamental requirement of the movement of inner organs, or the muscles. Movements can be described in the context of patterns and skills. A motor pattern is the movement involved in the carrying out of a particular task. This is different from a motor skill, which places emphasis on the accuracy, precision, and economy of performance of the task execution. One of the most fundamental tasks of early childhood is the development of the dominant movement patterns and motor skills through variety, increasing experimentation, and progressive learning. A major aim of motor development in the first two years of life, for example, is walking. Once initiated, proficiency in this basic motor skill develops at an exponential rate (Malina & Bouchard, 1991).

Education aims, through physical activities, to promote the understanding of regular systematic movement as a part and philosophy of life, with the idea that sport is a school for life. More specific movement, as required in sports performance, requires motor skill training to cultivate and refine highly skilled performance. Perceptual-motor skill training reflects the enhancement of those characteristics required for skilled performance. While the capabilities of a skilled athlete are numerous and sport-determined, there are identifiable aspects to expert performance, relating to economy of effort and precision of movement:

A complex, intentional action involving a whole chain of sensory, central and motor mechanisms which, through the process of learning, have come to be organised and co-ordinated in such a way as to achieve predetermined objectives with maximum certainty.

(Whiting, 1975, p6)

Defining skilled performance is important for the coach attempting to balance the amount of time dedicated to the various components of training. The practice of movement elements in open skill sports such as ball sports (particularly drill practice of basic skills) often takes up a disproportionate amount of time, despite the fact that perceptual and decision-making skills are regarded as highly influential in determining success (Abernethy, Wann, & Parks, 1999). The perceptual-motor skill is context-determined. With few exceptions, the expert performer in one sport will not demonstrate the same level of skill in another sport. There is virtually zero transfer from one sport to another (Lotter, 1960), although the learning process is transferable. Some sports, such as soccer, rely upon perceptual and decision-making abilities, with the uncertainty of opposition play, tactics, and timing. Other sports define expert performance by control and movement precision, for example artistic gymnastics, where actions can be planned in advance and performance conditions are predictable. The characteristics of each respective high-level performer differ enormously, yet each stands to gain perceptual-motor skill training.

PERCEPTUAL-MOTOR SKILLS TRAINING

An ability is a stable characteristic or trait, inborn and unaffected by practice and rehearsal. A skill is distinct. It can be developed or lost. Given this, the coach can assist the athlete through the development of skills central to movement technique, and ultimately performance. To do so using perceptual-motor learning theory in practical technique training, the coach emphasises first the sensory part of reactions or responses and, second, complete awareness and control over what is going on.

Sensory perception is a multi-dimensional construct blending external events with an accompanying interpretation of internal activity. Perceptual information is obtained via a collective process. An individual's ability to identify what is going on in the external environment, such as where a competitor is during a race; to interpret what is occurring internally, such as loss of concentration; to understand body positioning, such as trail-leg angle in hurdling; and to establish the actual relationship between the body and the environment, are accounted for by sensory perception. Perception is more than the body's reception of information by its various sensory systems. Associated sub-processes potentially limit performance. These are identified as detection, comparison, recognition, and selective attention. Whether a signal is present or not can be determined through detection. Comparison assesses whether two stimuli are the same or whether they differ. The identification of stimuli, objects and patterns known previously occurs by recognition, and selective attention ensures the appropriate allocation of processing resources where deemed relevant or ignoring distracting or less relevant information (Abernethy, Wann & Parks, 1999).

Every sport has sensory aspects. Where a hierarchy of sensory dominance is suggested, perceptual priority is afforded to vision. The dominant means of controlling skilled movement for the sighted athlete is via the visual system.

Kinaesthesis, audition and the remaining senses follow thereafter. Different sensory information is made available to facilitate 'reading' performance. The advantages of training perceptual motor skills are varied. Fatigue-induced distortion can be minimised, or the athlete can learn to anticipate requirements. Feed-forward – information sent ahead in time to prepare for the following sensory feedback – has been shown through research on visual perception to be of an advantage to the performer (Gallistel, 1980). A copy of the motor (efferent) command sent to the eye muscles is, in addition, sent to a location in the brain; the visual perception system is in this way informed about the imminent movement of the eye. This 'efference copy' mechanism may indeed exert similar parallel control over the movement of the limbs as well (Schmidt, 1988). Neurological evidence has indicated that sensory information to be received by the muscles is also sent to locations in the brain (Evans, 1973). Thus the aim of such activities may be to inform the sensory system and to prepare it for reception of feedback.

Fundamental to training are the sources of non-visual information and how they interact with vision. To develop sensory perception and necessary awareness, modified activities and games can be used to create a rich reservoir for understanding and perfecting techniques. The ballet dancer rehearsing movements before a mirror is educating the body in an entire movement range, teaching it through predetermined sequences and acquiring more knowledge of what is involved. The athlete must consciously make himself aware of responses and reactions, thereby accumulating movement information.

It is evident that this movement must be harmoniously controlled, a function carried out by the pyramid and extra-pyramid cells coming from the sub-cortex and connecting every part of the brain responsible for movement. Cooperation between pyramid and extra-pyramid nerves is very subjective where potential influences include feelings and emotions. A lack of coordination results in a certain mental state, expressed by a movement error during performance. Each small uncoordinated activity contributes to failure. Thus the aspect of self-control under a range of conditions faced by the athlete should be rehearsed where the athlete is to maintain a performance-facilitating equilibrium. The ultimate aim of perceptual-motor skills training is to ensure that the decoding of information being picked up by the sensory systems is attenuated and enhanced by accompanying learning.

Feedback and knowledge of results

The coach regularly provides the performer with feedback regarding athletic movement. Feedback is information from the environment that informs the athlete about performance efficiency during and/or following the movement. Feedback can be further classified into intrinsic feedback, which provides a basis for movement evaluation, and extrinsic feedback, information produced to augment intrinsic feedback. Both are of great importance to the athlete wishing to develop his performance. The value of feedback, however, would be severely limited without a dimension of external feedback known as knowledge of results (KR). KR, a verbal form of feedback, provides the performer with information comparing the actual performance with the intended goal. The athlete can use this information to improve performance. Another function of KR is that of motivation. The athlete's knowledge of results can motivate further performance improvement. Goals must be established for KR to be effective and meaningful to the athlete. A result without a predetermined goal offers little value.

THE LEARNING CONCEPT

A more complex model of events supersedes the concept of learning as a process of conditioned responses. This model might be represented as a type of self-regulating system (Bernstein, 1957) (fig. 62a). Although the terminology differs from that used in Bernstein's (1957) picture of things, Anochin (1967) and associates explained the underlying theory of learning a technique along similar lines (fig. 62b). This popular theory purports that two types of afferent supply incoming information.

(1) The situation afferent embraces all environmental stimuli and consequently includes stimuli that are both relevant and irrelevant via the sensory organs (proprioceptors). Recollected stimuli may also be included. This area of afference causes an integration of the nervous processes that precede the causal afferent.
(2) The causal afferent is the 'reading' of the situation afferent and selection of the relevant from the irrelevant.

This collective afference is referred to as the afferent synthesis and it concludes with the intention to act. Such intention is given expression by the effector apparatus. When afferent synthesis ends and action is effected, a specific afferent apparatus – the action acceptor – is formed. This compares the afferent synthesis (the plan of action) with the completed action on which information is brought back via situation and causal afferents. If there is agreement, the cycle is complete. If not, new reactions are formed as the difference between planned and achieved action is assessed, and corrections made as the effector apparatus modifies the original action until agreement is reached. In cybernetics, this concept of reafference is referred to as back-coupling or feedback. Principal types of reafferent may be classified as follows.

(1) Kinaesthetic afferents, which are represented by proprioception.
(2) Resultant afferents, which comprise all afferent characteristics which relate to the result of the completed action. All new actions, however, arise from previous

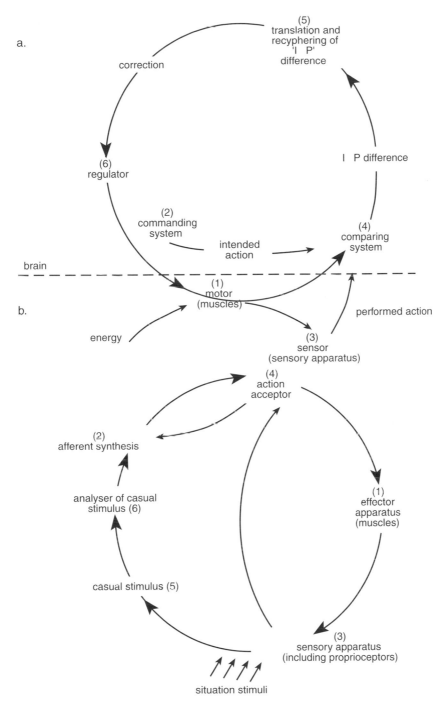

FIG. 62 Events in the learning process (a) based on Bernstein's model; (b) based on Anochin's model (numbered to help comparison)

actions, and those new actions will in turn form the basis for future actions. Hence Anochin's (1967) subdivision of resultant afferents:

- episodic reafferent, which provides information on intermediate actions
- final reafferent, which provides information on the final execution of the original plan of action.

The suggested existence of an afferent synthesis confirms the importance of factors such as training environment, motivation and a comprehensive under-standing of a given technique by the coach, while the action acceptor emphasises the importance of previous experience and a complete appreciation of a given technique by the athlete. It rests with the coach to ensure that such factors are carefully assessed if technical training is to be efficient.

Senses and the afferent syntheses

Although we traditionally recognise five senses: vision, audition, taste, smell, and kinaesthesis, a hierarchy of sensory dominance exists. The major sensory system utilised by humans is vision, where visual information is dominant over other received information (Posner, Nissen & Klein, 1976). Where a discrepancy may arise between visual information received and that offered by other sensory systems, the brain and nervous system resolve it by regarding the visual information as correct (Smyth & Marriot, 1982).

Internal and external proprioceptors register signals that form a complex support system often under-utilised by the performer in sport. While visual stimuli often lead the sensory complex, followed by kinaesthesis, other sensations affect the performer, such as the feel of the weight and size of the ball used by the footballer or basketball player, or the smell of the chalk on asymmetric bars. Established Soviet and Czech coaching methodologies have long made successful use of sport-specific leading senses within the sensory complex. This is known as the afferent synthesis, providing the performer with permanent information prior to, during, and following performance. The motor learning of an activity includes an appropriate breakdown of the skill, identifying and reinforcing the afferent synthesis. For example, a breakdown of high jump technique (Dick, 1993) can easily include the appropriate development of the leading analyser which will be athlete-determined (table 23).

During the movement series the leading senses are dynamically changed according to the demands of the movements of the body. If, for instance, the high jumper fails to clear the bar, knocking it off with the lower leg, then the afferent synthesis will automatically facilitate greater attention to the awareness of the activity of the lower leg in the next attempt. The performer is informed through this mechanism at every moment.

FOSBURY FLOP	PHASE	REFERENCE	CRITERION	LEADING ANALYSER SENSORY REINFORCEMENT	ASSESSMENT

	I Approach PENULTI-MATE STRIDE	A 1 foot plant
		   2 body/trunk
		   3 arms
		B 4 front supp.
		BC 5 supp. knee
		B 6 rear arm
		C 7 arms
			ball contact/curved path
			inclination/slight forward lean
			counter arm swing
			heel lead
			yielding
			held back
			parallel/behind trunk
				Visual as look for spot above the bar;
				Kinaesthetic as feel high knees to penultimate stride.	

	II Approach LAST STRIDE	D 8 trunk 9 supp. leg DF 10 take-off leg E 11 arms F 12 body/trunk F 13 foot plant EF 14 free leg	upright horizontal pushing action fast & active plant/pre-tension/'long' starting double swing inclination/backward lean 'through' the bar/optimal take-off pos. bending/forward-upward movement	*Kinaesthetic* as feel tall; *Auditory* as hear foot plant; signal then to initiate upward push; *Kinaesthetic* as feel arms then lean.	
	III TAKE-OFF	FG 15 take-off leg FH 16 arms FH 17 free leg GH 18 free knee H 19 arms H 20 shoulders H 21 body	minimal & passive yielding active double arm swing active knee drive 'opening'/block in horizontal pos. blocked/bent lifted/horizontal vertical/parallel to upright	*Kinaesthetic* as feel arm swing & knee drive.	

TABLE 23 Model technique analysis sheet for the Fosbury Flop (adapted from work by G. Tidow)

			Visual/Kinaesthetic
IV RISING	I 22 head	view; along the bar	*Visual as spot over the bar; Kinaesthetic as feel body opening; feel rising.*
	I 23 outside arm	'leading'	
	IK 24 body	longitudinal axis rotation	
OPENING	IK 25 arms	'opening'	
	IK 26 free leg	lowering	
	K 27 back	parallel to bar	
	K 28 head	backward movement	
V LAYOUT	KL 29 arms	extended/'diving action'	*Kinaesthetic awareness of back & hips; exaggerate arched feeling.*
	L 30 hips	hyperextended/elevated	
	L 31 legs	bent/directed downwards	
	L 32 back	'arched'	
	L 33 head	thrown back	
	L 34 longit. axis	rectangular to bar	
VI RECOVERY	LM 35 pelvis	active lowering	*Kinaesthetic acknowledgement of lowering of pelvis; Visual as see clearance of legs.*
	M 36 head/trunk	're-active' countermovement	
	M 37 hips	active bending	
	M 38 legs	synchronous active knee extension	
	M 39 arms	bending	
VII PREPARATION FOR LANDING	NO 40 head	raised	*Kinaesthetic with raised head; maintain 'L' shape feeling.*
	NO 41 hips	bent/blocked	
	NO 42 arms	spreading	
	NO 43 body	in 'L-position'	
	NO 44 legs	extended/directed upwards	

TABLE 23 Continued

Biofeedback

Biofeedback is a vehicle by which the performer can voluntarily control functions of the autonomic nervous system. It can be a powerful tool in assisting the attainment of self-regulation in competition, for example, reducing the debilitating effects of anxiety. It makes use of instrumentation to assist the athlete to control autonomic nervous system responses. From initial learning within a laboratory setting, the feelings and experiences associated with tuning into and reducing responses from the sympathetic nervous system are transferred into the athletic environment.

Under competitive conditions, emotions can block the awareness of the afferent synthesis. Given this likelihood, the athlete should take the opportunity to engage an appropriate mental training technique. Similarly, following error, the athlete can make use of a compatible technique such as successful imagery or relaxation. Useful mental training methods are integrated with technical training, optimising training conditions for the athlete. The athlete must be able to analyse the afferent synthesis so that he can read the appropriate sense and use it for anticipatory purposes. Beginners do not have this sense and so may find themselves stretched. For example, the young soccer player may pass the ball behind an oncoming team-mate. Anticipation together with the process of cognition gives the prediction and prognosis of events. It is sensible for the coach to include this type of training within the planning of competitive conditions.

An operational understanding of the benefits of various data collection techniques will enhance the value of specialised input in coaching/training. Irrespective of the analysis method undertaken, it is fundamental that a systematic approach is used in the analysis of sports movement (Marshall & Elliot, 1999). Predictive analysis methods use computer simulation to explore 'what if' scenarios. A model of a person or apparatus is created to predict changes occurring as a result of varying input parameters. Image analysis techniques, IT, movie photography and video photography capture complex movement sequences on film or videotape allowing notational analysis. While helpful, objectively, film or video techniques cannot provide movement measurements, only a means for the recording of movement and subsequent basis for discussion. In order to do so, specialised apparatus and procedures are needed.

Electromyography (EMG) also records movement, within the muscle. As muscle action is initiated by electrical activity associated with the contraction of muscles specific to a response, electromyography detects and catalogues this. The weak signal within the targeted muscle is amplified and then stored on a polygraph recorder for later analysis. EMG indicates levels of activity or inactivity. To establish the forces produced in a muscle, controlled conditions must be adhered to (Dainty & Norman, 1987). Such a procedure can also be used to identify any work by associated signals when using imagery (G. Tidow). Internal imagery is primarily kinaesthetic in nature as the athlete feels himself performing while 'seeing out' from within his own body. External imagery is considered to be visual as the athlete watches himself perform from the outside. Internal (kinaesthetic) imagery has been proven a superior method in that it results in actual subliminal muscle activity in the muscles associated with the imagined actions (Mahoney & Avener, 1977). Both internal and external imagery skills should be developed.

The kinaesthetic sense is often regarded as the dark sense, as it is difficult to know what the muscular apparatus senses. Appropriate skill breakdown where the sensory complex is managed and reinforced will enable the performer to exert control over this automatic process. In this way, the leading sensory channel, and the dynamic change of leading channels, are developed. The actual breakdown with an integrated series of practices helps the athlete learn control at a conscious level.

This type of sensory training shadows the athlete through his skill development. At the initial stages of games learning, activities for children involving throwing a variety of suitable objects such as soft miniature implements and balls will introduce sensory awareness. Likewise an elite javelin thrower can benefit from increased kinaesthetic awareness of the hand by changing the throwing implement with emphasis on good technical form. Where every activity has a specific complexity of afferent synthesis, both coach and athlete can explore training opportunities to reinforce appropriate sensory perception. Approaching the hanging ball from different directions will assist the footballer with the skill of heading; the tennis player maintaining a bouncing tennis ball on the racquet while keeping a balloon off the ground with his foot couples sensory awareness with the attention required for a specific activity. Patience is required as motor learning is not directly observable.

Learning

Learning is a process involving the acquiring of increased skill capability. A series of internal processes associated with practice or experience will influence this capability for skilled behaviour, resulting in relatively permanent change. An individual will learn from participation itself within an appropriate situation, and from the breakdown of skill. Whole and part approaches should be combined. To optimise later skill automaticity, part-skill practices may shape initial learning conditions. A learning ceiling is presumed when some success is experienced by a performer, yet there is evidence to suggest that further practice brings about continued skill enhancement due to 'over-learning' (Schmidt, 1988), as opposed to learning beyond the original learning goal. Given the possibility of further improvements in performance, the learning design should facilitate adequate opportunity: part skill – whole/modified; part skill – whole/less modified;

part skill – whole/realistic situation; part skill – whole/game situation. The approach is not prescriptive but tailored to the individual's response.

Unfortunately, simply accumulating time in the game does not eradicate sufficient bad habits and patterns acquired due to lack of a stable learning base. Basic skills should be mastered sequentially to arrive at precise task performance. At every competitive level, fundamental errors are apparent, particularly when the performer has to mobilise reserves in order to cope with changing conditions in a game or event. If an athlete succumbs to externally induced or self-perceived factors such as the opposition scoring and panic resulting, or celebrating a point and losing concentration as a result, the least established skill patterns are more vulnerable.

Associated with this notion is that of effort. As an athlete learns a motor skill, the subsequent execution of that skill requires less effort (Kahneman, 1973), leaving the athlete more freedom to attend to game/event-specific information. Learning should allow the athlete processing and movement efficiency. Every life activity is directed by a high level of automisation of the basic elements of sensory and motor control. Given that the athlete must be able to concentrate on a range of game/event-induced aspects if performance is to be successful, information processing should not be overloaded. Automaticity implies that skills do indeed become automatic, thereby interfering less with other tasks. Learning occurring in the over-learning phase reduces attentional load and allows more accurate secondary task performance (Schneider & Fisk, 1983). Such improvement can perhaps be attributed to less interference from the main task.

Standard situation learning

Given the need for sports literacy – the ability to read performance-related internal and external cues – practice variation is vital. Both athlete and coach will be aware of performance hot spots, regular incidents, most frequently used moves, techniques, or skill patterns. Statistical analysis reveals how such standard situations impact upon performance and thereafter can influence the content of the learning to be automated by the athlete. This does not mean that outlying possibilities are not considered when dedicating time to technical training, but that the athlete has a ready library response from which he can select what is required. The established learning process gives greater room to manoeuvre, freeing up space more easily for the allocation of reserves in the event of unexpected contingencies, or by helping facilitate further more economic (saving time) and efficient (reserving energy) learning.

AIMS OF TECHNICAL TRAINING

The general aims of technical training are as follows:

(1) **To direct the athlete's learning, and to perfect the most efficient technique(s) relative to a given sport.** This demands that the coach has a complete understanding of the sport and its particular technical demands; of the athlete's present capabilities and his potential development; of techniques used by other athletes who are enjoying success; of teaching and developmental methods. In short, the coach must establish a sound technical or biomechanical model, based on athlete and sport, towards which he must direct the athlete.

(2) **To direct the athlete towards a stable performance of the learned technique.** This implies a progressive 'opening' of the situation, in which the athlete must perform the given technique. One might visualise an initial stage in the process where all conditions for learning are perfect and totally without distraction. A final stage might also be visualised where, irrespective of the bombardment of distracting factors and within biological limits, the performance of a given technique is as perfectly reproduced as if the situation was without interference. Environmental interference may come from wind and weather, apparatus, altitude, spectators or other athletes.

(3) A further aim might be considered for sports where the athlete is forced **to make a rapid selection of correct technique from a reservoir of many**. To solve a situational problem the coach must direct the learning of this capacity. Thus, it is not only the techniques themselves that separate the weight lifter from the football player, but also the total nature of the competitions in which their techniques are executed.

Classification of technique

Attempts have been made to classify technique. The three classifications are determined by the nature of technique: single or multiple; and the performance/competition situation: constant or variable.

(1) Sports in which a single technique determines the performance, and which are based on a constant technical model, where the structure of competition is relatively constant. This includes most track and field events, swimming, bowling, shooting, and archery. Any variation within the structure of competition is restricted to factors such as weather, competition surfaces, facilities and equipment.

(2) Sports in which a multiplicity of techniques determines the total performance, and where the structure of competition is relatively constant. Within each sport there exists a similarity of technical model between certain techniques, but each technique is distinct. Constancy of technical performance is made possible by the structure of competition and the conscious differentiation of

techniques. Into this category will come artistic gymnastics, dance, figure skating, and diving.

(3) Sports in which a multiplicity of techniques may be demanded of a rapidly changing competition structure. Athletes here must select appropriate techniques to meet the changing demands of competition, but must also master each technique in the 'pool' at the athlete's disposal. Into this category come all team sports, combat sports, sports in which there are exchanges with an opponent (such as racquet games) and sports in which environmental demands other than the opponent (e.g. weather, terrain), necessitate rapid and/or accurate selection of the most expedient technique (sailing, climbing, golf or canoeing).

The development of technical training must follow a different course for each classification:

Class 1

- Develop the technique in a closed situation (e.g. without environmental or competitive interference) as a 'performance'.
- Introduce a progressively open situation (e.g. more variables) while maintaining the 'performance' approach.
- Introduce a progressive intensity of competition.
- The general progression is from performing a technique to applying the technique in competition. In some cases the latter demands greater application of strength, or speed, (e.g. long jump), while in others, accuracy of performance is essential (e.g. shooting).

Class 2

- Develop each technique separately and in an order which permits the learning of each to proceed without the interference of the other.
- Again, the situation for learning each technique must be closed.
- The situation is now opened through the use of other equipment or different facilities. It may also be opened through a combination of techniques in movement sequences.
- This progression may be pursued throughout the athlete's future development as new techniques are introduced and new permutations and combinations of these techniques are advanced.
- Introduce a progressive intensity of competition.
- Here the progression develops accuracy of reproduction in the performance of techniques.

Class 3

- Develop each technique separately in a closed situation and in an order which permits no mutual interference.

- The situation is opened primarily by applying the technique in a changing situation (e.g. active opposition, varying climbs, sets).
- The athlete must also be exposed to technical adjustments necessitated by varying playing conditions. A more complex opening is where the athlete in the face of active opposition or varying terrain may choose one of several techniques.
- Introduce a progressive intensity of competition or environmental stressor.
- Here the progression is from learning and developing each technique to learning to select the correct technique for given competition demands.

Technique may also be classified by considering the aim of each technique. On this basis, Dyatchkov (1967) offered the following classifications:

(1) Sports in which the aim of the technique is to express intensive strength of brief duration within the ideal technical model, such as sprints, jumps, throws, or weight lifting.

(2) Sports in which the aim is endurance development with an optimal expression of strength. This embraces middle and long-distance running, skiing, rowing, swimming, cycling.

(3) Sports in which the aim of technique is development of those physical abilities permitting accuracy of performance of movements within a prescribed programme. This includes gymnastics, trampolining, figure skating, and diving.

(4) Sports in which the aim is the solution of those complex problems associated with interplay of athletes and/or environment, i.e. team games, combat sports, racquet games.

Despite these attempts to classify technique, certain activities may fall within several categories. The aim of classification, however, is primarily to establish the planned technical development of an athlete. Consequently, it is sufficient that the coach identifies the specific aim of technique for an athlete in a given sport. Having done so, it rests with the coach's knowledge of anatomy, biomechanics, physiology, rules of the given sport, experience within that sport, and the performance status of the athlete, to formulate a plan of technical development.

Learning technique

In general terms, it would appear that the learning process can be shown to display a discernible pattern (table 24). It is recognised that the well-conditioned athlete arriving at stage 1, equipped with many (if not all) of the basic components of the total technique to be learned, is better prepared to advance through the stages than the athlete with little experience or conditioning to call upon.

stage or phase	morphological/ functional	regulative/neural	teaching/coaching methods and conditions
1. Irradiation of stimulation	First concept of movement is learned, followed by an attitude to its learning.		Previously acquired related knowledge plus general total concept of action influence this stage. Teaching objective
2. Irradiation of stimulation processes	First ability to perform action and first acquisition of the action i.e. the basic form of the action is performed.	There is a generalisation of motor reactions together with muscle tensions and unnecessary movement, brought about by irradiation of stimuli to neighbouring areas of the cerebral cortex.	is to produce an accurate basic action and eliminate unnecessary movements, etc. Demonstration and film accompanied by verbal instruction (simple) is indicated.
3. Concentration through development of inhibitory processes	Correction, refinement and differentiation. Finer co-ordination of movement.	Concentration of focus of cerebral cortex processes. Movement is accepted more fully into the consciousness and in greater detail. Individual phases of movement become stabilised. Proprioceptors begin to take a leading role.	Training must be concentrated but too frequent repetition within a training unit will fatigue the beginner and impede learning. Detailed learning of the movement is now worked on. Methods based on kinaesthesis (the feel of the movement) are used. Intervals between training
4. Stabilisation and automisation	High degree of precision in performing the action in a closed situation.	Complete harmony of neural processes where proprioceptors and cerebral cortex eliminate interference	units can now be increased, as can the number of repetitions within each unit. Stabilise action and perfect technical detail.

TABLE 24 Outline of learning stages in the acquisition of techniques

stage or phase	morphological/ functional	regulative/neural	teaching/coaching methods and conditions
		due to unnecessary movement; and rapid adjustment to changing conditions allows performance of a perfect action.	Training is designed to eliminate variables and give opportunity for 'perfect' execution of the action.
5. Stabilisation and automisation	Precision in performing the action in an open (more variable) situation.		Progressive development of physical capacities (e.g. strength, elastic strength, speed, etc.) necessary for long-term development in performance.

TABLE 24 Continued

Returning to the concept of the learning process, one might suggest that it is in the interest of the athlete to be exposed to an education of basic movement components in pursuit of providing a more sophisticated action acceptor. Physical education appears to have focused emphasis on increasing the scope of a child's 'movement experience'. If such experience moves from the general and extends along a specific avenue of activity, it seems logical to anticipate the natural evolution of 'fundamental components'. From these fundamental components, highly specialised techniques may develop (fig. 63). The concept of fundamental components, and the development of exercises based on them, has been successfully applied to sport, with the former German Democratic Republic (GDR) particularly benefiting from this methodology.

Establishing exercises based on components demands a detailed knowledge of the original technique used. Each of these exercises must have the greatest possible range of application in techniques within its sphere, yet the essence of the component must not be destroyed by further breakdown or modification of parts. This suggests the possibility of derivatives. Derivatives of the first degree coincide with the essential parts of the component, while derivatives of the second degree are characterised by comprising only some of the essential parts of the component. The role of these components in the former GDR research was in two parts.

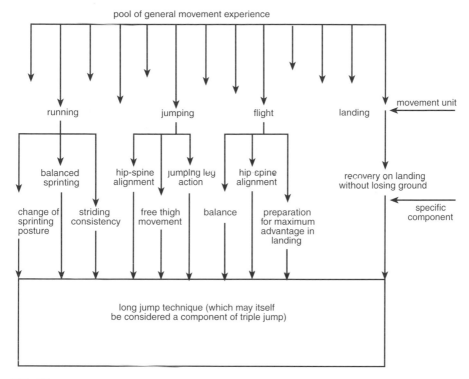

FIG. 63 The development of specific technique via fundamental components

(1) The integrating role (establishing the complete technical model from the components).

(2) The differentiating role (establishing stability of the technical model by ensuring an ability to clearly separate one technique from another, correct movement from wrong movement). From this, and similar work, some important points emerge:

- when the first component learned is one that unites as many parts as possible of the final technique, learning time is reduced
- learning time for differentiation is also reduced by this approach
- the use of first degree derivatives does not demand stability of the component, but second degree derivatives must not be introduced until the component is stable, otherwise there will be negative interference.

Each component must be constantly related to the whole technique. This is most important where the derivative is of the second degree, or where the derivative of the first degree contains a limited range of essential parts. Harre (1982) noted that athletes who learned derivatives of the first and second degree, by conscious acquisition of fundamental exercise, and who were made to differentiate consciously, proved, when learning new movements, to be more capable of distinguishing the details of the movement and performing them with accuracy. A progressive development in ability was noted with the increasing mastery of varying exercises. The athlete must be offered the benefit of expert guidance during the learning of technique. Consequently, the practice of providing instruction for beginner athletes via novice coaches might be the basis of a poor technical education which will make itself evident at a later date in faulty technique.

Faults and corrections

Without the assistance of sophisticated equipment, the coach offers instruction based upon the comparison of a 'mental' technical model and what may be readily perceived. There are very obvious limitations to what can be perceived at any one time, so the coach relies mainly on experience of cause and effect. The immediately apparent problems are that coaches have varying amounts of experience and, even with experience, cause and effect are not always easily identifiable. It is nevertheless essential to the athlete's development that accurate information be readily available when kinaesthetic impression and concept of movement are fresh in the athlete's mind. If there is no immediate feedback for the athlete, there is considerable risk of stabilisation of faults. The use of photosequence cameras, video tape, film, kinographs, videographics, print-outs on force components, velocities, photo-electric apparatus, notational analysis, virtual reality, software packages which allow real time technique comparison, or computerised segmental analysis can provide such feedback. Even if some of this equipment is not readily available for showing the athlete's own performance (e.g. video), it should still be possible to show the correct technique where the athlete is not matching the technical model. The efficiency of technique might be evaluated in one or several of the following broad categories of method.

(1) As implied above, **evaluating the athlete's technique against the technical model**. This approach is used in many so-called 'skill tests', with the athlete 'scored' against norms. It is also used in comparative analysis of the athlete with another athlete known to be technically proficient, or of the athlete with a film of himself performing a technically proficient jump at some previous date. Filming techniques, photo-sequence techniques, light-track photography techniques, dedicated software packages, or standard testing techniques may be applied to this type of evaluation.

(2) Another type of method is the **comparison of actual performance with theoretical performance**. For example, a comparison of the height through which the athlete raises his centre of gravity with the height actually jumped in a high jump competition. This method may be extended to include comparison of performance with related criteria in standard tests. Thus, the long jumper may compare competition long jump performance with, on the one hand, standing long jump, sargent jump, 30 m sprinting speed; or on the other hand, the horizontal velocity and parabola of flight of the athlete's centre of gravity. Again, filming techniques, dedicated software packages, and a knowledge of related standard tests may be applied to the evaluation.

(3) A third class of method **evaluates a particular technique relative to its success or failure against opposition**. Technique is evaluated on the basis of gaining advantage in attack over defence or, conversely, in gaining advantage in defence over attack. It could be argued that tactical input rather than technique is being evaluated in, for instance, team games. Filming techniques and notational analysis are essential to this class of evaluation for it to be more effective.

Despite detailed and expert planning, it is nevertheless possible for faults to arise. Before any attempt is made to correct such faults, the exact cause or causes must be determined. This is emphasised due to the fact that 'effect' is more readily recognised; the coach may occasionally reduce the effect of a fault rather than eliminate the cause. It is also important to assess how well established the fault has become. Faults that come to light during the early stages of learning are less difficult to correct than those which have become stabilised to such an extent that they are almost a part of the athlete's technique.

Correction should always ensure the athlete understands the technical model, the fault and the correction. This is vital because frequently athletes who are technically lacking in proficiency may produce superior performances and the novice may seek to follow that technique because it produces favourable results.

Faults must be discovered and corrected early. To delay will stabilise the fault and possibly cause stagnation in performance. Moreover, should the athlete 'grow with the fault' then any attempt at correction becomes more difficult. This is due to the basic inertia of an entrenched pattern and also because performance in general will fall below that recorded when the 'wrong' technique is used, thereby causing a loss of confidence in the process of developing a correct technique. Finally, the additional time required to correct a well-established fault is hard to justify when the time should be directed towards improving an athlete's performance. Getting it right will always prove less expensive than putting things right.

Correction may be pursued by contrasting a faulty and correct technique component. Arranging that faulty performance is impossible so it might prove a useful exercise to practise the movement with, for example, the other leg or arm. The progressive replacement of a faulty technique with a correct technique appears to advance in four stages. The time span involved varies with the stability and nature of the fault.

Stage 1: the faulty technique asserts itself whenever concentration is lost. The correct technique is occasionally reproduced.

Stage 2: neither the faulty nor the correct techniques are strong enough to dominate, so there is frequently a confusing or mixing of techniques. The correct technique is reproduced more frequently.

Stage 3: there is a conscious differentiation, with the correct technique only occasionally lost, in fatigue or stress.

Stage 4: complete stability of correct technique.

Opinions differ on the relative merits of massed and distributed practice as the athlete learns technique. Personal experience, in the absence of conclusive evidence, suggests an initial massing of practice until the whole activity can be put together, then a gradual separation of practice units. Even when well established, time must be taken to realign technical models at least annually following the competition macrocycle.

General points on technique training units

There must be flexibility in determining exact durations for technique training units because individual athletes vary not only in their capacity for concentration, but also in their status of physical abilities. Several points might be made, however, as a basis for establishing suitable unit construction in technique training.

(1) Concentrated technique work should not go beyond 20 minutes without a break.
(2) The prospect of a long unit of technique work prepares the athlete for an extended distribution of effort. Consequently, a prolonged unit must be divided into subsections, possibly with each section having a separate emphasis.
(3) Reduction of fatigue improves motivation, not only within the session, but also from day to day. Thus, within a training workout, a technique-training unit must come before a conditioning unit and a heavy 'conditioning day' should not precede a 'technical day'.
(4) A compromise must be effected between maintaining the excited state of the neuromuscular system and allowing recovery from a previous effort. This will be individually arrived at. It would appear that during recovery from technical training there is a perseveration of neural processes. This may be because when intense external stimulation ceases, internal consolidation occurs. It has also been suggested that organisms are refractory to (resist) early repetition of an act.
(5) During recovery there may be a tendency for incorrect associations to be 'forgotten' faster than correct ones. This could be due to the non-existence of positive reinforcements.
(6) In technical development, unit construction should be so arranged that all practices are related to the given technique, unless the objective of the unit is to develop the ability to differentiate techniques, select appropriate techniques, or put together a sequence of techniques. Practices may be related by similarity of content, technique, principles, etc. It should be appreciated that these practices are techniques or sports in themselves and are not to be confused with components.
(7) Only one technical point should be considered at any one time.
(8) Adapt sport to athlete before adapting athlete to sport. This principle should be followed unless adapting the sport creates a wrong basis for development. For example, hurdles should be reduced in height and spacing, and 'mini' ball games developed for early learning.
(9) For sighted athletes, approximately 80% of what is learned is from visual stimuli, so a correct demonstration or a well-explained film is more appropriate

than words alone. Auditory and kinaesthetic stimuli are the key learning conduits for blind athletes.

(10) It is important to note that the novice athlete must be given expert technical instruction when being introduced to sport. Conversely, the novice coach must not be used as teacher of the novice athlete.

(11) 'Repetition is the mother of learning.' The athlete must know the correct technique(s) to repeat and be sufficiently conditioned to perform sufficient repetitions without fatigue-induced compensations creeping in.

(12) The progressions of adding endurance, resistance or speed to development of technique can only be introduced within the limits of keeping the technical model intact. To continue technique work without an intact technical model can lead to 'chronic' rather than 'acute' technical errors.

(13) When technique breaks down, it is essential that 'rebuilding' be done at a slower overall speed. The speed should be such that the athlete can feel the correct sequence of individual body segment contribution to the technique.

(14) Conditions must be favourable, as concentration and freedom of movement are fundamental to learning technique. A warm, windless environment without interfering variables such as noise or distracting movements must be available. Once the technical model is well established, the athlete must learn to keep technique intact in a climate where hostile variables increase in number and degree.

(15) There appears to be little difference in the methods used in teaching techniques to men and women. There can be variance in the techniques of men and women, however, even in the same discipline.

(16) Children may not be equipped to learn techniques used by mature elite performers. It is the basic technical model that the young athlete learns, and not some sophisticated elaboration of that model.

(17) When working to correct a technical fault, the best advice is to go back one or even two steps before the appropriateness of the exercises selected to effect correction. For example, if selecting specific drills for foot movement in tennis, work first on conditioning exercises to develop those muscles on which efficient performance of those drills depends.

SUMMARY

Fundamental to the athlete's long-term development is the learning of sound technique. The coach directs such learning and works towards stability of technique through technical training. The classification of technique determines its course of development but, broadly speaking, coaching methodology is geared to various learning stages. An interpretation of cybernetic theory affords an explanation of the concept of learning. Within the framework of this concept the coach will identify the role of fundamental components, the need for accurate identification and speedy correction of faults, best relevant technology, and the importance of providing the beginner athlete with the best available technical expertise.

12 PSYCHOLOGICAL CHANGES AND THE GROWING CHILD

Perceptual skills impact upon performance. Given that simple kinaesthetic skills, body movement sensations arising from musculoskeletal sensors, develop during childhood, the coach should be aware of the various stages of development through which the child is required to progress towards adulthood. The trainability of a range of performance-influencing factors is age-determined. The following age divisions are offered as guidelines. Their appropriateness will vary according to many factors, including individual rates of development, male/female differences, and the differential effect elicited by society.

GENERAL PATTERNS

Early primary school (5–7 years of age)

By the age of five the child has developed a wide range of abilities and skills, and individual differences are already apparent. While heredity plays a major role in this individuality, the seeds from which many psychological functions and characteristics of the developing personality have grown (and will grow) are to be found in the many forms of play which constitute the major activity of the child through the early primary school years. He is emotional, thinks graphically, seems to live in a world of half fantasy and half reality, has mastered a wide vocabulary and its use, and thinks rapidly in short, intense bursts which is a mark of mental agility rather than a lack of ability to concentrate. The roles he adopts in play are drawn most accurately from his immediate social environment and, towards the end of this period in primary school, relationships with other children become more stable.

During these formative years, the importance of play must be stressed in the introduction of sport because it is through play that the child develops. His imagination must be stimulated, with success attainable. Above all, activities must be intrinsically enjoyable. Award schemes (and variations) are extremely valuable at this stage for they offer a framework within which it is possible to shape the pupil's behaviour. Finally, it is worth noting that psychological characteristics developed by the age of five may be dampened by the imposition of school discipline at that age. In most other cultures, school is postponed at least one year. It becomes clear then that the play concept must be the key to maintaining the impetus of developing in a broadening social world, as represented by the school. A guided play approach achieves better results when learning motor skills than does free play. The teacher plays an important part in the child's life at this time. Possibly the coach could come to fulfil a parallel role in terms of an early introduction of the child to coaching in certain sports (e.g. gymnastics).

Primary–secondary school bridge (8–11/13 years of age)

This period may be described as a gentle shift from naive realism to critical realism. At the beginning of this period, the child is acquiring knowledge of the world without understanding relationships or trying to see what lies behind reality. Nevertheless, he concentrates on the detail of his environment and can be analytical in perception, memory and thought. His power of concentration is still unstable, so the teacher or coach should avoid lengthy explanations. Variety both in content and method are prerequisites to successful instruction. Throughout this period, the child often requires guidance in the stabilising of social relationships and experimentation in group situations should be encouraged and observed.

As the period progresses, the child becomes capable of concentrating on specific tasks for longer periods of time and begins to seek logical connections and generalisations. As intellectual development progresses, so does his play. Early play experiences (before five years of age) are to gain mastery over his environment and, having achieved this, past successes are re-enacted in a symbolic manner as play develops towards the formality of the game situation. The trend, then, is away from imagination and towards logical thinking. Also worth noting is that towards the end of this period children will have a well-developed ability to memorise. This period also marks the separation of the sexes, in that acceleration towards maturity is greater in girls. One consequence of this is that interests become extremely varied between the sexes. Emotions, while well-balanced and optimistic early in this period, can begin to shift towards a less carefree profile. Consequently, at the end of this period the child has completely altered physically, intellectually, socially and emotionally. Most children will already have entered the period of adolescence.

Mid-/post-secondary (11/13–16 years of age)

The start of this period is a whirlwind of change in every characteristic mentioned earlier. Learning becomes an intellectual exercise and productive activity assumes a major role. More social opportunity is now available and relationships within the family unit assume a different form. Social and physiological changes result in emotional imbalance and instability of mood. The young person's uncritical self-assurance is replaced by a fluctuation between esteem and doubt as he gradually pieces together a concept of himself from the collective impression he has of how others see him. This situation is a crucial factor in the information of attitudes that the young athlete in this age range will have towards participation in sport. How he sees himself in the eyes of his peers may influence whether or not he will continue his commitment to pursuit of competitive advantage.

This phase over, the adolescent moves to the final phase in this period. The agitation and disharmony of the first phase gives way to inner assurance that is linked with a visible increase in social capacity. Hopefully, the society in which he grows will not only make high demands of him, but will grant him the right to, and every possibility for, an all-round development of personality and, in particular, progressive situations demanding responsibility. Intellectual development reaches a near-adult level and his attitudes are consciously critical and searching in pursuit of independence of opinion and judgement. A continual awareness of this developmental continuum is important if the child is to grow within the social framework of the 'club' in particular, and the sport of his choice, in general.

Throughout his development, the sport should be adapted to the child before the child is taught how to adapt to the sport. The spirit, not the letter, of both constitutive and regulative rules and regulations should be applied to afford an attractive and flexible framework within which the child will be attracted to express himself. Gradually, by careful planning of his programme of sports education, the official rules will replace this flexible framework without prejudicing his interest, enthusiasm or enjoyment. As the adolescent moves towards the 17–22 year age group, the personality fills out around those basic characteristics evolved up to this period. More and more, however, that personality will seek to stamp itself upon the society about it, and our society (i.e. sport) must learn to accommodate rather than contain it.

MOTOR LEARNING CHARACTERISTICS

Early primary school (5–7 years of age)

The period of development probably begins around 3–4 years of age, when a few basic forms of motor patterns are at his disposal. He can crawl, walk, pull, swing, climb, clamber, jump down, run, throw from standing, jump low heights and short distances, and can both catch and kick a ball. These actions represent each of the three forms of movement: locomotor, in which the body is moved through space, walking, running, jumping; non-locomotor, where specific body parts are moved via pushing, pulling, twisting; and manipulative, through which objects are moved, catching, throwing, striking. Already a preference to left or right is evident. In the course of development, all these forms of movement are improved in quality and their repetition seems endless. The first combined movements (rather than movements in sequence) can be seen, i.e. running and jumping, high throwing and catching, running and throwing, running and slinging, running over low barriers in balance, jumping onto objects, running to swing on a rope. Consequently, by the end of this period it is possible to carry out all-round exercise with plenty of variety and intensity of movement.

For many reasons, little is known of the development of physical abilities (e.g. strength) in this age group. It has been shown, however, that speed of movement is only very slightly developed and does not reach more significant values until 9–10 years of age (e.g. up to eight years of age, reaction time is in excess of 0.5 seconds). Also, as far as can be assessed, strength and agility are not well developed at this stage. On the other hand, mobility and aerobic endurance are well developed towards the end of this period. The explanation of the former lies in the elasticity of the movement apparatus and the looseness of joints, while the latter is well developed due to the varied and active play activity. At this stage, a general approach serves to improve strength by using body weight and apparatus together with light resistances such as medicine balls and sling balls, as well as to improve the coordination of movement at speed. The introduction of many skills is quite practicable and the following may be borne in mind. These youngsters:

- have a powerful but uncontrolled and non-directed joy in movement
- concentrate for very short spells
- remain undeveloped in their direction of effort
- are limited in their capacity for motor learning
- display a weak retention for what has been learned
- exhibit a limited group consciousness. Exercising individually or in very small groups is recommended.

Primary–secondary school bridge (8–11/13 years of age)

This is without doubt the most important period in the progress of motor ability. It is that phase of development in which already familiar forms of movement are vastly improved and many new ones learned and stabilised, often without instruction, demonstrated in activities such as roller skating, ice skating, skateboarding and cycling. New movement patterns are frequently mastered at the first attempt, following suitable demonstrations, concise explanation and one or two trials and accurate corrections. This period has been termed 'the age of specific achievement' or 'the child's best age for learning'. Almost all measures of physical achievement have their greatest rate of improvement at this stage, with speed, agility and aerobic endurance showing the most outstanding rises. Mobility, however, will decline shortly after this period begins and considerable work must be done to improve upon, or even maintain, the levels already acquired.

During these years, the youngster may develop a keen interest in sport, an enthusiasm for learning sport skills, a love of activity, an uninhibited attitude in the learning situation, and an increasing ability to embrace the value of learning athletic skills. The educator is in a favourable position as the youngster wants and has the ability to learn, and enjoys an activity and its related practices. There is a longing for achievement and for challenge. Consequently, training loads can already be quite high, provided the principle of gradual progression to sub-maximal loading (80–90%) has been strictly followed. Particular caution is urged in speed endurance and strength training. The former is known to be among the most severe stresses of athlete training and would certainly seem inadvisable at this stage. In addition it is debatable whether the youngster is well equipped to tolerate lacticanaerobic stressors. Maximal strength training is not advisable on the grounds of an unconsolidated skeletal structure to which only sub-maximal work should be offered as a load. With initiative and intelligent use of equipment and apparatus, the youngster should find sufficient resistance in the handling of his body weight. Certainly there is no justification at this stage for loading the spine by taking weights on the shoulders. Legwork is best done by other means and time would be better spent exercising the spine's own muscular apparatus.

Mid-/post-secondary (11/13–16 years of age)

The majority of physical ability statistics continue to show improvement through the traumatic phase of puberty (fig. 64). The neuromotor system should now have achieved full capacity and be able to offer a store of movement from which more and more complex permutations and combinations can be produced. The increased trainability of the strength components of speed is a consequence of the augmentation in muscle mass resulting from naturally increasing levels of testosterone or oestrogen during puberty.

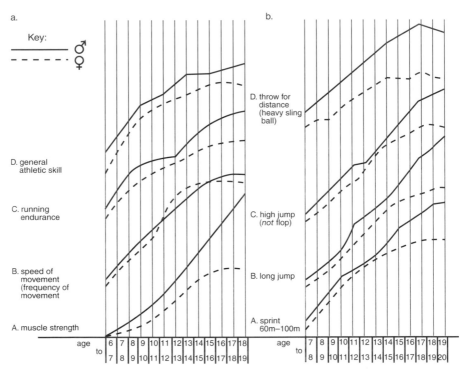

FIG. 64 (a) Non-parametric representation of development, specific to age, of some physical characteristics (from Smedley, Farfel, Jokl and Winter, 1959); (b) non-parametric representation of development, specific to age, of some basic athletic events (from Peters, Stemmler and Janeff, 1959).

From now on, development will mean the increasing sophistication of technique, despite interference of environmental variables. The athlete learns by instruction and experience to reproduce perfect movement despite wind, rain, temperature, or opposition tactics. Problems may arise in the shifting relationships of limb proportions in the early years of this period. Such problems, should they occur, will affect coordinative ability, harmony of movement, ability to learn new skills, and motor adaptability. Agility suffers under these circumstances. The problems will manifest themselves in a temporary lack of performance stability, particularly where movement patterns were not learned in the 8–11/13-year-old stage. This emphasises the importance of that stage, and it is suggested that when such problems arise, no new skills be introduced but that work be done on the improvement and consolidation of known skills. It would be ill-advised, for example, to start working on hitch-kick, but right to spend time on stride-jump, in long jump, if this flight technique had been used up to this point.

Gradually the youngster concludes the period of pubescence and slides gently into adolescence, which takes him towards adulthood and the relatively conclusive appearance of all physical and motor characteristics. A second opportunity exists here to introduce new patterns of movements, and progress towards sophistication mentioned earlier begins. Harre (1986) summarises this period as one of 'harmonisation, increased individualisation, relative stabilisation, and sex differentiation'.

With the relative conclusion of physical growth, untrained youngsters gradually reach their individual best achievements. Girls mature at 15–16 years of age, in contrast with boys at 18–20 years of age (fig. 66). Strength, elastic strength and endurance capacities are all highly trainable during this period and will continue to be so for several years. However, speed improvements become more difficult unless speed has been temporarily stagnated due to habitually low levels of stimulus (e.g. running with slower athletes, running solo, or running on slow tracks).

SUMMARY

The coach clearly has a role to play in contributing to the education of the growing child. This brief outline of psychological and motor learning characteristics provides a basis for planning this contribution. Development of play constitutes an essential vehicle of total development and the concept of a progression from informal individual play through group games to the formality of organised sport, serves as a framework within which the coach will develop the child's ability to express himself. The most critical period of technical development is suggested as 8–11 years of age (girls) and 8–13 years of age (boys). Sound technical expertise interpreted through play must be available in these years. As coaching does not occur in a vacuum, more than technical efficiency is required. This more holistic approach ensures that the coaching exchange is much more than mere skill acquisition.

SUMMARY OF PART 3

The coach works to improve the efficiency of energy production and of energy expression. At a simplistic level, this means getting the right fuel to the engine and making sure the engine can use it. But athletes are adaptable and creative and, unlike engines, become involved in their own development. The coach must understand and be able to apply not just the 'technical business' but the 'people business'. Both are essential for the coach to be effective. Consequently, the coach requires a sound working knowledge of education and self-education when developing the athlete towards an independence in delivering a quality performance, whether in an individual sport or a team sport and whether in a contributory role or a cooperative role within a team. The coach should understand the learning process, from the specific components which are moulded into a whole in developing an athlete's particular technique(s), through to the climate of emotional arousal, motivational environment, tentative maps of personality, and psycho-regulative phenomena which make every coach-athlete contact period far more unique than generic.

REFERENCES FOR PART 3

Abernethy, B., Wann, J. & Parks, S. (1999) Training perceptual-motor skills for sport. In *Training in Sport*. B. Elliot, Wiley, England

Allport, G. W. (1961) *Pattern and Growth in Personality*. Holt, Rinehart & Winston, New York

Allport, G. W. (1937) *Personality*. Holt, Rinehart & Winston, New York

Allport, G. W, Vernon, P. E. & Lindzey, G. (1951) *A Study of Value: A Scale for Measuring the Dominant Interests in Personality*. Houghton & Mifflin, Boston

Amrose, A. & Horn, T. S. (1997) Relationship between perceived coaching behaviours and motivational climate in college athletes. *Journal of Sport & Exercise Psychology*, 9, June

Anochin, D. K. (1967) *Das Funktionelle System Ais Grundlage Der Physiologischen Architektur Des Verhaltensaktes*, Veb Gustav Fischer Verlag, Jena

Apitzsch, E. & Berggren, B. (1993) *The personality of the elite soccer player*. Sweden: Lund University

Apter, M. J. (1982) The experience of motivation. In *The Theory of Psychological Reversals*. Academic Press, London

Arkes, H. R. & Garske, J. P. (1982) *Psychological Theories of Motivation*. 2nd Edn. Brooks/Cole Publishing Company, Monterey, CA

Balson, P. D., Elcblom, B., Soderlund, K., Sjodin, B. & Hulfan, G. (1993) Creative supplementation and dynamic high intensity intermittent exercise. *Scandinavian Journal of Medicine & Science in Sports*. 3. 143–149

Bandura, A. (1977) Self-efficacy: Toward a unifying theory of behavioural change. *Psychological Review*, 84, pp191–215

Bangsbo, J. (1994) The physiology of soccer with special reference to intense, intermittent exercise ACTA *Physiologica Scandinavica*, 151, Suppl 619, 1–115

BarEli, M., Hartman I. & LevyKolker, N. (1994) Using goal-setting to improve physical performance of adolescents with behaviour disorders: The effect of goal proximity. *Adapted Physical Activity Quarterly*, 11, 86–97

Bauersfeld, M., and Voss, G. (1992) *Neve Wege im Schnellgkeitstraining*. Philippka, Munster

Beggs, A. W. D. (1993) Goal setting in sport. In *Stress and Performance in Sport*. Jones, G. J. & Hardy, L. (eds). Wiley, Chichester

Bernstein, N. A. (1957) *The Coordination and Regulation of Movements*. Pergamon Press, London

Biddle, S. J. H. (1995) Exercise motivation across the life span. In *European Perspectives on Exercise and Sport Psychology*. Biddle, S. J. H. (ed). Human Kinetics

Blanchard, K. & Johnson, S. (1983) *The one minute manager*. In K. Blanchard, P. Zigarmi & D. Zigarmi (1986) *Leadership and the one minute manager*. Willow Book, London Blanchard, K. & Schula, D. (1995) *Everyone's a coach*. Harper Business, New York Bloomfield, J., Ackland, J. & Elliott, B. (1994) *Applied Anatomy and Biomechanics in Sport*. Blackwell Scientific Publications, Melbourne Bolton, B. (1992) In F. Dick, *Winning: Motivation for business, sport and life*. Abingdon, London Boutcher, S. H. (1993). The role of performance routines in sport. In *Stress and Performance in Sport*. Jones, G. J. & Hardy, L. (eds). Wiley, Chichester

Buhrle, M. (1989) MaximalkraftSchmellkraftReeaktiukraft. *Sportsswissenschaft*, 3, 311–325

Burton, D. (1990) Multimodal stress management in sport: current status and future directions. In *Stress and Performance in Sport*. Jones, G. J. and Hardy, L. (eds). Wiley, Chichester

Carbonaro, G. (2001) *Motor Coordination in Sport and Exercise*, Fidal, Rome

Carron. A. V. & Ball, J. R. (1977) Cause and effect characteristics of cohesiveness and participation motivation in intercollegiate ice hockey. *International Review of Sport Sociology*, 12, pp49–60

Carron, A. V., Widmeyer, W, N. & Brawley, L. R. (1985) The development of an instrument to assess cohesion in sport teams: the Group Environment Questionnaire. *Journal of Sport Psychology*, 7, pp 244–267

Cattell, R. B. (1965) *The Scientific Analysis of Personality*. Penguin, Baltimore

Cohen, F. and Lazarus, R. S. (1979) Coping with serious illness. In *Health Psychology*. G. S. Stone, F. Cohen and N. E. Adler (eds.). Freeman, San Francisco

Côté, L, Salmela, J, Trudel, P., Baria, A. & Russell, S. (1995) The Coaching Model:

A grounded theory assessment of expert gymnastic coaches' knowledge. *Journal of Sport and Exercise Psychology*, 17, 1, pp 1–17

Covey, S.R. (1992) *Principle-centred leadership.* Simon & Schuster, New York

Cox, R. H. (1998) *Sport Psychology. Concepts and Applications.* 4th Edn. WCB/McGrawHill

Counsilman, J. E. (1977) *Competitive swimming.* Prentice Hall, Englewood Cliffs, NJ

Dainty, D. A. & Norman, R. W. (1987). *Standardising Biomechanical Testing in Sport.* Human Kinetics Publishers, Champaign, IL

Davidson, R. J. and Schwartz, G. E. (1976) The psychobiology of relaxation and related states: a multiprocess theory. In *Behavioral Control and Modification of Physiological Activity.* D. Mostofsky (ed). Prentice Hall, Englewood Cliffs, NJ

Dick, F. (1992), *Winning – Motivation for Business, Sport and Life.* Abingdon, London

Dick, F. W. (1993) *High Jump.* British Athletic Federation, Birmingham

Dick, F. W. (1995) *Players Guide.* West Hartlepool Rugby Football Club

Doherty, J. K. (1963) *Modern Track and Field: Promotion, History and Methods.* Bailey & Swinfen, London

Donnellon, A. (1996) *Team talk: the power of language in team dynamics.* Harvard Business School

Dyatchkov, N. V. (1967) *Soversenstsvovanie Techniceskogo Masterstva Sportsmenov.* Fiskultura i Sport, Moscow

Evarts, E. V. (1973) Motor cortex reflexes associated with learned movement. *Science*, 179, pp501–503

Eysenck, H. J. & Eysenck, S. B. G. (1968) *Eysenck Personality Inventory Manual.* University of London Press, London

Fredenburgh, F. A. (1971) *The psychology of personality and adjustment.* Menlo Park, CA: BenjaminCummings

Freud, S. (1931) Libidinal Types. In *Sigmund Freud: Collected Papers, Vol 5.* Strachey, J. (ed). Basic Books, New York

Frankel, L. P. (1997) *Overcoming your strengths.* Harmony Books, New York

Fromm, E. (1941) *Escape from Freedom.* Holt, Rinehart & Winston, New York

Fromm, E. (1947) *Man For Himself.* Holt, Rinehart & Winston, New York

Fuoss, D. E. & Troppman, R. J. (1991) *Effective Coaching: A psychological approach.* Wiley, New York Gallistel, C. R. (1980) *The Organisation of Action.* Erlbaum, Hillsdale, NJ Galtanus, G. C., Williams, C., Boobls, L. H. & Brooks, S. (1993) Human muscle metabolism during intermittent maximal exercise. *Journal of Applied Physiology*, 75, 712–719

Galvin, P. (1999) Applying an organisational developmental model to a sports set-ting. In *Sport Psychology in Performance* (1999). ButterworthHeinmann, Oxford

Geese, R. & Hillebrecht, M. (1995) *Schnelligkeitstraining.* Meyer and Meyer, Aacheon

Gollnick, P. D. & Hermanisen, L. (1973) *Biomechanical adaptations to exercise:*

anaerobic metabolism exercise and sport science reviews (ed. Wilmorg, J. H.) Vol. 1, Academic Press, NY, USA

Gould, D. & Krane, V. (1992) The arousalathletic performance relationship: Current status and future directions. In *Advances in Sport Psychology*. T. Horn (ed.). pp119–141. Human Kinetics, Champaign, IL

Gruber, J. J. & Gray, G. R. (1981) Factor patterns of variables influencing cohesiveness at various levels of basketball competition. *Research Quarterly for Exercise and Sport*, 52 pp19–30

Gruber, J. J. & Gray, G. R. (1982) Responses to forces influencing cohesion as a function of player status and level of male varsity basketball competition. *Research Quarterly for Exercise and Sport*, 53, pp27–36

Harre, D. (1986) *Trainingslehre*. Sportverlag, Berlin

Harris, D. V., & Harris, B. L. (1984) *The Athlete's Guide to Sport Psychology*: Mental skills for physical people. Leisure Press, New York

Hendy, H. M. & Bower, B. J. (1993) Gender differences in attribution for triathlon performance. *Sex Roles*, 29, 527–542

Hill, K. L. (2001) *Framework for sport psychologists*. Human Kinetics, Champaign, IL

Hollander, E. P. (1971) *Principles and Methods of Social Psychology*. Oxford University Press, New York

Horne, T. & Carron, A. V. (1985) Compatibility in coach-athlete relationships. *Journal of Sport Psychology*, 7 137–149

Huber, V. L. (1985) Effects of task difficulty goal setting, and strategy on performance of a heuristic task. *Journal of Applied Psychology*, 70, pp492–504

Ickes, W. J. & Layden, M. A. (1978) Attributional styles. In *New Directions in Attribution Research* Vol. 2. J. H. Harvey, W. J. Ickes & R. Kidd (eds.). Erlbaum, Hillsdale, NJ

Iso-Ahola, S. E. & Hatfield, B. (1986) *Psychology of sports: A social psychological approach*. Wm. C. Brown. Dubuque, Iowa

Jacobson, E. (1929) *Progressive Relaxation*. University of Chicago Press, Chicago

Jones G. J. (1990) A cognitive perspective on the process underlying the relationship between stress and performance in sport. In *Stress and Performance in Sport*. Jones, G. J. and Hardy, L. (eds). Wiley, Chichester

Jones, R. L. (2000) Toward a sociology of coaching, In *Sociology of Sport*. Jones, R. L. and Armour, K. M. Longman, Harlow Katzenbach, J. R. (1995) *Real change leaders: how you can create growth and high performance at your company*. McKinsey & Company, NY Kinlaw, D. C. (1993) Coaching for commitment. *Managerial strategies for obtaining superior performance*. Pfeiffer & Company, Oxford Komi, P. V. (1973) Measurement of the force-velocity relationship in human muscle under concentric and eccentric contraction. *Medicine of Sport*. Vol 8: Biomechanics III, pp. 224–229, Kargo Basel

Komi, P. V. & Bosco, C. (1978) Utilisation of stored elastic energy in leg extensor muscles by men and women. *Medicine and Science in Sport and Exercise*. 10, 261–265

Kozlov, I. & Muraveyev, I. (1992) Muscles and the sprint. *Fitness and Sport Review* 6, 192

Krech, D. & Crutchfield, R. S. (1962) *Elements of Psychology.* Alfred A. Knopf, New York

Kyllo, L. B. & Landers, D. M. (1995) Goalsetting in sport and exercise: A research synthesis to resolve the controversy. *Journal of Sport & Exercise Psychology*, 17, 117–137

Landers, D. & Leuschen, G. (1974) Team performance outcome and cohesiveness of competitive coacting groups. *International Review of Sport Sociology* 2, pp57–69

Lenk, N. (1969) Top performance despite internal conflicts: An antithesis to a functionalistic proposition. In *Sport, Culture and Society: A reader on the sociology of sport.* J. W, Loy and G. S. Kenyon (eds), pp393–397. Macmillan, New York

Locatelli, E. (1999) The Energetics of the short sprint: Influence of Morphological Characteristics – Doctoral Thesis.

Lopez, V. (1991) An approach to strength training for sprinters. *Track technique* 115, 3668–3695

Lotter, W. S. (1960) Interrelationships among reaction times and speeds of movement in different limbs. *Research Quarterly*, 38, pp202–207

Mahoney, M. J. & Avener, M. (1977) Psychology of the elite athlete: An exploratory study. *Cognitive Therapy and Research*, 1, pp 135–141

Malina, R. M. & Bouchard, C. (1991). *Growth, maturation, and physical activity.* Human Kinetics Books. Champaign, IL

Marshall, R. N. & Elliot, B. C. (1999) The analysis and development of technique in sport. In B. Elliot, *Training in Sport.* Wiley, Chichester

Martens, R. (1987). *Coaches' Guide to Sport Psychology.* Champaign, IL: Human Kinetics

Massimo, J. (1980) The gymnast's perception of the coach: Performance competence and coaching style. In R. M. Suinn, *Psychology in sports: Methods and applications.* Macmillan Publishing Company. New York, pp229–237

McAtee, R. (1993) *Facilitated Stretching.* pp 13–92. Human Kinetics Campaign, Ill. USA

Miller, T. W. (1982) Assertiveness training for coaches: The issue of healthy communication between coaches and players. *Journal of Sport Psychology*, 4, 107–141

Moritani, J. (1992) Time course of adaptations during strength and power training. *Strength and Power in Sport.* (ed. Korni, P. V.) pp 266–278, Blackwell Scientific Publications, Oxford

Murray, P. E (1994) IS4, *Integrated Sport Science Support Strategy.* International Coaching School of Canada, August, Victoria, B.C.

Murray, P. E (1995) *Integrated Sport Science Support Strategy.* BASES.

Murray, P. E (1996) Cohesion, a perspective from operationalised coaching styles in coacting and interacting sports. Educational Research in 1995, Working papers in education. Educational Research Unit, University of Wolverhampton

Murray, P. E (1999) The construction and validation of the Facilitating Coaching Styles Questionnaire. University of Wolverhampton, University Press

Murray, P. F. & Krastev, A. M. (1992) La ejecucion élite y el comportamiento del entrenador. Estudios del Entrenador; apoyo academico para la maestria en las ciencias del deporte. Universidad Autonoma de Chihualiua, Prensa Universitaria

Nolan, T. (1997) A walk on the wild. *Coach and Athletic Director*, April, pp51–58

Ozolin, E. S. (1990) The sprint. Soviet Sports Review, 2, 57–60: 3, 142–144, 4, 195–199

Pollard, A. (1998) Sociology and teaching: A new challenge for the sociology of education. In P. Woods and A. Pollard (eds). *Reflective teaching – The Sociological Contribution*. London: Croom Helm

Pope, W. (1998) 'Emile Durkheim'. In R. Stones (ed). *Key Sociological Thinkers*. Basingstoke, Macmillan

Posner, M. I., Nissen, M. J., & Klein, R. M. (1976) Visual dominance: an information-processing account of its origins and significance. *Psychological Review*, 83, pp157–170

Pousson, M., Van Hogeke, J. & Goubel, F. (1990) Changes in elastic characteristics of human muscle induced by eccentric exercise. *Journal of Biomechanics*, 23, pp343–348

Schmidtblgicher, D. (1992) *Training for Power Events. Strength and Power in Sport.* (Ed. Komi, P. V.) pp 381–395 Blackwell Scientific Publications, Oxford

Smyth, M. M., & Marriot, A. M. (1982). Vision proprioception in simple catching. *Journal of Motor Behavior*, 14, pp 143–152

Steiner, C. (1999). *Achieving emotional literacy*. Bloomsbury, London

Sternberg, R. J. (1999) *Thinking Styles*. Cambridge University Press, Cambridge

Tellez, T. (1991) In D. Hemery, *Sporting excellence; What makes a champion?* Harper Collins, London

Verhoshansky, Y. V. & Lazarev, V. V. (1989) Principles of planning speed and strength; speed endurance training in sport. *Journal of National Strength and Conditioning*, 2, 58–61

Westre, K. R. & Weiss, M. R. (1991) The relationship between perceived coaching behaviours and group cohesion in high school football teams. *Sport Psychologist*, 5, (1), pp41–54

Whiting, H. T. A. (1975) *Concepts in skill learning*. Lepus Books, London

Wilke, K. (1992) Analysis of sprint swimming; The 50 m freestyle: *Biomechanics and Medicine in Swimming* (eds. Maclaren, D., Reilly, T. & Legs, A) pp 33–46. E. & F. M. Spon, London

Wilson, G., Elliott, B. & Wood, G. 1992) Stretch shorten cycle performance enhancement through flexibility training. *Medicine and Science – Sports and Exercise*, 24, pp116–123

Zimmerman, B. J. & Kitsantus, A. (1996) Self-regulated learning of a motoric skill: The role of goal setting and self-monitoring. *Journal of Applied Sport Psychology*, 8, pp60–75

BIBLIOGRAPHY

Hickson, R. C. (1980) Interference of strength development by simultaneously training for strength and endurance. *European Journal of Applied Physiology*, 42, pp372–376

lmgjer, F. & Myhere, K. (1992) Physiological Effects of altitude training on young elite male cross-country skiers. *Journal of Sports Sciences*, 10, 49–63

Legs, A. & Arthur, S. (1988) An investigation into anaerobic performance of wheelchair. *Ergonomics*, 31, 1529–1537

Wadler, G. R., & Haimling, B. (1989) *Drugs and the Athlete*. F.A. Davis, USA 104

<<

<<

PART 4

THE LANGUAGE OF TRAINING THEORY

In parts 1, 2 and 3, relevant aspects of the sports-related sciences have been reviewed. Parts 4 and 5 seek to draw together the practical implications of this review and, by considering these against a backcloth of experience, to apply them to the development of the athlete.

One of the greatest problems in studying training theory is the diversity of terminology. The most obvious examples of this are in the area of fitness and its components. In part 4, a framework of definition and explanation is set out to establish a sound basis in this aspect of training theory. The concept of *fitness* is examined as it applies to all lifestyles. The major components of fitness, seen here as *strength, speed, endurance, mobility*, and their derivatives, are brought into focus in separate chapters. The technical component is covered in chapter 11. An understanding of these components is fundamental to the construction of training programmes specific to athlete and discipline.

The final chapter of part 4 deals with *evaluation*, a process critical to the ordered progression of training and, consequently, of fitness.

<<

13 FITNESS

Fitness may be defined as the level of adaptation to the stressors of a given lifestyle. It is an essential component in the concept of 'wellness', which might be defined as a persistent endeavour to achieve the highest probability for total well-being (fig. 65). A scientifically based and systematic training programme is fundamental to the athlete's fitness. Training provides the athlete with the basic means to adapt to his particular stressors through controlled exercise. Training theory may supplement the coach's practical knowledge to help him formulate a balanced training programme. The principles of training which apply in designing fitness programmes apply equally to elite performers, recreational performers, developing performers and those whose lives are not orientated towards sport or physical recreation.

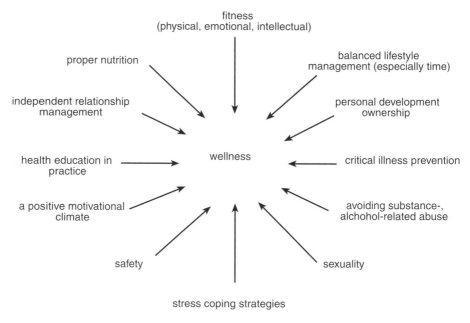

FIG. 65 Critical components of 'wellness'

THE GENERAL PICTURE

If a fitness programme is to be relevant, three questions must be answered. What is the lifestyle of the person involved? Is that person fit for that lifestyle? How can that person become more fit, or maintain present fitness levels?

To answer the first question one must review the stressors of the lifestyle: work, social, family, leisure pursuits, and so on. The review becomes more complex when such factors as ambition and anxiety are taken into account. Without a detailed answer to the first question, it is impossible to consider the second. The review is seldom easy, because not all stressors are obvious. Issues become confused as there is temptation to focus only on those factors which can readily produce the effects of stress-related problems. The fact that a person appears to have the measure of his cumulative stressor climate, as determined, say, by a favourable testosterone/cortisol ratio, should not be interpreted as meaning that one may dismiss the relevance of any component stressor within that climate. Each stressor must be considered – and the athlete's status relative to that stressor evaluated before addressing the final question of how to ensure that the athlete remains in control, or can regain control.

One's lifestyle might be thought of as a three-lane motorway along which a person travels through life (fig. 66). The 'Highway Code' is one's values framework. There is overall purpose for the journey variously determined by religious beliefs or philosophies of life. Each lane represents a broad avenue of progression: one's occupation or means of earning (career); one's social and family responsibilities (family and social); and the avenue of one's personal expression or creativity (you). Each person is continually on the move along the 'motorway', meeting the demands of pursuing objectives in any or all of the lanes at any time. There are many possible stressors in pursuit of these objectives (fig. 68).

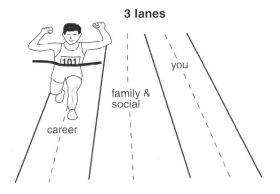

FIG. 66 A balanced approach to personal development requires planning to achieve goals in all three lanes

Career

Most careers have their own in-built set of stressors. On starting a new career, one is more aware of what they are. The majority are soon accommodated as routine is established and they consequently represent a low-level package of stressors. However, crises have to be managed, personal emotions must be suppressed despite provocation, and routine must be pursued despite peaks and troughs of general health and instability in the non-working environment.

For the committed athlete, whether professional or amateur, full time or part time, 'career' embraces the 'career' that is outside sport, such as study and business, plus the 'career' that is sport. Because performance is competitive, sport is a total expression of an athlete's complex profile of competence and motivation, and pursuit of achievement represents a considerable range of stressors. They include the physical demands on the organism when training to develop those conditioning characteristics relevant to a given sport. These are represented in figure 67. As the athlete progresses through a year plan, the effects of physical stressors vary according to how the athlete's conditioning status matches the

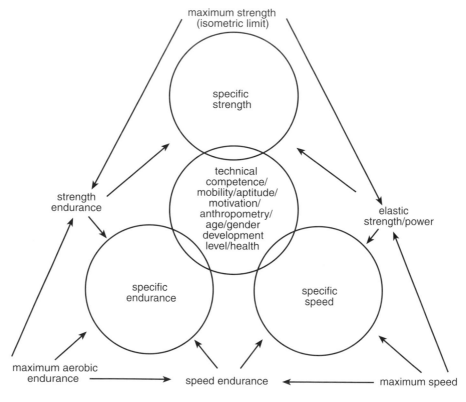

FIG. 67 Schematic representation of the relationship of basic fitness characteristics and their involvement in the specific fitness required of individual disciplines/sports.

specific demands of cumulative training loads. The range of stressors also includes those associated with varied fortunes in pursuit of high ambition, especially when sport is 'career'!

Family and social

Home and social situations also have their own stressor profile. Family bereavement not only represents an immense immediate stressor of emotional trauma, but also the shock waves can last months, or even years, putting health at risk. Moving house is also a most stressful experience as its disorientation drains reserves of physical and emotional energy. Other states of transition can have high potential as stressors. They include shifting from school to university or school to employment; from childhood through adolescence; from a stable to an unstable relationship; from employment to unemployment; from having children at home to having them leave; and from a comfortable economic scenario to one where there is seldom enough to meet the round of bills.

You

Most people seldom attend to addressing those stressors that impact on personal life. Personal development can too readily be considered relative to 'career' rather than the 'real you'. In the interest of emotional, intellectual and physical health/fitness/wellbeing, there should be a strategy for coping with the total environment of stressors and for delivering on personal development. The key to achieving the right strategy is understanding that there is only one pool of adaptation energy available to cope with cumulative stressors (fig. 68).

Running across these three broad areas of stressor is a person's profile relative to the impact of their personal interpretations and delivery of other 'wellness' components in practice. The total complex of the stressor environment is, then, substantial and unique to a given person. Each person is located somewhere on a lifelong fitness continuum. What fitness means in personal terms reflects where someone is on that continuum, which might be thought of as a progression of roughly 10 year stages.

Age →5–14	Learning skills, developing conditioning base and forming attitudes to use over the next 20 years to development advantage.
15–24	Fitness relates to pursuit of development/competitive advantage.
25–34	Cosmetic fitness; weight control; peak competitive years (in sport).
35–44	Wellness focus to protect from coronary disease.
45–54	Balancing lifestyle to avoid stress-related illness.
55–64	Maintaining energy levels to keep pace with 35–54-year-olds.
65 →	Living that pace of life which lets you enjoy it.

5–14 years

Family, school, local authorities and activity-focused clubs build on the personal talents/abilities one is born with, plus early life experience, motivational climate and early attitude framework. These years, which bridge primary and secondary school years, are more development-centred than achievement-centred. They are critical preparation for the next 20 years and, therefore, for life. They prepare young people for what they will do and how they will do it in the challenging and competitive years to come. They are the fitness foundation years for a healthy life.

15–24 years of age

Even if one is not committed to becoming a 'sports star', these years could be vital in establishing a pattern of physical recreation. Sports centres, sports clubs, sports councils and governing bodies of sport will be able to advise on where and when one may participate in sport and recreation at one's own level. Regular exercise is the best form of preventive medicine against fitness and health problems in the following years.

25–34 years of age

Problems in this age group find their origins in the previous decade. Difficulties in weight control are derived from indiscriminate eating habits and lack of exercise. By reducing the daily calorific intake, weight will be lost but muscle tone will not improve. Only exercise will improve muscle tone, but it must be aimed at the appropriate muscles. Exercises fall mainly in the strength endurance, heart endurance and mobility areas. However, if one is pursuing continued involvement in sport, all the characteristics mentioned for the previous decade will be developed, and to an appropriate level. Regular aerobic exercise is a vital form of preventive medicine to introduce in this age group.

35–44 years of age

The accumulation of stressors may lead to the possibility of a heart attack in this period (fig. 29, p. 90). If people in this age group have done very little exercise, they may have one or several of the following problems:

- being overweight, which puts an extra load on the heart and is unattractive
- poor muscle tone, which endangers joints in sudden exertion (especially the back). It also leads to postural problems
- joint stiffness, which limits movement in the joints and consequently discourages exercise
- poor condition of the oxygen transporting system. This leads to breathlessness in even slight exertion, is related to coronary problems, and generally discourages active recreation.

Twenty years or so of inactivity will make it very difficult and even dangerous to launch into vigorous exercise now! The best policy is to start by improving the joint mobility, then the oxygen transporting system, and then move on to muscle tone. Low impact exercise will help avoid the demotivation which comes with muscle and joint aches. So instead of jogging, try mountain biking, roller blading, langlauf, etc. This, combined with dietary control, will reduce weight. As a result new life will be put into these years with the physical, social and mental benefits of physical recreation.

45–54 years of age

Many problems of the last decade still exist here and the exercise programme should be similar to that of the preceding age group. Oxygen transport may be improved by jogging, walking and swimming, etc. Muscle tone improvement can come through strength endurance work, and mobility through exercise with or without apparatus. Regular review of stressor climate and stress management is essential.

55–64 years of age

Major emphasis is now on efficiency of the oxygen transporting system, with a continuation of gentle mobility work. Strength is not a factor to be emphasised and any work in this area should be light. Again, management of the impact of the stressor climate is essential. It is a time for broadening those fields of personal interest and aptitude which will enrich not only the regeneration process in a world of challenges, but life as a whole.

65+ years

'The third age' sounds more appropriate to the concept of fitness in these years, than for 'retirement'! Broadening of personal interests and doing something with them has been prepared for in the previous 10 years. Now it's time

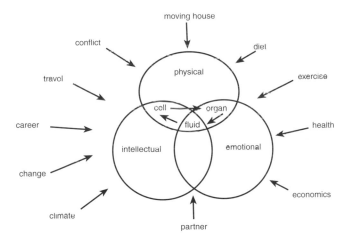

FIG. 68 Stressors persistently bombard us. Our response is stress-increased agitation in the cycle of interdependence between cell–organ–fluids. Because the pool of general adaptation energy required for that response is finite, the stressor effect is cumulative. The total stressor 'package' must then, be identified and managed.

to live them and enjoy them to the full by being fit to do so. All the better if, in doing so, there is a real sense of continued personal value within the family, the community and/or other 'teams'. When self-awareness affords any suggestion that personal value is reducing, self-belief ebbs and that constitutes a big negative stressor.

Where competitive sport is the focus of personal development, fitness must be approached as a process commencing early and continuing through and beyond peak performance years. Of course, the peak performance years vary between sports. The fact is, however, that the components of each development phase must be addressed if athletes are to deliver their true potential in those peak performance years. Forcing the pace of development cannot be considered as reflecting a sense of responsibility for a young person's preparation for a healthy life. Emotional, social and even intellectual development can be compromised. This said, commercial aspects of top-level sport may alter perspective. The ethical issues here must be thought through

BASIC PRINCIPLES IN TRAINING

The principles, or 'laws of training', of specificity, overload and reversibility are basic to the theory and practice of physical development, but will be more fully appreciated when related to the basic physical characteristics (see p. 225–6).

Specificity

Adaptation is specific to a stressor and the effect of a stressor is specific to an individual athlete. The importance of this should become apparent if we consider two athletes (a), and a training unit (b).

(a) John: best 200m = 22.0 seconds; Angus: best 200m = 23.0 seconds
(b) Unit = 6 x 200m in 24.0 seconds with 90 seconds recovery

This unit cannot have the same effect on each athlete because it represents a different % max intensity for each.

Reversibility

When intensity, extent or density is reduced, the degree of adaptation brought about by the training loads will gradually weaken. Strength losses are faster than mobility losses. Status improvements brought about by special methods over a short term are lost quicker than those brought about by 'slower' methods over a long term. Yet there are occasions when loads are reduced deliberately in special preparation for a major competition. The coach must decide the extent to which such training should be cut back and for how long.

EFFECT OF TRAINING

Training might be considered as having three levels of effect.

(**1**) Immediate: the immediate effect of training is the body's reactions to the stressor of the training stimulus. They include increased heart rate, perspiration, increased blood lactate, heightened endocrine system involvement and fatigue. This is the catabolic effect of training.

(**2**) Residual: the residual effect of training is what might be considered as the body's recovery and preparation response. The recovery response is seen in a raised general metabolism for some time after exercise is concluded. During this time the body's resting state is restored with the waste products of energy expenditure removed, and other stressor-related effects gradually eliminated. The preparation response is seen in the heightened level of adaptation to future training stimuli. Having been stressed by a training stimulus, the body organises itself to ensure that next time it will not be 'stressed' so much by the same stimulus! Put another way, this effect of training ensures that the body is prepared for a greater training stimulus next time. This is the anabolic effect of training.

(**3**) Cumulative: the cumulative effect of training is the body's progressive adaptation through the preparation response. This is what is measured in fitness monitoring tests over a period of months or even years.

The effect of training will be considered again in chapter 21.

BASIC PHYSICAL CHARACTERISTICS

The interpretation of specificity is clear when one considers the type of fitness required for a given lifestyle. Whereas the athlete works to increase fitness towards some level of excellence, the non-athlete may work to compensate for the damage his lifestyle is causing. Thus, the lorry driver slumped at his wheel uses few abdominal or back muscles and should therefore attempt to improve muscle tone in these areas.

The definition of overload chosen by the coach depends upon the particular physical characteristics that need to be developed.

Strength: overload is increasing the resistance in terms of kg, etc.

Strength endurance: overload is increasing repetitions of an activity with a resistance ranging from the athlete's own body weight, to adding weighted belts, etc. to the athlete, to light and sub-maximal loads. The lactic anaerobic energy pathway has high involvement.

Aerobic/heart endurance: overload is increasing the amount of time that the person can continue a low strength demand in a steady state of work of low-intensity repetitions. The aerobic energy pathway is involved exclusively.

Speed endurance: overload is increasing the number of high-quality repetitions of an exercise per unit of time; or increasing the quality of repetition while keeping the number at or above a fixed threshold; although this may take place in a climate of cumulative lactic anaerobic pathway by-products, the alactic energy pathway has critical high involvement.

Speed: overload is performing (and or selecting) a given task faster.

Elastic strength/power: overload is increasing the resistance without loss of speed; or increasing speed of moving a fixed sub-max → max resistance.

Mobility: overload is taking effective joint action beyond its present limit.

Clearly there are several subdivisions and variants of these broad areas of characteristic. Reversibility interpreted for the non-athlete or athlete will give an indication of how much exercise is required each week to maintain a reasonable degree of fitness. It is believed that a minimum of 2–3 units per week is necessary for the non-athlete, while the athlete is often involved in 2–3 units of training per day. The minimum will be used by the majority of non-athletes, e.g. day 1: jogging and mobility exercises, day 2: circuit training and jogging, day 3: some form of physical recreation. On the other hand, it would be ideal if some form of physical activity and regeneration training became part of daily routine.

POINTS ON FITNESS AND TRAINING

The following are some general points on fitness and training for both the athlete and non-athlete:

(1) Before beginning any exercise programme, both athlete and non-athlete should have a full medical check-up. It is good practice to make this the start of regular annual or biannual check-ups. Some medical conditions may suggest a modified programme.

(2) Children will not damage a healthy heart by exercising – quite the opposite. When children are tired they stop!

(3) There is no upper age limit for exercise. The right exercise programme supported by relevant medical advice will keep the heart, muscles, joints, vascular and support systems healthy to provide and use energy required to enjoy one's lifestyle.

(4) The starting focus of all exercise programmes is low intensity training – general all-round aerobic activity to prepare a foundation for developing a programme. General activity in terms of strength should focus from the outset on postural muscles – spine (core strength) and those responsible for balance, stability, etc.

(5) Stiffness following exercise is natural – and not serious. Sharp pain rather than discomfort during the next bout of exercise may be cause for alarm. It might

be due to slight muscle strain, and rest followed by low-intensity exercise and gentle stretching – or a prescribed rehabilitation programme – should return things to normal. If the pain persists, a physiotherapist must be consulted. If exercise is being commenced after a long period of inactivity, it should be low impact (e.g. aqua-jog) and gentle mobility.

(6) Too much training does not shorten life, but too little may. It cannot be said that training will necessarily lengthen life, but it will help make one's 'allotted span' more enjoyable.

(7) There is no such thing as 'overtraining'. Physical, mental or emotional 'burnout' is due to the cumulative effect of *all* the stressors in one's life. Rather than compromise the training programme, the overall picture must be reviewed with the various objectives and tasks prioritised to create 'space' for adaptation to take place.

(8) Women are able to train as hard as men. Following pregnancy, women's training load capacity increases and competitive performance in most cases improves above that of the accepted normal progression curve. Women may train hard throughout the menstrual cycle. However, in the 2–3 days prior to menstruation high intensity elastic strength work (i.e. jumping routines) which focus sudden high loads on the hips/lower-back should not take the athlete towards fatigue. The sacroiliac joint is less stable at this point in the cycle and can be strained.

(9) People do not 'go to fat' when they finish serious training. The fact is that their appetites often stay high while their energy expenditure is now lower, and, consequently, weight increases. Such athletes should maintain a programme of lighter training as part of their personal fitness programme and review eating habits. This approach will also help maintain general muscle tone.

(10) Training does not make people 'muscle-bound'. This is an obscure expression which reflects the fact that certain types of strength training will considerably increase the size of muscles – for example in body building. This will only happen if this is the objective of training and specific diets or exercise are pursued to this end. Normal exercise programmes do not have this effect. In fact, by reducing fat around the muscle, and improving muscle tone, a more attractive definition of the limbs will result.

(11) Exercise machines are sound and safe for non-athletes to use provided their use is properly explained by a qualified instructor.

(12) For personal safety, neither athlete nor non-athlete should work alone with loose weights or exercise machines.

(13) Isometrics should not be used indiscriminately, especially by those aged 35 and over. They *may* overload the heart.

(14) Because fitness is specific, so also are fitness programmes. The objectives of each phase of a training programme should be clearly defined and the programme planned to meet those objectives.

(15) Personal fitness programmes, whether for athlete or non-athlete, must on the one hand set out details of physical activity and regeneration and, on the other, afford advice from fitness-related areas such as nutrition, sports psychology and sports medicine – relevant to the individual's needs.

(16) No fitness programme can be seriously considered without a definite time commitment on the part of the person for whom the programme is designed.

(17) Once a regular routine of training is established, there should be a balanced mixture of exercise machines and free weights exercises in the programme. This should be a well-planned programme, to ensure that those muscles acting as synergists in controlling movements are not neglected.

(18) Because habitual posture and activity patterns can lead to imbalances and compensatory stress in the joint complexes, it is sensible to consult a chiropractor or osteopath at least once a year for monitoring and corrective treatment.

SUMMARY

The meaning of fitness is specific to a given individual. Against the background of fitness to tolerate the stressors of day-to-day living, the athlete seeks to develop a fitness specific to the demands of his sport. It must be borne in mind that just as the demands of each sport are diverse, so are the day-to-day lives of the athletes. If the athlete becomes 'unfit' for life outside sport, due to an inability to adapt to its stressors, then there will certainly be an overlap into sport, and his capacity for developing fitness for his sport will be impaired. The coach must view the development of fitness as unique to athlete and situation, and consequently the totality of the athlete's life must be taken into account in identifying his 'uniqueness'.

14 THEORY AND PRACTICE OF STRENGTH DEVELOPMENT

STRENGTH

Strength, or the ability to express force, is a basic physical characteristic that determines performance efficiency in sport. Each sport varies in its strength requirements and, in the interest of specificity, we should examine its relationship to speed and endurance.

There are three main classifications of strength, namely maximum strength, elastic strength and strength endurance. The last two are most pertinent to sport in general, but maximum strength does have its place in some sports (e.g. weight lifting) and is clearly a component of elastic strength and strength endurance. When designing the strength portion of an athlete's personal fitness programme it is specific to athlete and sport/discipline. It will draw variously, then, on these three main classifications of strength (figure 67, page 220).

Maximum strength

Maximum strength (gross strength) is defined as the greatest force the neuro-muscular system is capable of exerting in a single maximum voluntary contraction. Consequently it will determine performance in those sports where great resistance has to be overcome or controlled (e.g. weight lifting).

'Controlled' means here that the muscles may be required to remain in a state of static contraction (isometric) at maximum or near maximum static strength demands. It is possible to combine demands for maximum strength with a high speed of contraction (e.g. in hammer and shot put) or with high demands on endurance (e.g. rowing).

The smaller the resistance to be overcome, the less the involvement of maximum strength. Accelerating the body from rest (sprinting) or propelling the body from the ground (jumps) means a greater resistance must be overcome than maintaining uniform motion, as in medium and long endurance sports. Figure 69 helps to bring this concept of maximum strength involvement into perspective.

Maximum strength is the product of three factors: biological, neuromuscular and mechanical.

Biological refers to muscle cross-sectional area, the amount of contractile elements within the muscle and fibre types:

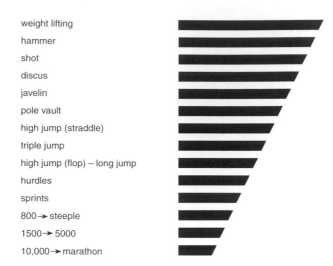

weight lifting
hammer
shot
discus
javelin
pole vault
high jump (straddle)
triple jump
high jump (flop) – long jump
hurdles
sprints
800 → steeple
1500 → 5000
10,000 → marathon

FIG. 69 Schematic representation of maximum strength contribution to various athletic events (adapted from Harre, 1986)

Type I   (slow-twitch for long-lasting, low force level production)
Type IIA   (fast-twitch for prolonged high force production)
Type IIB (IIX)   (fast-twitch for short duration, high force production)

Neuromuscular refers to firing rate and motor unit recruitment. The last fibres to be recruited are Type IIB (IIX) (see also page 113).

Mechanical refers to the mechanisms of muscle action, the velocity of contraction and the muscle length. Maximum force production is delivered in eccentric contraction. These values exceed isometric maximum values by 10–40%. Isometric maximum values exceed concentric maximum values by 10–15%.

Elastic strength (power, speed strength)

The ability of the neuromuscular system to overcome resistance with a high speed of contraction is defined as elastic strength. The neuromuscular system accepts and expels rapid loading at high velocity through the coordination of reflexes and elastic and contractile components of muscle. The adjective 'elastic' is very appropriate and a key to avoiding confusion between 'speed of contraction' or 'strength of contraction'. Although this mechanism involves both, it is their complex coordination and the involvement of reflexes and elastic components that defines it as a most specific area of strength. Elastic strength determines performance in all of the so-called 'explosive' sports, i.e. jumping, throwing, sprinting, striking, etc.

Strength endurance

This is the capacity of all or part of the organism to maintain strength expression through fatigue. It is characterised by a relatively high application of strength, together with mental and physical perseverance.

Age-old tests of 'strength', such as maximum press-ups or holding a weight at arm's length for as long as possible, are, in fact, tests of strength endurance. It determines performance principally when considerable resistance is to be overcome for a fairly long period of time. Thus in rowing, swimming, cross-country skiing and track events between 60 seconds and 8 minutes duration, one would expect to find strength endurance a critical factor. This may explain the relationship in track and field athletics between hill running and 800 m improvement demonstrated by Viru, Urgenstein and Pisuke (1972).

Absolute and relative strength

In sports where maximum strength is the principal component (fig. 69), body weight and performance are closely correlated. In other words, heavy athletes can, in absolute terms, achieve greater strength expression than lighter athletes. The maximum force that an athlete can express, irrespective of body weight, is therefore referred to as absolute strength. On the other hand, the maximum force that an athlete can express in relation to body weight is known as relative strength. This is of obvious importance to athletes who must move their own body weight in, for instance, jumps and gymnastics. It is calculated by dividing absolute strength by the athlete's own body weight, and reduction in body weight will increase relative strength.

Shot-put athlete (male) weighs 100 kg : leg press (90° knee) = 300kg
        Therefore relative strength = 3.0 kg/kg body wt.
Long jump athlete (female) weighs 60 kg : leg press (90° knee) = 200 kg
        Therefore relative strength = 3.3 kg/kg body wt.

Absolute leg press strength favours the putter, but relative leg press strength favours the jumper.

In some sports it is important for an athlete to have high absolute and relative strength. For example, in rugby union, a prop forward must have high absolute strength and body weight in the scrum, but must also be fast over short distances and have the level of endurance necessary to positively influence the pace of the game. This would suggest that relative strength must be high. Strength training for such a player should then reflect the fitness requirement of all aspects of his 'total' game. A similar situation exists for rugby league, Australian rules, NFL, Gaelic football, etc.

Additional strength parameters

Interest in strength development in academic institutions has produced further parameters defined in the first instance by specific measurement criteria. Tidow listed several following the Freiburg 'Symposium on Strength' (1983). They include:

Parameter	Area of Definition
Absolute Strength	Electric-stimulation-maximum value, computer tomography of muscle cross-section.
Maximum Strength	Maximum voluntary contraction against an eccentric loading* (140% maximum isometric).
Strength Deficit	Difference between maximum strength (as measured above), and isometric maximum strength (in %).
Strength Maximum	This is the maximum load which can be lifted.
Explosive Strength	Maximum rate of strength increase per unit of time (isometric/dynamic).
Starting Strength	Strength score achieved 30 milli-seconds after start of contraction.

The athlete's status relative to such parameters may be used as a guide to the review of training programmes on the basis that such parameters are considered usable as indices of specific strength relative to the athlete's discipline or phase of training.

External resistance and the athlete's ability to express force

The athlete expresses force (or strength) through the body's lever system by converting chemical to kinetic energy, and by neuromuscular coordination. In all physical activity, the athlete expresses this force against external force (or resistance). Resistance may take the shape of weights, throwing implements, water, air, the athlete's own body weight, momentum, and so on. Sometimes the athlete's ability to exert force is referred to as internal force, as opposed to the external force of the resistance. The relationship between the two is critical because it determines different classes of muscular activity (see chapter 6). These classes are apparent in the components of individual sports techniques. In the interest of specificity, exercises must develop efficiency of appropriate muscular activity in those muscle groups involved in specific joint actions. This means identifying the muscular activity and the actions. Is the muscular activity elastic strength, strength endurance, etc? Is the action postural/synergic, protagonist, etc?

Static (or isometric) muscular activity

This is frequently, but mistakenly, thought of only as maximum force of contraction. Measurements of isometric strength have perpetuated this belief, with tensiometer and dynamometer tests being used to evaluate maximum strength in a specific area of joint action. However, the ability to balance on one foot, to maintain an upright posture, to counter the hammer's pull in the turns, or to hold a vertical alignment of shoulder/hip at long jump take off, are all examples of static contraction.

During static muscular activity the force expressed by the athlete equals the force expressed by the resistance. In other words, the greater the resistance, the greater the strength required by the athlete to maintain the relationship between levers at a given joint. This implies that the athlete has sufficient reserves of strength to do this, which in turn implies an ultimate maximum for that athlete in a given joint action. When the resistance exceeds this maximum the muscular activity is no longer isometric, but a type of eccentric activity.

The range of isometric strength expression is obviously very great, yet the need for discrete neuromuscular adjustment to hold levers in critical alignment is essential to a successful performance in technical sports. Consequently, training should embrace work to develop specific isometric efficiency, focusing on the role of certain muscles as postural and/or synergic, or holding a particular position of spine extension, flexion or lateral flexion or rotation while performing upper or lower limb complex actions. Weakness in muscles which act to maintain posture or which are synergists can increase the possibility of technical errors or injury. Whether an athlete is beginner or elite, the training programme must include work for development of these muscles. For example, standing on one leg and simply swinging the other leg forwards and backwards, then across in front of the standing leg and high to side, then 'drawing a figure of eight out to the side', etc., helps develop those muscles supporting the foot, ankle, knee and hip of the standing leg. This kind of work is embraced by the notion of 'general/all round/basic strength' as 'core strength', when targeting spine postural stability.

Dynamic muscular activity

Dynamic muscular activity can be sub-divided into concentric and eccentric.

Concentric muscular activity

Joint movement will take place when the force expressed by the athlete does not equal that imposed by the resistance. In concentric work, the athlete is expressing more force than the resistance and consequently the muscle shortens to pull the levers it connects towards each other. Individual muscles, or groups of muscles, can be developed by resistance training which corresponds to this type of activity. Biceps curls, for instance, will develop the flexors of the elbow. This type of activity is very common in sport, but developing the ability to perform with greater strength will not necessarily lead to improved performance. The coordination and role of each joint action must be considered in its entirety and the whole must be developed.

Eccentric muscular activity

Elastic concept: like concentric activity, this results from a disparity between force expressed by the athlete and force represented by resistance. It operates at two quite different levels. First, the resistance may be less than the maximum strength which the athlete *can* express. This will occur when lowering a weight to the floor, or accepting body momentum as the athlete moves into the basic discus throw position, or with each landing/take-off in triple jump. The need to develop the athlete's ability to perform such muscular activity has given rise to training methods such as jump decathlons, Verhoshansky's (1971) depth jumps, Endemann's (1975) weights jacket work from boxes with throwers, and the Bulgarian system of mixing concentric work with eccentric work. This might also be referred to as elastic eccentric work (plyometrics).

Plastic concept: the second level is where the resistance imposed is greater than the athlete's maximum isometric strength. Here, the athlete can only attempt to control a losing struggle with the resistance. Because loading effect is maximum throughout the whole range of movement in this type of activity, the tone or quality of muscular contraction is constant and is referred to as isotonic. It is not technically correct to so describe all muscle activity where movement takes place, as the load effect alters along the range in a given joint action. The 'isokinetic' devices developed in the late 1960s allowed muscular activity to be more truly isotonic than other exercise methods at that time. Exercise employing this type of loading is used in progressive physiotherapy units, both to develop strength through a period of post-injury or post-surgery rehabilitation, and to measure strength throughout the full range of a given joint action. This may be referred to as plastic eccentric work and such exercise should be performed under supervision.

STRENGTH RELATIVE TO MOVEMENT

Figure 70 schematically represents a biceps curl. If X units of strength are required to move from position A, more units of force must be employed to maintain movement with the increased resistance at B (note the increased length of the load arm). In moving towards C, however, the load arm diminishes and consequently so does the resistance. The movement will now be faster if the same number of units are used.

This variation implies that once initial inertia is overcome, the 'value' of the resistance will be less effective in the development of strength elsewhere in the range. In other words, only the beginning of the movement will be overloaded. Ideally, each point in the range of movement should be offered a similar overload, which could be assessed from graphs such as that in figure 71. However, isolating specific parts of the range may well interfere with the natural pattern of acceleration associated with movements through the full range.

'resistance'
= load x (a)

'resistance'
= load x (c)

'resistance'
= load x (b)

FIG. 70 The change of 'resistance' at different points in the range of movement of flexion at the elbow

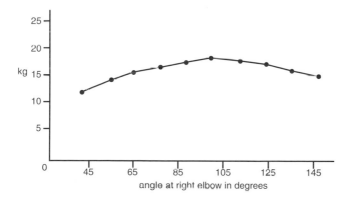

FIG. 71 Kinetic strength measured at different joint angles for flexion at right elbow (schoolgirl aged 13)

Auxotonic muscular activity

Auxotonic activity is the particular neuromuscular pattern associated with a given sports technique. It involves the complex programming of static and/or dynamic activity at different joints, the control of muscle contraction against muscle relaxation, and the movement-specific speed that is both absolute in terms of the whole movement and relative in terms of synchronisation of different joint actions. In other words, it is a specific pattern dictating which levers are used, and how, when, and where they are used. To develop various strength requirements the athlete must load the various actions in accordance with that pattern. Consequently, orthodox weight training exercises can only contribute to improved performance in the sports technique if regularly channelled through special exercises and competition specific exercises. Auxotonic activity must be clearly understood in order to differentiate between general, related and specific exercise, and to develop relevant practices.

DEVELOPMENT OF STRENGTH

Development of this physical ability, like all others, must obey the three laws of training – specificity, overload and reversibility (see chapter 13). The athlete's strength requirement for a given sport, although specific to the sport and his status relative to that sport's demands, will in almost every case cover a range of strength classifications and sub-classifications. All sports bring something to the 'party' of strength development and, therefore, strength training. But that 'something' must be carefully interpreted and synthesised to meet the specific needs of a given athlete in a given sport. Weight training units, in particular, must be considered in this light.

Strength demands of sports

Sports may be classified according to the demands of the discipline/sport.

1. Long duration force application
These sports cover a wide range of duration and of applied force level. The force is, at its highest level, sub-maximal and may be either:

(a)   concentric with alternating relaxation and tension (e.g. rowing)
(b)   concentric but predominantly isometric with brief periods of lower tension (e.g. downhill skiing/skating)
(c)   near maximum isometric contraction for relatively short duration (e.g. gymnastic apparatus work). Energy supply is as much a limiting factor as strength.

2. Short duration, high force application
These sports again cover a wide range between maximum strength and maximum speed. For example, consider the extremes of discipline and sport, and the 'middle ground'.

(a) Maximum strength. In weight lifting, maximal weight must be accelerated over a given distance.

(b) Maximum speed. There is very little load/resistance to be moved at maximum speed – e.g. cricket ball, foil in fencing, tennis racquet. There are three different objectives under this heading:

(i) accelerating the implement to a maximum, e.g. tennis serve, volley ball spike

(ii) a given distance must be covered as fast as possible to counter an opponent's move e.g. judo, boxing, fencing. Also included here is acceleration from a stationary position. This may be preceded by a counter movement (e.g. jumping to block a volleyball) or without (e.g. ski jumping, sprint start)

(iii) optimal speed imparted to moderate resistance. These disciplines/sports include the throws in athletics each enjoying a pre-acceleration of the entire body or implement (turn, swings, shift, approach run). Synchronised 'strengths', the contribution of body limb complexes in sequence from feet to fingers, is key to performance.

3. Eccentric/concentric combination force application
These sports clearly involve elastic, ballistic, plyometric strength activity. All jumping activities in track and field; basketball lay-up shots; javelin and discus throw, hip and shoulder action, are included here.

Strength development training

From the discussion of theory, it should be evident that for each sports technique there will be a selection of exercises for the development of relevant strength. In a list of these exercises, broad classification would group exercises as *general*, *related* and *competition specific*. These terms are used throughout discussion of physical development and strength training, and may be described as follows.

General exercises

These exercises do not relate closely to specific technical models in sport. They must, however, provide the foundation upon which the more specific training for strength and technique are built. For this reason they have a greater share of an athlete's training load in his or her early development years and in the first 4–12 weeks of the annual cycle at all levels of development. They are used primarily:

• to ensure that the athlete does not develop disproportionately, i.e. by using a general conditioning circuit where all parts of the body are systematically exercised. Overuse injuries may be reduced by incorporating such sessions

- to offer a high level of active recovery, i.e. using general exercises during the competitive season where a total but light loading is of physiological benefit
- to establish a broad basis of general strength on which to build higher levels of specific strength. For example, the strength of the back muscles may limit loading in hip/knee extension work, therefore the back must be exercised
- to develop maximum strength in those muscles which are broadly related to the sport, i.e. in the use of power-cleans for jumpers. Here muscle areas involved in the events are developed, but not according to the time/force pattern implied by the sports techniques themselves
- to provide that level of strength in postural/synergist muscles which allows those muscles involved in the major joint actions of a given technique to operate optimally
- to afford a basis for athletes to perform more specific exercise. For example, exercises to develop foot speed in tennis require that the player is generally strong enough in the foot/ankle/calf to perform the exercises required.

These exercises may involve whole body movement as in cleans, or single joint movement as in biceps curls. Where whole body movement is involved then other aspects of physiological adaptation are also affected, for example, the oxygen transporting system.

Related exercises

These exercises relate to the specifics of *joint action* or *muscle dynamics* involved in the techniques of the athlete's sport. They take components of the sport's technique and develop them according to the type of strength required. Whereas general exercise for the discus thrower may be bench press, or dumbbell flying, related exercises might include slinging a medicine ball 'explosively' from kneeling with hips extended. A wide selection of such exercises is absolutely vital in an athlete's development.

Technically it may be desirable to employ sophisticated methods of electromyography to determine which related exercises are most suitable in terms of their relationship to a particular technique. Ivanova (1967) has examined these possibilities in a comprehensive comparison of the activity of muscles in rowing with related strength exercises. For example, if one considers muscle activity of the quadriceps in rowing as 100%, full squats scored 420%, whereas standing long jump scored 258%.

Specific exercises

These strength exercises are essentially whole technique exercises, but the movement may be given added resistance. Throwing with heavier hammers, training for rugby or football with a weighted jacket, sprinting from blocks in harness, playing tennis with a weighted racket, running with ankle weights and so on, reproduce the movement and relevant speed patterns. Only the absolute speed of movement is decreased. However, one important word of caution is if the resistance causes extraneous compensatory movements in the body, then the correct movement pattern will suffer. Athletes should work on a varied resistance unit when doing such work so as to avoid the development of wrong patterns of movement.

Development of strength for static muscular activity

It is now well-established that in strength training the principal type of training used should correspond to the type of contraction used in a given technique. It follows then that isometric or static methods are employed in the development of static or isometric muscle activity. It does *not* follow that isometric exercise will develop eccentric or concentric activity but some improvement can be expected as table 25 illustrates.

	static strength increase	*dynamic strength increase*
isometric-type training	15.1%	11.5%
concentric-type training	9.2%	18.1%

TABLE 25 Isometric and concentric-type contraction training compared (adapted from Brunner 1967)

Isometric activity mainly occurs in the maintenance of posture and such conditioning may be developed in related or specific exercises where whole or part of the technique is loaded isometrically. Functional isometric exercise may also contribute at this level. These isometric exercises are executed at various points throughout the range of movement involved in technique, the theory being that the strengthening effect throughout the range is achieved by 'irradiation'. However, isometric training methods, as advanced by Hettinger and Muller (1953), have a limited application to sport. Their value will almost certainly be with sports requiring great maximum strength and, even then, their use must be supplemented by dynamic work.

Finally, muscle groups should be trained in their postural or synergist roles. Leg swinging routines target the postural or synergist functions of the supporting leg. The postural role of the muscles of the spine is rehearsed by being supported face down on a bench only to the hips: holding the upper body horizontal, move the weighted arms forward, down, side (crucifix), down back (towards legs), down. This movement is repeated several times obliging the muscles of the spine to retain postural alignment while adjusting to changing forces.

Development of strength for dynamic muscular activity

This is the most frequently used type of exercise in the development of strength in sport. Variations of loading intensity, extent or density will dictate the relative contributions to maximum, elastic, or endurance strength. Even if absolute speed of movement is reduced, the relative speed variations within the movement should reproduce as closely as possible that of the particular action at a particular joint when it is incorporated in a given technique. Consequently, attempting to develop an efficient hurdle trail leg recovery or tennis forehand against elastic resistance is not advised. When elastic is stretched the resistance increases, thus decelerating the lever in a joint action. This does not happen in the actual event. Working against a pulley resistance, or throwing heavier implements, would allow a scaled-down pattern of acceleration closer to the pattern of the event.

Kusnezov (1975) suggests that, whether or not technique action is dynamic or static, occasional units which include the other will aid development in the principal action, especially in general exercises for strength development. This may be related to the concept of active recovery.

Development of strength by eccentric activity

Resistance can be greater than the maximum strength which the athlete can express. When this is the case there will be very distinct gains in maximum strength because the system will be overloaded throughout and the stimulus will be of long duration (Gundlach, 1968). Strength in all three types of muscle activity will increase by this method. Where the resistance is less than the maximum strength of the athlete, considerable strength gains can be expected in those aspects of technique where eccentric activity is followed by concentric. Various types of rebound, loaded rebound and depth jumps fall into this category.

Development of strength by ballistic activity

Ballistic activity refers to that type of exercise where there is rapid exchange between eccentric and concentric contraction. Skipping, hopping, rebound jumping, catching and returning medicine balls, and jump press-ups are all examples of this. The term 'plyometrics' was coined in the United States to cover this sort of training. Although it has become most closely associated with 'related exercises', it has now increased its contribution within the 'general exercises' programme. Verhoshansky (1971) first introduced depth jumping within a systematic progression of strength training. His emphasis was at 'general' rather than 'related' training – with a view to a more effective maximum strength programme. His exercises were based on the body's momentum loading the legs.

Kusnetsov carried this further by considering how to similarly load the arms by catching and returning heavy weights on a sloping ramp. His work then progressed to the use of machines such as pendulums where athletes were swung at walls and were obliged to 'kick' off the wall with either legs or arms. Once into the use of technology to provide a level of loading not previously available, he postulated that if machines could oblige athletes to express strength faster, by recruiting elastic and reflex mechanisms, then human potential would break new ground. In the year of his death (1986) he was working on a machine which would react to pressure by 'kicking back' faster than the athlete's muscles were eccentrically contracting – forcing the neuromuscular system to 'learn' to move through the eccentric-concentric exchange even faster. More recently, exercise programmes using a vibrating resistance have proved effective in strength development.

Komi (1990) has pointed out the importance of pre-activation of the extensor muscles before ground contact in jumping – like a pre-impacted compression of the 'bio-spring'. Komi and Bosco as early as 1978 stated that reactive strength is dependent on the storage of energy in the muscle's elastic component.

In many sports, improved performance depends on expressing sound technique with greater force at greater speed. The most difficult aspect of this is coordinating that greater force at greater speed. There is little doubt that it is related to elastic strength but it also involves that sophistication of technique where the existing synchronisation of a specific neuromuscular pattern is challenged. In many cases this leads to reduction in performance as the new timings are learned.

Development of maximum strength

The optimal stimulus for the development of maximum strength is related to the following factors:

- the intensity of the stimulus relative to the maximum strength of the athlete. (This may be interpreted as a recruitment of maximum available motor units.)
- the duration of that stimulus
- the frequency of recruitment of maximum available motor units.

Loading to create such a stimulus will be that which will allow exercise to be performed once only. This load is referred to as maximum or 100%, for a particular exercise. Such intensity, however, cannot be considered acceptable in the following cases.

(1) Where the athlete has an unstable technique when performing the exercise. Here, the athlete must work with many repetitions of lighter loads until technique is stabilised. The possibility of injury is therefore very slight. However, should these lighter loads be repeated to the point of fatigue in training units, the load will again tend, in effect, to approach maximum, bringing associated problems. As a guide, the number of repetitions should be 12–15 and should not take an athlete to the point where exercise technique deteriorates.

(2) Where the athlete has not quite reached maturity and the muscle/bone/joint system is not yet completely stabilised. To work an athlete to maximum under these circumstances may interfere with muscle/bone connections and disturb the complex integrity of a system of joints. The contractile force potential of the big muscle groups would be completely out of sympathy with the development of bone and joint, and the juncture of tendon and bone. This is especially relevant where loads are taken on the shoulders while also attempting maximum loading of the knee and hip extensors. This then places the lumbar spine and sacroiliac region at risk.

(3) Where maximum strength development is not relevant to sports technique.

(4) In mesocycle 1_2 (see p. 324), where 3–5 sets of 15 repetition max. are used to establish a maximum strength base.

In terms of the training unit then, where maximum strength development is sought, optimal effects will result from working over several sets at an intensity which allows the exercise to be performed 1–5 times, i.e. 85–100% maximum (table 28, p. 252). Recovery periods of up to five minutes between sets are almost essential to avoid cumulative fatigue.

Where isometric training methods are being used, and the load may be varied, contractions against 80–100% maximum, held for periods of 9–12 seconds, should be used for advanced athletes, while intensities of 60–80% held for 6–9 seconds seems adequate for the novice. Using a lighter loading and repeating an exercise to the point of fatigue will also improve strength, but to a limited extent as such work moves into the area of endurance training. For the young athlete, this type of work over many exercises will establish a sound general basis of strength.

Eccentric work with loads in excess of maximum isometric strength will also develop maximum concentric strength. Specific intensities are not available from most research authorities, but personal experimentation suggests that loadings from 105–175% of the maximum concentric load can be used over specific ranges of movement. If, for example, an athlete's half squat was 100 kg, the eccentric load will range from 105 kg to 175 kg. To achieve this, the staggered sets, as advanced by Lay (1970), are used, but in reverse. Safety must be emphasised here and pins *must* be able to accept the load at the bottom end of the exercise.

The isokinetic machines, while offering a considerable duration and maximum intensity of contraction, may interfere with the natural patterns of acceleration–deceleration in the muscle. On the other hand, where there is less emphasis on acceleration–deceleration in the muscle due to specific demands of a sport, this method offers considerable advantage. The case for inclusion in the programme will be stronger then, for rowers, swimmers and cross-country skiers, than for hurdlers or tennis players.

Several strength development systems focus on mixing the strength training stimuli. This is programmed at the inter-unit and intra-unit levels.

For example, inter-unit mixing may take the form of alternating 3–5 x 5 x 85% with 3–5 x 10 x 65% with one day rest between. Intra-unit mixing may take the form of 'sandwiching' 5 x 85%; 10 x 65%; 5 x 85%; 10 x 65%. Again, the intra-unit mixing may, in order to provide a very rapid acceleration of maximum strength levels, mix 'orthodox' weights loadings with elastic or plyometric loadings. An example of this would be 5 x 85% half squat; 5 x 5 hurdle rebounds; 5 x 85% squat; 5 x 5 hurdle rebounds. This latter example is applied on a base of several weeks of 'orthodox' strength training units, or inter-unit alternation of intensities as suggested above. When applied it is usually for no more than three weeks.

Electronic stimulation of muscle to develop strength is a further option, but there is varied opinion on its application to elastic strength – specific activity.

Finally, it has been suggested that just as there is some optimal frequency of stimulus within a training unit, there is also an optimal interval of recovery between units where maximum strength is being developed. This interval is variously set at 36–48 hours for natural recovery to take place. This said, by varying the 'target areas' on alternate days, maximum strength units can be worked on daily, e.g. day 1, 3, 5, upper body; day 2, 4, 6, lower body.

Development of elastic strength

Broadly speaking, elastic strength can be developed by improving maximum strength and/or speed of coordinated muscle contraction. The problem lies in effecting an optimal compromise of development that can be translated to the sports technique. This is a problem because if the athlete works with a heavy loading then both strength and speed of contraction will develop for that specific exercise. However, there is not necessarily an increase in the speed of muscle contraction in the sports technique where loading is much less. On the other hand, if loading is very light there will be an improvement in speed of working against that load provided that load is within a certain range – variously stated at 5–20%. If outside this range, compensatory movements interfere with technical precision, so a programme which varies the intensity and consequently the speed of movement is recommended. It is therefore suggested that maximum strength work and light resisted related exercises must be used within each microcycle (see chapter 21) if specific elastic strength is to be developed. Moreover, within units for maximum strength, a lower intensity set or sets should be included in the exercise regimes. Experimental programmes have been tried to develop maximum strength first over several months, then followed by a training programme to develop speed. However, this attempted development of elastic strength in series has far less value than if both areas of development are advanced 'in parallel'.

In terms of training units the intensity of stimulus should be around 75% maximum, using 4–6 sets of 6–10 repetitions. As with maximum strength work, up to five minutes rest should be allowed between sets. Using this particular format, Harre (1973) and associates believe both maximum and elastic strength can be advanced at the same time. If maximum strength work is being done with training units, then elastic strength supplementary work is proposed by Harre (1973) at loadings of 30–50% maximum. Personal experimentation has shown increases in both elastic and maximum strength by alternating loads of 55–60% with 85–100%.

Strength training for the development of elastic strength, where relative strength is critical, should not be accompanied by muscle hypertrophy and consequent increase in body weight. According to Bührle (1971) hypertrophy is optimal where loadings of 65–80% maximum are repeated 6–10 times in 3–4 sets or more. Body builders have been known to work 6 sets of 12 repetitions at 60–65%. This work is not recommended for athletes requiring increased relative strength. Harre (1973) suggests that preference be given to working in specific movements with body parts weighted at 3–5% body weight in total, as used by gymnasts (wrist weights, jackets): 'The high muscle tension necessary for an increase of strength, is thus generated by the "explosively" quick muscle contraction.'

Without doubt the greatest single contribution to improved elastic strength is via ballistic/plyometric routines which focus on related and specific exercises. Such work is with body weight, limb weights, weighted jackets using varied weight, light resistances such as medicine balls, logs, sand sacks and gymnastic equipment. It can take 1–2 hours of fairly concentrated work, but with sufficient recovery periods included to ensure that fatigue does not take the 'elasticity' out of the athlete's movements. It is this repeated 'elastic' neuromuscular control of impact which provides the training effect. However, for the long bones and joints this may set the scene for damage. The extent of loading must, then, be carefully controlled to avoid fatigue.

Development of strength endurance

It is quite clear that an athlete with maximum strength of 200 kg in one exercise, will repeat the exercise with greater comfort at 50 kg than the athlete who has maximum strength of 100 kg. Also, if two athletes have the maximum strength of 200 kg, the athlete with a well-developed oxygen transporting system will endure more repetitions at 50 kg than the athlete with poor oxygen transport status. However, the exact relationship between these poles and the characteristic of strength endurance is not clear. It would appear that the foundations of training in strength endurance lie in the ability to perform the highest possible number of repetitions against a loading which is greater than that normally experienced in the event. Moreover, according to Saziorski (1971), maximum strength ceases to be a critical factor if the strength requirement is less than 30% of maximum. While at the other end, according to Astrand (1970), oxygen transport efficiency is a necessary precursor of the anaerobic development required for development of strength endurance (see chapter 5).

A complex form of training appears to be the key, with resisted exercises preferably of the competition specific or special variety being employed. Thus, the athlete may run in snow, sand, uphill, in plough, in surf, or dragging a sled, while the oarsman may row pulling a drag and the swimmer may likewise swim pulling a resistance. Where general exercises are employed, circuit-type training is used and repetitions of approximately 50–75% of maximum, with a loading of 40–60% maximum and optimal recovery between, seems a sound rule of thumb.

Unit construction for strength development

A detailed account of unit construction was presented in six articles by Lay in *Athletics Weekly* 1969/70, which examined simple sets, super sets, pyramids, circuits and so on. The detail of these systems is beyond the scope of this book but, for reference, figure 72 suggests a relationship between intensity and extent.

FIG. 72 Pyramid relating intensity and extent of loading, suggested by Bührle in 'Die Lehre Der Leichtathletic' – 26.1.71. He suggested maximum strength depends upon (a) cross-sectional areas of muscle (reps. of 6–10); (b) intramuscular coordination (reps. of 1–3); (c) inter-muscular coordination (Technique and Standard of Performance). (Modified – Dick/Arbeit, 1996).

Microcycle construction

In designing the strength training detail of microcycles/macrocycles, a coach must have a feeling for the situation summarised by figure 73. Each athlete has his specific development requirement with the 'specific strength' demands of a given sport, event or even position within a team. For example, in rugby the specific strength demands of a prop forward are not the same as those of a wing three-quarter. So the detail of strength training units must reflect this. But more than this, any given microcycle is put together to meet not one but several training objectives and very careful value judgement must be applied to ensure that each objective is constructively pursued without compromising progress of the others. In short, strength training units cannot be seen in isolation.

Moreover, the practical implications of developing and monitoring strength are rather greater when applied to athletes who have relatively long competition seasons, e.g. soccer, rugby, hockey; where double periodised years are pursued; or where the nature of the sport and related lifestyle includes several irregularly spread tournaments throughout the year e.g. tennis, squash, golf and to a certain extent Formula 1.

Of course, such variations in relationship of preparation and competition periods also influence development of other areas of conditioning such as endurance – but the greatest problems are in the strength programme.

General strength development will focus on an all-round balanced increase in the area of maximum strength, strength of synergists, stabiliser groups, compensatory work, and therapy or rehabilitation according to the demands of the sport/event and needs of the athlete.

Related and specific strength will focus on the specific joint actions and muscle dynamics required for the sport, its techniques and its competition framework and detail. It is the developmental bias implied by this kind of work which makes it essential that a general strength programme is spread, albeit with shifting overall load priority, throughout the year.

To construct an individual athlete's strength training microcycles then, the coach must know:

- the general all-round strength balance of the athlete
- maximum strength demands of the sport and the athlete's status in this area
- related/specific strength demands of the sport and the athlete's status in this area, e.g. a sprinter requires: starting strength via harness running; sprinting strike strength via skip drills; sprinting stride strength via bounding; sprinting arms strength via speed ball routines.

Evaluation of strength status

There is a wide variety of tests to evaluate strength, but not all are relevant to the assessment of strength for a sport. Selection must take into account the specific quality to be measured. If eccentric, concentric or isometric muscular activity is being measured, then it is logical that any testing procedure should involve that activity. If the strength is maximum, elastic or endurance then, again, the testing procedure should measure that type of strength. The testing procedure must be valid, reliable and objective and, furthermore, must be validated against performance, or some test, in a given technique. If possible the testing procedure should involve the dynamics of movement typical of the event.

This said, it has become common practice to create specific strength controls. These controls are designed to monitor status of that type of strength which the coach associates either with progress at a particular phase in the training year or with level of preparation for optimal performance. So, for a long jumper in mid-preparation phase, a control might be standing long jump – whereas in early competition season it might be distance covered in 10 bounds against the time taken.

This approach has been applied by the former Soviet Union sprint coaches in linking the target 100 m times to particular jumps tests, as is shown in the table below.

target time	standing long (m)	jump reach (cm)	3 bounds* (m)	5 bounds* (m)	10 bounds* (m)
10.20–10.65	2.90–3.20	76–85	9.20–10.00	15.90–17.10	29.50–39.50
10.70–11.10	2.70–3.00	68–77	8.50–9.10	14.60–15.60	27.00–37.00
11.20–11.70	2.60–2.90	60–69	7.90–8.50	14.00–15.00	25.00–35.00
11.80–12.20	2.50–2.80	53–61	7.50–8.10	13.40–14.40	23.00–33.00
12.30–12.70	2.40–2.70	46–54	7.20–7.80	12.80–13.80	21.00–31.00
12.80–13.20	2.30–2.60	39–47	6.80–7.40	12.20–13.20	19.00–29.00

* From standing.

TABLE 26 Bounding controls

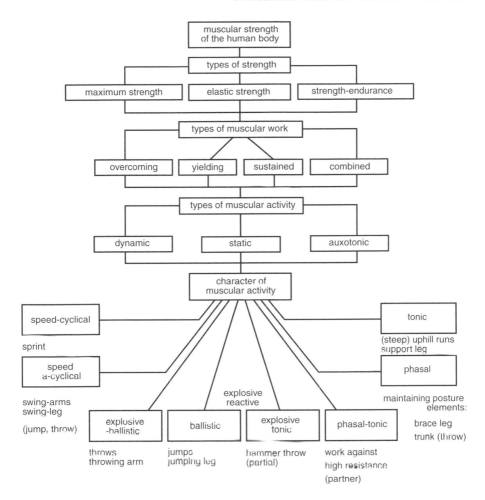

FIG. 73 Summary of different forms of muscular strength

Figure 73 is offered by way of a summary of muscular strength and its various forms expressed to meet the demands of individual sports. Development of strength to meet these demands is a unique blend of general, related and specific strength training programmed according to the athlete's status relative to these demands; the time available to train; and the quality of the training environment.

In concluding this topic on strength development, table 28 provides a summary of suggested training loads.

Notes on strength training

(1) Emphasis in strength training is obviously on development of specific contractile properties. It is essential that mobility and stretching work is also included to ensure that a full range of movement is possible in all joint actions and that normal growth and development may proceed naturally.

(2) In young athletes and novices it is advisable that a broad basis of general strength training is used, involving medium intensity over sets of 8–10 repetitions.

(3) In strength training for women, while strength objectives, training load extent, intensity and frequency can be as for men, progression should be more gradual and over a longer period. (Note: female athletes should avoid jumping activities or any exercise which puts sudden impact on the sacroiliac joint in the 2–3 days pre-menstruation period – see note 8 page 227.)

(4) In young and novice athletes considerable attention in training should be directed at development of those muscles which stabilise the spine on the pelvis (abdominal and back muscles) and the rotators of the spine.

(5) Maximum training must maintain a natural balance of protagonist: antagonist strength ratio, e.g. building up the quadriceps and neglecting the hamstrings creates an imbalance.

(6) Maximum strength programmes must not be attempted when an athlete is already fatigued or has not warmed up.

(7) Passive mobility work must *never* follow maximum strength training.

(8) Activity should cease whenever there is sharp pain in the exercising muscles.

(9) In pursuing a maximum strength programme for a particular joint action, there should be variety in the exercises used. This not only enhances the strength development process but contributes to a healthy motivational climate. For example, although squat work might be the focus of exercise for developing the quadriceps and hip extensor, it should be interrupted and augmented from time to time with such exercises as leg press, hack lifts, front squat, knee extensions, step-ups, slide squat, single leg squats, etc.

(10) In all strength work, the range limits should be determined by neuromuscular control – *not* by the body's skeletal structure. For example in squat work, the 'full squat' limit should be as deep as the controlled eccentric contraction of the quadriceps will allow – *not* the collapsing of thighs against calves.

(11) Strength training in the growing years should be progressed in stages (table 27a).

(12) Elastic strength work in the growing years also progresses in stages (table 27b).

(13) Until the growing athlete has stabilised in bone/joint development, it is inadvisable to load the spine when exercising. As a rule, weights should not be taken on the shoulders until 16 or 17 years of age, unless the athlete has an extensive background of general strength work which has systematically developed the musculature supporting the spine.

(14) When loads are taken on the shoulders, strain is placed on the spine. The spine *must* therefore be kept straight, with no exaggerated lumbar curve nor rounding of the shoulders as either will put the joint complex of the spine at a serious mechanical disadvantage and consequently risk of serious injury could be considerable.

age	training
5–7	Introduce a wide variety of strength-related basic exercises with little or no weight; develop the concept of a training unit; teach sound exercise techniques; progress from body weight work through partner exercises to lightly resisted exercise. Volume kept low per exercise.
8–10	Gradually increase number of exercise repetitions; techniques for those weights exercises which do not load the spine; resistance remains low with very gradual increase; volume gradually increased; monitor exercise stress. Use a circuit approach.
11–13	Develop weights exercise units without spine loading; emphasise exercise technical exactness; increase resistance within a volume limit of 12–15 reps; introduce more advanced exercises with little or no resistance; the object is not muscle hypertrophy; use a circuit approach.
14–15	Develop more advanced weights exercise units without spine loading; ensure sound exercise techniques; mix resistance in exercises; introduce sport-specific components; increase volume via sets. Use a stage approach.
16+	Move into programmes which are senior athlete variants, including spine loading only when athlete has a foundation of strength training experience similar to that described here.

TABLE 27a Progression of strength training in stages according to age groups

age	training
10–14	Variety of movement experience and rhythm training: alternating jumps, light hops, two-legged bounces. Varied rhythms in a series of jumps. Jumps on/off low boxes/benches. Emphasis must be on speed not maximum height/distance. Surfaces should be no more cushioned than for senior athletes, or the reactive/elastic strength dynamics are not developed.
15–18	Programmes should progress from the 10–14 stage in terms of speed and volume. Reactive/elastic strength at the highest level does not appear to be maximum strength-dependent. However, parallel development of maximum strength ensures programme progression.

TABLE 27b Progression of elastic strength work

(15) All related/specific exercises with resistance must be well schooled from a technique point of view and kept close to the timings/accelerations of the technical models required by the athlete's sport or event. This implies learning with lighter loads, and fairly tight supervision through early progressions.

(16) Exhausting anaerobic endurance work should not follow maximum or elastic strength work, as this will create a climate for connective tissue injury.

(17) The general progression of strength should take the following shape:

- carefully selected activities and games to develop all-round balanced strength
- circuit training focused on all joint complexes for a balance of strength
- stage training using the same exercises as circuit training
- stage training using resistances such as weighted jackets; wrist/ankle weights; weight belts; medicine balls; sand sacks, etc.*
- weight training based on multiple repetitions (up to 12) on foundation of sound technique*
- progressive loading weight training with periodic tests for maxima*
- special programme mixing intensities inter and intraunit
- special programmes using machines and/or electronic stimulation, etc.* (Note: not all athletes will be suited to this area of progression.)

(18) Women's strength training programmes should be continued, if at a slightly lower extent, throughout the competition season. This is not such a necessary requirement with men.

(19) There is a time lag between achievement of new best results in control tests for strength, be that general, related or specific, and best performance in the athlete's sport. The time lag will vary according to the strength characteristic measured and the athlete involved. Coaches should be aware of this and plan the phasing of strength training and introduction of competition accordingly.

(20) In those sports where there is high maximum strength dependence, a strength unit is often introduced the day before competition. The theory behind this practice is that the neuromuscular system will remain in a state of high excitation for 24 hours after such a unit. The key is to avoid units where strength training is in pursuit of maximum values, or where the athlete is fatigued by the unit.

(21) Elastic strength units require a longer period of recovery than orthodox concentric strength work with weights, etc. Consequently, it is *not* advisable to include elastic strength units in the 3–4 days before competition.

(22) Each exercise or movement requires an adjustment of balance to stabilise body parts. Strength training programmes must, then, include a variety of exercise and movement through the equipment and methods used, as much as through the combinations of training ratios and structures of loading. Strength training machines, orthodox weight training equipment, medicine balls, water resistance, partner work, heavier sport – specific implements, weights jackets, etc. *all* have their place somewhere in the athlete's year-round programme.

(23) In team games, the specific strength requirement of players varies according to the demands of their respective positions. For example, in rugby union, the strength programme for props differs from second row or back row, etc.

*parallel development of specific strength

objective	intensity of training load	repetitions in each set	sets in each unit	training system	recovery between sets	time holding isometric	evaluation procedures contraction	(possible event app.) probable event app.
Development of maximum strength in events where single expression of maximum strength is required.	Concentric 85%→100% Eccentric •105%→175%	1→5	A 5→8 N 2→4	Simple sets Super sets Stagger sets Pyramids-5 x 85%→1 x 100% Mixed sets (ecc-concisom)	4→5 mins	A 9→12 secs 80%–100% N 6→9 secs 60%–80%	Max. lift dynamometer	e.g. weight lifting shot discus hammer javelin (jumps) rugby front 5
Development of maximum strength in events where multiple expression of maximum strength is required.	70%→85%	5→10	2→5	Simple sets Super sets Pyramids-8 x 75% ↔6 x 80% ↔5 x 85%	2→4 mins		Max. lift dynamometer	e.g. (circle throws) javelin high, triple, long sprints hurdles, rowing
Development of elastic strength where work is also done in other units for maximum strength.	30%→50% or 55%→65% or 3%→5% body	6→10 5→8 6→10	4→6 4→6 3→5	Simple sets Super sets Pyramid by intensity only. 10 x 30%: 10 x 40%: 10 x 50%: 10 x 55%: 10 x 60%: 10 x 65%	3→5 mins		Standing long, triple, vert. jump etc.	All explosive sports

TABLE 28 Summary of suggested training loads

objective	intensity of training load	repetitions in each set	sets in each unit	training system	recovery between sets	time holding isometric contraction	evaluation procedures	(possible event app.) probable event app.
	weight resistance exercises involving whole technique (e.g. gymnastics, jumping, etc.) or related plyometrics specific & special strength exercises	5→10	Performed as stage training 3→5	Performed as stage training				A advanced athlete N Novice athlete *Advanced athlete only
Development of elastic and maximum strength simultaneously	a 75% or b 3%–5% bodyweight resistance exercises involving whole technique	6→10	4→6	Simple sets Super sets	3→5 mins		Standing long, triple, vert. jump etc.	All explosive sports e.g. hockey, rugby, soccer

TABLE 28 Continued

objective	intensity of training load	repetitions in each set	sets in each unit	training system	recovery between sets	time holding isometric	evaluation procedures contraction	(possible event app.) probable event app.
	or c alternating between 85% and elastic/plyometric equivalent			Performed as stage training	3 →5 mins			General for all sports especially young or novice athlete
Development of maximum strength base or strength endurance for all events.	N 30%→40% A 60%→65%	25%→50% Max. 15	4→6 3→5	Simple sets circuit Simple sets stage	Optimal 4→5 mins		Max. repetitions Max. holding time, etc. Max. lift	All sports e.g. rowing, wrestling swimming cross-country skiing
Development of strength endurance in those events with high demands for it	40%→60% Max according to activity loading the basic technique (e.g. hill running, swimming, rowing dragging resistance, etc.)	50%→75%	3→5	Circuit training	30→45 secs	Not isom. but controlled lifts with 30%→50%, max. e.g. 6 secs flex. Performed as stage training	Max. repetitions per unit of time	swimming cross-country skiing ice hockey steeplechase

TABLE 28 Continued

SUMMARY

Broadly speaking, the athlete develops strength to make available a greater potential force of energy expression. This force may be used against external resistance in pursuit of performance objectives where speed, strength, endurance and mobility are variously, and separately, the criteria of success. The role of strength for a muscle group assumes a unique character according to the technical demands of a sport. This role ranges from dynamic to static and from relative to absolute in pursuit of specific performance objectives. Methods used in development of strength reflect the demands of these objectives.

15 THEORY AND PRACTICE OF SPEED DEVELOPMENT

SPEED IN SPORT

Speed in training theory defines the capacity of moving a limb or part of the body's lever system or the whole body with the greatest possible velocity. Maximum value of such movements would be without loading. Thus, the discus thrower's arm will have greatest velocity in the throwing phase if no discus is held and velocity would be reduced as the implement's weight is increased relative to the athlete's absolute strength.

Speed is measured in metres per second, as, for example, in quantifying the value for speed of moving one part of the body's lever system relative to another; the forward speed of the body in sprinting or at point of take-off in jumping; and the velocity of implements and balls at release or on being struck. The time taken to achieve a certain task may also be considered a measure of the athlete's speed. So controls for sprinting speed might be time taken to sprint 30 m. Or again, the number of repetitions of a task within a short period of time might be considered an index of speed. For example, the number of repetition runs in a shuttle run over 5 m in 20 seconds. Measuring equipment includes stop watches video-linked to relevant IT and software, photoelectric cells coupled to print-out devices, cinematographic techniques based on film speed, force plates, and so on.

Speed is a critical component of that complex requirement for achievement in competitive sport. It has four strands (fig. 74).

Strength in itself will not influence maximum speed of limb movement, but developing greater strength and applying it at speed will certainly positively influence performance. There is a critical sequence in the progression of developing performance in this respect.

- Develop the general strength and mobility consistent with the technical model(s) required.
- Learn sound technique(s) (technical models).
- Develop related and specific strength.
- Learn to perform these at optimal speed.
- Develop general/related/specific strength to apply at optimal speed.

'Optimal' speed is as close to maximum as possible without compromising the technical model(s). In endurance sports, speed's role on the one hand expands the range of tactical variants. On the other, it is, as in the progression suggested above, within development of related and specific endurance.

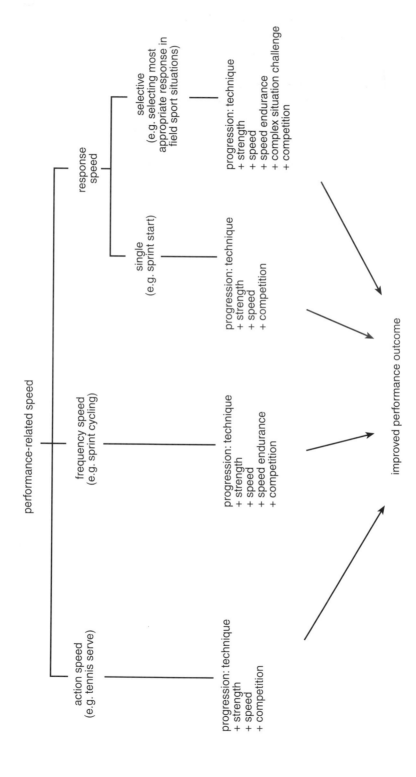

FIG. 74 Four strands of speed

Speed may be a determining factor directly, as in, for example, reacting to the starter's pistol, or indirectly, as, for example, in the development of kinetic energy in jumping. The difference between direct and indirect is that, with the former, 'optimal speed' is close to maximum, whereas with the latter, 'optimal speed' is a critical percentage of maximum which allows maximum expression of relevant strength. It is therefore important to bear in mind that speed increases may not necessarily lead to improved performance. The pattern of speed and acceleration of relative movements must be synchronised so that each part of the lever system can make an optimal force contribution. For example, there would be no point in making the discus arm so fast that it began to make its contribution before the legs and trunk, nor would it benefit the long jumper to have so much horizontal speed at the board that there was insufficient time for the take-off leg to express the strength required for vertical lift. Speed development is, then, very much a matter of learning how to use it.

SPEED DEVELOPMENT

Speed in practice

There are seven areas in sports performance where training will enhance speed.

(1) Response to a signal as, for example, in the sprinter's reaction to the gun, or the tennis player's reaction in volleying.
(2) Capacity to accelerate: this is of particular importance to those athletes who must beat opponents across the ground or who must quickly reach a particular point on the court/pitch to execute a technique.
(3) Capacity to rapidly adjust balance following execution of one technique in order to prepare to execute another. This applies to every games situation.
(4) Achievement of maximum speed: the athlete here is executing a given technique as fast as he can without breakdown of that technique's effectiveness. Often speed is mistakenly thought of as an entity in itself. It is not. It is a sophistication of technique, where all demands of the technique are performed at the highest speed consistent with the general synchronised framework.
(5) Capacity to maintain maximum speed once it is reached. This also is a coordination issue, and is seen, for example, in 100 m where an athlete such as Bailey* can maintain his maximum speed of 12.05 m/sec for only 20 m. This is not followed as one might expect by a gradual loss of speed for the balance of the race. Rather there is a breakdown of coordination for 10 m (Bailey – 11.76 m/sec) before a gradual deceleration will commence through to the finish.
(6) Capacity to limit the effect of endurance factors on speed: the rate at which fuel reaches the working muscles and waste products are removed, eventually represents a limiting factor to producing the high intensity muscle

*Donovan Bailey – Canada – Olympic 100 m champion 1996

contraction and quality coordination necessary to maintain maximum or near maximum speed.

(7) Capacity to choose correct action options: in many sports, the difference between success and failure is the speed at which the correct action option is chosen by a player or players to solve a problem posed by the opposition; and a problem is then set for the opposition. The better the opposition or higher the level of competition, the less time a player has to make those choices.

These areas are embraced by the four strands of fig. 74.

Strand	Areas			
Action speed	(2)	(4)		
Frequency speed	(2)	(3)	(5)	(6)
Single response speed	(1)	(2)		
Selective response speed	(3)	(5)	(6)	(7)

The development of speed is dependent on several factors, the main ones being as follows:

(1) Innervation (fig. 39, p. 109): a high frequency of alternation between stimulation and inhibition of neurones, and an accurate selection and regulation of motor units, makes it possible to achieve a high frequency of movement and/or speed of movement, married to an optimal expression or deployment of strength. This is the fundamental ability to move limbs at maximum velocity.

(2) Elasticity (fig. 41, p. 111): the capacity to capitalise on muscle tone via the elastic component of muscle has relevance to those sports demanding high starting acceleration (as in sprints and most field sports) or 'rapid strike' (as in sprinting and jumping). The precise mechanisms involved are not clear but there appears to be a complex coordination of motor units, reflexes, elastic component and the ability to contract muscle at high speed. The characteristic is, however, identifiable and has been referred to in sports jargon as 'bounce'. Elasticity is connected to relative strength and elastic strength.

(3) Biochemistry: speed would appear to rely specifically on the energy supplies within muscle, i.e. alactic anaerobic pathway (see chapter 6), on the speed of its mobilisation, and, where speed is the determining factor beyond approx. 15 seconds (e.g. 200 m sprint), the lactic anaerobic pathway kicks in. Short duration maximum intensity work appears to be the training stimulus for development of this area, via changes in glycolitic and mitochondrial enzymes (Costill et al 1979; Helsten et al 1993, 1994; Sharp et al 1986), and in fibretype composition of muscle (Costill et al 1979; Jacobs et al 1987; Helsten et al 1993, 1994).

(4) Muscle relaxability: the ability of the muscle to relax and to allow stretch in speed exercises is fundamental to perfect technique and to a high frequency of movement. Harre (1973) has said: 'If these qualities are insufficiently developed, the required range of movement cannot be achieved in the course of the movement, particularly at the points of reversal of movement, as the synergists

have to overcome too great a resistance.' Training which obliges the athlete to relax all muscles not directly involved with a given series of joint actions, even in fatigue, is of the utmost importance. Mobility work and focused application of psychoregulatory techniques for physical, mental and emotional relaxation are also clearly indicated here.

(5) Will-power: the athlete must concentrate on maximum voluntary effort to achieve maximum speed. However, unlike the weight lifter who has a quantified target as the focus of his concentration, the athlete has nothing more to go on than physical sensation, comparison with another athlete, and the evidence of a stop watch. Human error may occur with the latter, so the coach must ensure that all possible information on speeds and times is given to the athlete. Moreover, to provide a suitable stimulus or target, speed work may be performed in groups, using handicaps, competitions, etc.

(6) Action acceptor: many situations, especially in combat sports and field games, etc., demand rapid selection of relevant cues and the technical ability to do so accurately will influence speed of movement or reaction.

(7) Environment: warm climate, altitude, footwear, running surface, low air resistance, clothing which enhances aerodynamics, or anything which may oblige an athlete to learn how to move faster will assist speed development.

(8) Aptitude, early development and optimisation of development stages.

- Speed athletes have an above average population of fast-twitch muscle fibres.
- Optimal trainability of reactive/responsive and frequency speed abilities and optimal preconditions for motor learning are 8–11 (girls), 8–13 (boys) – with a 'peaking' at 9–10 (girls), 10–12 (boys).
- During puberty (11–15 girls; 13–17 boys) there is improved trainability of the strength component of speed. Initial training of fast strength/elastic strength should be with low resistance. Maximum strength appropriate to speed per- formance is introduced later.
- High-quality early technical schooling is essential in creating the right physical and timing framework(s) of coordination through which speed, then strength, then endurance may be applied.
- Anticipation is the capacity to read situations ahead of the game – (psychological precognition). It permits earlier choice of action options and so reduced response time whether for single or multiple action responses to the challenge of the situation. It profoundly influences Action Speed, Single Response Speed and Selection Response Speed.

Training for speed development

Speed development for track events has been extensively documented and will provide a useful base for the practice of speed development for other sports.

Intensity

The intensity of training loads for speed development commence around 75% maximum. Here, the athlete is learning, at relatively high intensity, those adjustments necessary to maintain the pace or rhythm of a technique while 'timing' is put under pressure. Gradually, the athlete moves towards 100%. However, progression demands that the athlete attempts to surpass existing speed limits. Rehearsal of technique at intensities which break new ground is clearly not possible in great volume for reasons ranging from mental concentration through to energy production. It is for this reason that measures are taken to facilitate the learning process such as training athletes at altitude; pulling the athlete on an elastic rope or pulley system; reducing the weight of implements; reducing the time scales for making choices of action; in fact anything which requires a speed beyond the existing 100%.

The sequence to developing performance set out below is not a once only sequence. It belongs to a continuing cycle which operates over a year and even through mesocycles (see chapter 21). This also applies where endurance is part of that sequence. The sequence of development is:

• develop a level of general conditioning which permits learning a sound basic technique
• learn a sound basic technique
• develop a level of related and specific conditioning which permits progressive sophistication of technique
• develop technique at speed.

Technical components should be learned and stabilised at slower speeds. Nevertheless, from the outset the athlete should be encouraged to consolidate technique by accelerating the level of intensity. This is necessary because the transfer of technique learned at a slow speed to the demands of maximum speed is usually very complex. To this end, practices are used in sprinting where the athlete runs a distance of, say, 75 m, concentrates on the perfection of running action for 40 m and then raises the speed of running for 35 m. Or a technical component, such as those rehearsed in sprinting drills, is worked for 25 m and then the athlete gradually accelerates to near maximum intensity over the next 50 m. A hurdler strides over three hurdles with 5–7 strides between, then sprints over three hurdles with the normal three stride pattern. A tennis player brings the speed of service down to that which allows him to place the ball accurately in the service court, and to 'feel' the synchronisation of each element in the technique. The idea is to relate to the timing of the technique as a basis for development; *then* to progress pace but within the constraints of sound technique. Finally the athlete masters that level of speed which permits him to select a given pace within his range, and which is sufficient to overcome the challenge of his opposition.

There should be no fatigue factors in speed training because it is essential for the nervous system to be in a state of optimal excitement. Consequently speed training will follow immediately upon relevant warm-up. Endurance or strengthening work may follow, but never precede, speed training.

Extent

A relationship exists between intensity and extent of loading. If the athlete is working at maximum intensity, the extent of loading cannot be great. On the other hand, it is necessary for the athlete to rehearse a technique frequently at high intensity, if new levels of speed are to be stabilised. The following points may serve as a useful guideline to making decisions on extent.

(1) Techniques can be repeated in high volume *and* high intensity only if presented in small 'learning packages'. This ensures the highest speed of execution *and* recovery periods which permit athletes time to consolidate neuromuscular memory patterns. So a large number of sets with small numbers of repetitions of very high intensity would be most suitable.

(2) In sprint training the minimum distance to develop acceleration is that which allows the athlete to achieve near maximum speed. For most athletes this is around 30–40 m. However, in other sports there are constraints imposed by the confines of the playing area. In some sports, then, the athlete must learn to achieve maximum acceleration over a very short distance (5–10 m) and 'arrive' at the conclusion of such a burst of speed, prepared to select and execute a high precision technique. Soccer, tennis, and basketball are examples of such sports.

(3) Where maximum speed is being practised, a limiting factor to effective rehearsal can be the exhausting process of accelerating to maximum speed. For example, in long jump and in games where passing must be practised at the highest speed, the athletes must lift their pace from being stationary to the pace required. This is very tiring. To overcome the problem, some athletes practise from longer rolling starts or with the assistance of downhill starts. This means that although the athlete will look to distances of 10–30 m to practise maximum speed itself, it may be necessary to have 40–60 m roll-in to reach that speed.

(4) Optimal values can only be determined by individual testing on how long maximum speed can be held. The initial problem is, of course, to achieve maximum speed. It has already been pointed out that Bailey could only maintain his maximum speed for 20 m. Coordination and concentration are the keys to extending this distance, but it is unlikely that it will reach 30 m or further without the assistance offered by altitude, following wind, etc., and then over distances of around 25–40 m.

(5) In sprinting, most athletes require 5–6 seconds to achieve maximum speed. This suggests that distances of 50–60 m are required to develop the linking of initial acceleration and the 'pick up' to maximum speed.

Density

Recovery periods between runs at maximum speed must be long enough to restore working capacity, but short enough to maintain excitement of the nervous system and optimal body temperature. Given a reasonably warm climate, the interval between each run should be 4–6 minutes, which creates problems for athletes living in countries with long cold winters.

In the interest of gaining optimum advantage from each run, it might be advisable to allow this interval and to 'warm-up' before each run. Sets should again be used with, say, 3–4 runs per set and 2–3 sets per unit.

For 100% recovery from a maximum speed or elastic/fast strength or speed endurance unit, approximately 48 hours is required. A further 24–36 hours is required for the peak of over-compensation (fig. 88) (Grosser 1991).

Units

The total number of runs per unit, as indicated above, should lie between six and 12, although individual variations exist. The number of units per weekly microcycle (microcycles, macrocycles and units are explained in chapter 21) will vary throughout the year, but at least one unit per microcycle must be included in mesocycle 1 of the annual cycle (see p. 306) with 2–3 in mesocycle 2, and 2–4 in mesocycle 3, irrespective of the sport. With endurance sports, speed work will range in intensity from maximum to racing pace and unit distribution will vary according to racing distance, phase of the year and the athlete concerned.

Against this background of sprint speed development, six basic principles (Stein 1998) may be considered as the foundation of speed training method.

1. **Quality first** All speed training is at the near maximum and super maximum level. This places high demands on neural and hormonal systems. That means low overall training volume and long regeneration time.
2. **Technical precision without compromise** Whether as a whole technique or as a drill, the technical execution must be precise, since feedback mechanisms are at the spinal level of the central nervous system rather than the peripheral.
3. **Speed develops according to specific actions and requirements** Speed component of performance is the focus of specific exercise rather than related or general. 'These special exercises should simulate the spatial, temporal, dynamic and energetic characteristics of competition as closely as possible.' (Stein 1998). This does not negate the value of drills which isolate speed of particular joint actions (e.g. sprint drills programmes of Seagrave, Mach). They facilitate learning and execution of the full technical model which must be performed at speed *early* after drills training to ensure no breakdown in the temporal aspects of full technique performance.
4. **Speed development depends on several factors** The eight factors set out on pages 258–9 must be understood and built into a speed development programme.
5. **Speed training must include constant feedback** Both objective (e.g. recorded times, video access); and subjective (e.g. perception of maximum speed) estimated times in completed trials are critical to the learning process of speed development.
6. **Speed development depends on high motivation** The athlete must be actively involved in affording intellectual contribution to speed development.

This demands a rich and focused motivational climate in maintaining the highest levels of concentration and the will to go beyond comfortable limits.

These principles help design speed development in any sport. The following are specific examples:

For acceleration development

- Different starting positions sprint to 50 m/60 m.
- Facilitated movement – sprinting downhill, pulled by elastic/pulley system.
- Resisted movement* – uphill sprint, resistance towing.
- Competitions – handicap starts.
- Varied speed runs – sprint drive – 20 m; hold form 20 m; lift pace 20 m; etc.
- Extreme short sprints – 5 m; 10 m; 15 m; 20 m.

For developing capacity to maintain maximum speed

- 'Flying' sprints.
- 'Build-up' sprints – getting faster each 25 m from 0–75 m, then hold max speed for 25 m.
- Coordination light stride runs (running on hot bricks).
- Isolation and elastic drills – hopping, high knee running, 'prancing horse' (skip) runs, heel flicks, skip drills fast ankle flexes on spot.
- Sprinting downhill on 10–15% gradient.
- Facilitated (pulled) sprints – elastic rope, pulleys, superspeed motorised treadmill.

For frequency speed

- Maximum speed frequency repetitions should be worked for 8–10 secs (elite performer); 6 secs (youth) in these practices.
- Active ankle work – isolation and elastic drills.
- Skipping rope workouts maximum speed.
- Low obstacle or ground marking precision/speed movement – sprints on flat, uphill, downhill.
- Alternate side speed hopping across a line.
- Alternate forward/backward hops across a line.
- Sprints/fast foot movements across hoops/tyres on ground; rope/stick ladder on ground; speed grid – 3 m x 6 m (18 x 1 m x 1 m squares) – stepping/hopping challenges.
- Speed change sprints.
- Direction change sprints through a cone grid (3 m separating cones in any direction.
- Contrast method (Matveyev 1981) – resisted activity immediately followed by normal or facilitated activity.

(*When resistance is used it should not exceed 5% of the normal situation in these or other technical/ strength speed practices. If it does, the technical model is compromised and compensatory movements are introduced.)

Young athlete speed development

When developing speed in young athletes, the learning situation should be modified to permit maximum speeds by:

- using lighter equipment
- using smaller equipment
- using body weight supports
- using reduced dimension areas
- using isolated action speed then building towards multiple action and selective response. Response speed may be developed by challenging response speed to optic, acoustic or tactile signals.

Throwing: speed in throwing can be developed by using lighter implements. Insufficient research data is available to provide detailed information, but the following points may serve as guidelines.

(1) If the implement is too light, there is the risk of injury and disruption of the normal motor patterns of technique. Using implements approximately 5% heavier for a set of repetitions followed by 5–10% lighter, and then the normal weight on a set-for-set basis, improves speed. This mix can be extended to include specific strength work with implements heavier than the normal implement.

(2) Rebounding work or plyometrics should be considered as speed-related training. Work in this area may effect a faster transition from yielding to the power of approach, shift or turn, to overcoming the load of impetus when moving levers (legs, hips) through the throw. This is particularly so for javelin, where increased speed of approach will place a considerably greater load on both legs. It is as if the athlete must concentrate on 'bouncing' out of the entry into the throw, rather than accepting the momentum of approach or shift. The danger is that to 'accept' is often to 'cushion' and this decreases speed and the elastic use of kinetic energy.

(3) Speed should only be pursued within the limits dictated by the athlete's technical ability. The fundamentals of technique must not be abandoned in the pursuit of speed.

Jumping: the development of speed in jumping should be considered in two parts: development of approach speed (e.g. sprinting), and development of ability to use kinetic energy of increased approach speed. The previous discussion of sprinting speed should be applied to the development of approach speed, bearing in mind that the approach run must be consistent, even with advances in speed. The problem of using this increased speed is best solved by learning the new motor pattern of a faster passage over the take-off foot, and then progressing to the application of strength at this increased speed. The high-energy cost of acceleration means that flat-out approach runs from scratch are inadvisable. The areas of practice that should be explored are:

- downhill approach to take-off
- fast 'touch-off' take-offs

- rolling start approaches
- pole plant in sand following the above (landing area placed over long jump pit-pole vault)
- faster high jump approach onto extended landing area
- increasing the speed of the non-jumping limb movements relative to the jumping limb.

Ultimately, the ability to use the kinetic energy of the approach is strength related and consideration must be given to elastic strength work, rebound work, and depth jumping. *Relative* strength rather than *absolute* strength is critical.

In some sports, speed development offers a different type of challenge:

Swimming: Specific endurance is the single most important conditioning requirement in competitive swimming. The 50 m sprint event brought to the sport speed demands within the traditional technique–strength–endurance framework previously only associated with water polo. When 50 m sprints were introduced, maintaining speed and maximum speed required focus and improvement.

The process sequence for speed development training is:

- a foundation of swimming specific basic strength and aerobic endurance
- increased related strength (therefore hypertrophy) via the weights room and in the water
- increased specific strength by swimming against resistance (therefore increased fibre recruitment)
- facilitated (via pulley, etc.) super-maximum speed training to oblige increased stroke/impulse frequency
- to build-in speed endurance.

Individual repetitions within sets in a speed-training unit last 6–8 seconds max.
Intervals are between 3–5 minutes.
Total repetitions within a training unit are 4 minimum–20 maximum.
In other sports it represents a very complex challenge.

Tennis: Tennis is one of the most demanding and complex sports in terms of top competitive performance. A player's abilities are a mixture, requiring high levels of specific competence at technical, tactical, strategic, psychological levels and in strength, endurance and speed.

The modern game changed quite dramatically in the 1980s and 1990s; of course commercial pressures and the shape of the competitive year changed, but technology also accounted for new speed demands.

Materials were optimised in areas such as stiffer racquets, changing court surfaces and ball technology. On top of this there has developed a more aggressive playing attitude and changing anthropometry and physical condition in both men's and women's tennis.

As a result, speed has become a key component in a player's performance armoury. A player is dependent on speed for:

- returning the ball on court one more time than the opponent
- sprinting to get to the ball
- reading the game better than the opponent
- psychological construction of a tactical plan and for changing it
- preparing for and executing a stroke then moving to reduce the opponent's choice of response
- the pace of the player's game and response to the opponent's
- speed given to the ball; taking the ball earlier; response in volleys, etc.

Energy production/demands is also an issue, of course, as shortcomings in meeting energy demand shifts the game from one of speed/strength to one of strength/endurance. The average duration of rallies is 10 seconds and time between 20 seconds. Maximum sprinting distance is 14 m – but the average is around 4 m. There are also two minute pauses after every other game. So the energy requirements are in the main closer to those of a sprinter than an endurance athlete. That said there must be a sound aerobic base to reduce the possibility of cumulative fatigue.

So what sort of speed work does a tennis player require?

- short sprints to optical/acoustic signal – 2 m-15 m. Varied distance short sprints 5-20 m in 10-90 seconds sets of sprint/skip-walk-jog
- court sprints over marked routes
- shadow/mirror sprints
- volleys under pressure in 5-15 seconds sets, with two feeders; with a 360 degree turn between, or sitting/squatting/kneeling between; with back to feeder and responding to sound; standing or covering 2.5 m right and left, etc.

Sprinting exercises

- Sprinting drills.
- Flying sprints 10-30 m.
- Standing start sprints; sprinting from 'dancing' on the spot 2-10 m.
- Facedown lying sprints 2-10 m.
- Fast feet drills for 6-8 seconds in one position, with turn, etc.
- Plyometric/elastic strength routines – hopping, bounding, two-feet jump.
- Multidirectional 'sprints' – side, forward, back, diagonal, etc.
- Fan sprints.
- Potato races; shuttle sprints.
- Performing these practices with racquet to play strokes either shadowing or actual.

Tennis-specific speed

- Rapid serves, forehands, returns under time pressure (10-20 seconds).
- 12 repetitions of 3-4 winning shots hit either forehand or backhand from half court.
- Tennis strokes with squash/badminton racquet and soft balls.

- Fast shots in specific situations – fast lobs, smashes, returns on the run.
- Working through 3–4 identical tactical sequences under time pressure.

The speed barrier

Saziorski (1971) suggests that a 'speed barrier' can arise if the young athlete trains exclusively on sprint exercises, or if the advanced athlete neglects the use of special exercises for the development of elastic strength. Osolin (1952) tends to agree by stating that due to establishing a 'kinetic (motor) stereotype' by working at maximum intensity (e.g. training with the same group at all times) the development of speed may be made more difficult, or even prevented. However, he offers a note of optimism by suggesting that practices such as 'forced speed' (e.g. catapulting the athlete with the use of an elastic rope), or 'assisted speed' (e.g. altitude sprinting, downhill runs, or wind-assisted runs), or lighter implements, or increased competition demands, etc., will break an athlete's existing speed barrier.

Upton and Radford (1975) appear to support this and explain: 'The benefits of teaching methods which stress fast limb movements and the sensation of speed (e.g. by towing) may well result from improvement of neuronal programmes, increased motoneuron excitability and more synchronous firing of motoneurons.' This observation highlights an often neglected cause for speed barriers – the failure to involve efficient 'neuronal programs . . . and more synchronous firing of motoneurons'. The introduction of sprint drills to the conditioning programme may be an attempt to establish motor unit programming. In fact, Ballreich (1975) goes as far as stating that '. . . sprinting for top level sprinters can probably best be improved by developing its technical (coordination) rather than its conditioning (power) component'.

Endurance and speed training

The basis of specific speed endurance appears to lie in a certain measure of aerobic endurance developed by suitable loading. Although the absolute extent of this loading is low in the endurance programme of an endurance athlete, the relative extent can be high and may reach 90% in phase one of the preparatory period. Williams (1974) has suggested that this type of training improves aerobic capacity and glycogen concentration in red muscle fibres. This has a positive effect not only on speed endurance, but also on the capacity to recover after loadings of sub-maximum and maximum intensity. Thus, the athlete will be able to attempt *more* repetitions at the maximum and near maximum intensities of speed training.

Once a foundation for the development of aerobic endurance has been established, the athlete must be exposed to specific loadings similar to those of competition conditions. This work will be introduced in mesocycle 2 and continued in mesocycle 3. Broadly speaking, units for the development of competition speed endurance may be listed as follows.

(1) Repetition runs at sub-maximum to near maximum intensity. Long recovery periods are necessary between runs of near maximum intensity to ensure that quality is maintained, while shorter intervals are required where runs are of sub-maximum intensity. Sets of runs with 2–4 minutes between runs are recommended, but these will of necessity be short sets (e.g. 2–4 runs) to maintain quality. Between sets, longer intervals of 10–15 minutes should be introduced and it is recommended that at least half of this interval is active.
(2) Stress loading at maximum or near maximum intensity (for the distance used) over distances between $^2/_3$ x and 2 x the racing distance.
(3) Stress loading at maximum racing speed over stretches of up to 10%–20% longer than the racing distance.
(4) Varied speed runs where the tempo or intensity varies in the course of the run, e.g. 150 m of 50 m acceleration, 50 m hold, 50 m acceleration.
(5) High repetition, short distance sprints (30–60 m) where maintaining maximum striding rate is emphasised, e.g. 6 x 6 x 40 m – incomplete recovery in sets.
(6) Competitions.

A microcycle of 2–3 units per week should be used in mesocycle 2, but 1–2 units per microcycle will be adequate as the competition density assumes an endurance training role of its own.

Speed endurance practices for sports other than pure sprinting are poorly documented, but the endurance factor must be borne in mind. Five sets of top class tennis frequently exceed five hours (McEnroe–Becker, Davis Cup 1987, 6 hours 38 minutes); vault and high jump competitions can last over six hours; qualifying throws/jumps may be separated by 60 minutes; athletes declining to jump may cause an athlete to have several jumps/vaults in rapid succession; a qualifying contest and final in one day can necessitate nine throws/jumps at maximum intensity; field games last from 60–90 minutes; boxing (professional) may last 75 minutes; sailing lasts hours, etc. In Formula 1 races, the heart rate of drivers is, for approximately 90 minutes, in the range of 175–185 beats per minute. These factors may mean speed endurance and strength endurance work for all sports where there is a demand for speed in the presence of fatigue. For example in throwing:

• rapid succession throws with normal implements being fed to the athlete (full throws, isolated action and standing throws)
• rapid succession throws with medicine balls or lighter implements, as above
• single throws separated by 15–60 minutes, etc.
• track workouts followed by throws
• maximum repetition simulation throws per 30 seconds, etc.

Or in jumping:

- rapid succession short approach jumps
- rapid succession 'stepdown' jumps (e.g. 21 stride, 17 stride, 13 stride, 9 stride) with walkback recovery
- speed bounding/hopping, etc., over 30 m
- jumping circuits over 400 m (50 m bound, etc.)
- single jumps/vaults separated by 15–60 minutes, etc.
- fast agility work on ropes, bars, etc., for simulated work on the pole.

Or in games:

- rapid succession strokes in tennis/squash
- continuous pressure passing/lay-up practice in basketball
- unopposed non-stop rugby/soccer/hockey
- high speed games without breaks at altitude
- conditioning work followed by continuous speed work under pressure.

Attitude and speed training

In the intensely interactive world of team games, combat sports, racquet games, etc., in order for speed of individual or team performance to be delivered instinctively under the pressure of competition, it must be repeatedly rehearsed in training. Successful performance is not only due to speed of movement across the ground and speed of choosing correct action options, but also speed of thought and interpretation of situations. Just as a typist thinks in 'phrases' rather than 'letters and words', these players must think and act in 'action phrases'. A player giving or passing the ball to a colleague must be thinking about, and moving immediately to, a position to support the person receiving the ball. This means having this attitude in even simple practice situations. Without doubt it contributes immensely to the rhythm and speed at which a given team will play in competition.

Risk of injury

Speed work must be preceded by a full warm-up. Some 35–50% of warm-up mobility work must be dynamic mobility exercise. Maximum speed training will be developed on a basis of sound technique and relevant strength. In other words, speed training is introduced only when the athlete has been prepared for it. In cool/cold weather athletes should wear tights and warm but non-restrictive clothing. The advice of a physiotherapist should be sought to agree use of embrocations/ creams. At the earliest signs of cramp or pain, activity should stop.

SUMMARY

Speed of whole body movement, or of individual joint actions, is a decisive factor of successful performance in many sports. While speed is frequently the product of a coordinated sequence of strength expression of joint actions, the development of speed is not synonymous with the development of strength. In speed-dependent sports, it is important that speed of technical performance is introduced early. However, this must not compromise the basic technical model. Speed is considered under the heading of 'conditioning training' in many programmes, due to the possible combination of speed with strength, endurance and/or mobility. However, it may equally be considered as a sophisticated extension of technical training. Practices for development of speed are specific to the technical demands of a sport. Such demands vary according to the involvement of strength, endurance and mobility, the synchronised use of varied speed of joint action, and the requirement for optimum or maximum speed.

16 THEORY AND PRACTICE OF ENDURANCE DEVELOPMENT

TRAINING METHODS

It has already been suggested that a scientifically based and systematic programme of training is fundamental to the pursuit of high-level performance in sport. Of all sports, the endurance events of track and field and swimming are the best documented in these terms. Certain types of exercise *increase* certain bodily functions, while others *decrease* them (table 20, p. 148). Williams illustrated at the 1974 Meadowbank Convention that the effect of training is directly related to the duration and intensity of training load. The purpose here is not, however, to labour the 'scientific bases' but to examine the type of training included in the systematic programme. Various references to physiological measures are more in the nature of comment than detailed argument.

All training methods for the development of endurance can be divided into three groups: duration, repetition, and competition and testing methods (fig. 75).

Duration

Continuous method: this is running at a steady pace or intensity where the heart rate lies between 130 and 160 beats per minute. The duration of such running will be over 30 minutes for the young athlete and from 60–120 minutes for the mature. Improvement in VO2 maximum (aerobic capacity) is achieved here via long-term loading under aerobic conditions. This method is recommended especially for the long distance endurance athlete.

Alternating pace method: this is long duration running, with the speed of successive stretches alternating according to a plan. At the simplest level, one might have a slow pace (HR = 130-150 beats/minute) for 1.0 km alternating with a fast pace (HR = 170-180 beats/minute) for 0.5 km. The forced entry into anaerobic work and consequent oxygen debt demands repayment within the next 1.0 km and this situation acts as a strong stimulus for the improvement of VO2 maximum. This method is used extensively both by middle and long distance athletes.

Fartlek: this is running with varying intensity according to the requirements of the athlete and the dictates of terrain. The athlete will use a terrain which undulates and makes varying demands upon him (e.g. hills, woodland, plough, sand). Like the alternating pace method, anaerobic periods provide a strong stimulus for

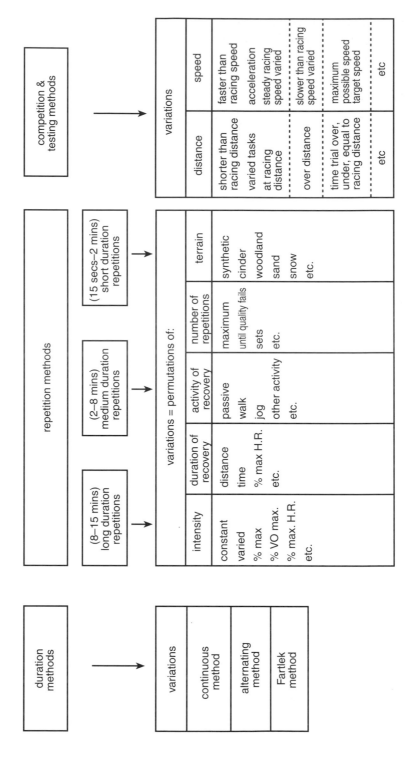

FIG. 75 Summary of endurance training methods (adapted from Harre, 1973)

the improvement of VO2 maximum. In addition, the demands of terrain stimulate strength endurance development and proprioceptive balance adjustment of ankle, knee and hip.

Repetition

These methods offer a wide variety of possible training effects, due to the number of variables.

(1) Duration of the training run (in distance *or* time: classified as short, medium or long).
(2) Duration of the recovery period (distance *or* time).
(3) Intensity of the training run (m, seconds, % VO2 maximum, speed, etc.).
(4) Number of repetitions and sets.
(5) Activity of recovery (walking, jogging, passive).
(6) Terrain for training (uphill, track, sand, surf, etc.).

Training is geared to the type of endurance required for a given sport and the difference in effect of adjusting these variables is quite startling. For example, the following are worth noting.

Interval training

This is training for the rapid development of aerobic endurance and has proved successful. Returning to the variables, interval training might look like the following.

(1) 200 m.
(2) 200 m.
(3) Intensity sufficient to raise HR to approximately 180 beats/minute.
(4) Progressive increase in repetitions.
(5) Jogging for 90 seconds – returning HR to approximately 120 beats/minute.
(6) Track.

This session is known in sports jargon as slow–fast 200s, and makes a more rapid improvement in aerobic capacity compared with duration methods (long steady distance), but its effects are lost quicker.

Speed endurance training

This develops the athlete's ability to produce high quality performance despite the by-products of anaerobesis. There are an infinite variety of units for this objective and their value may only be truly assessed by studying their place in a training plan. For example, in the month of August, a girl running 4 x 200 m in 27 seconds with 30 seconds recovery may have progressed in intensity and density, but regressed in extent from a unit performed in January of 10 x 200 m in 30 seconds with 75 seconds recovery. Of all types of track training, the control of these units is the most difficult, and coaches tend to use past experience as the main key for adjustment. Broadly speaking, the following general rules apply.

(1) Increase the total extent (number) of repetitions (e.g. 4 x 200 m → 12 x 200 m).
(2) Using a given recovery time, standardise an intensity of run over the training distance (each run aims at a given time, e.g. 12 x 200 m in 34 seconds with 75 seconds recovery).
(3) Gradually increase intensity (make runs faster, e.g.12 x 200 m in 34 seconds → 30 seconds with 75 seconds recovery).
(4) Reduce the total extent (number) of repetitions (e.g. 12 x 200 m in 30 seconds with 75 seconds recovery → 2 x 4 x 200 m in 27 seconds with 75 seconds recovery and 15–20 minutes between sets).
(5) Gradually increase density (shorten the recovery, e.g. 2 x 4 x 200 m in 27 seconds with 75 seconds → 30 seconds recovery).

This type of work seeks to maintain quality and striding rate, and work sets are often used. If the times for repetitions fall off in the course of the unit, the training is moving towards strength endurance rather than speed endurance. Consequently, all progression must guarantee the maintenance of quality. It should be noted that within a unit, varying pace may be used in separate sets – hence units such as 'stepdowns'. For example:

> 3 x 300 m in 48 seconds with 100 m jog recovery in 60 seconds
> (jog 100 m in 60 seconds between sets)
> 3 x 300 m in 45 seconds with 100 m jog recovery in 60 seconds
> (jog 100 m in 60 seconds between sets)
> 3 x 300 m in 42 seconds with 100 m jog recovery in 60 seconds

Or again, varying distances may be incorporated with varying pace within a unit. For example, the following comprises one set of a three set unit, with 100 m jog between sets and repetitions:

> 600 m in 108 seconds
> 400 m in 68 seconds
> 300 m in 48 seconds
> 200 m in 30 seconds
> 100 m in 14 seconds

These two unit variations are means of educating the athlete in pace judgement *and* in the physiological demands of pace change. Speed endurance training, in making complex demands upon the athlete in terms of energy provision, coordination, and strength, creates a stimulus for the complex adaptation required of middle distance athletes.

Strength endurance training

This is training to develop the athlete's ability to apply force in the climate of lactic anaerobesis. Quality demands are reduced and replaced simply by the task of completing the training unit. Recovery periods are normally very strict and, although the intensity of the run is seldom monitored, the athlete must run as hard as possible. Thus we have units such as:

circuit training
2 x 4 x 100 m 'back to back' (30 seconds recovery)
2 x 5 x 80 m 'turnabout' (shuttle running)
6 x 150 m hill run (jog recovery 90 seconds)
5 x 80 m sand dune climb (walk down recovery)
6 x 200 m in surf (passive three minute recovery)
4 x 200 m Skip B (high knee and clawing action; passive three-minute recovery)
resisted performance of a given activity in the climate of endurance factors, i.e.
6 x 50 m swimming and towing a drag, 8 x 500 m rowing and towing a drag.

Strength endurance training causes considerable wear and tear in the athlete's organism and it is possible that a saturation of microcycles with units of this type would cause a loss of mental and physical resilience. However, these units help the athlete to keep going when lactate is high and, although annual training plans vary, such units may be best inserted between mesocycles 1 and 2, and/or late in mesocycle 2 (see chapter 15).

Competition and testing

Without doubt, competition and testing methods are the best stimulus to develop specific endurance qualities. This is especially so if the actual competition duration is used for this purpose. Embraced by this type of endurance training method could be:

- time trials at distances equal to, less than, or in excess of the racing distance
- specific task runs where the athlete must reach a certain point in a given time, then meet the demands of a maximum intensity finish (e.g. 600 m where the athlete must reach 400 m in 60 seconds, then sprint to finish)
- standard training units where the athlete attempts to perform a given unit prior to being tested for various items significant to a bioprofile
- competitions themselves, e.g. indoor, cross-country, etc. It is also possible to give an athlete a specific task within a competition – say in one mile, to reach the bell in 3 minutes 3 seconds – then break four minutes for the final mile time
- maintenance of high rate of execution and accuracy of a given technique in the climate of endurance factors.

However, the intention here is not to advocate one method over another since each method and variation brings about psychological, physiological and biomechanical reactions. It is not sufficient to rely on one choice for the optimal development of the specific endurance capacities in a given athlete. Perhaps this point is best illustrated by referring to the study undertaken by Viru, Urgenstein and Pisuke 1972 (fig. 76). They trained nine groups of students using different training units. The difference in training effect was quite marked. For example, (1) interval training increased heart volume, while duration methods (continuous/Fartlek) were more effective in increasing the oxygen carrying capacity of the blood than interval training; and (2) the greatest improvement in 800 m performance was noted in the hill-run group (15°) and least improvement was noted in the complex method group. They concluded that no single method provided development of the total organism, and suggested that to use one method only may ultimately impair performance. Only by the skilful integration of the principal training methods, and their variations, will the required level of adaptation be approached, let alone achieved.

The training plan for an athlete must be dictated by:

- the competition demands of the sport
- the individual athlete's training status
- the stage of development of the athlete (age, gender, anatomy, physiology, etc.)
- the long and short-term objectives of training
- the limitations of the training environment
- the demands of the non-athletic environment
- the athlete's own personality.

The competition demands of the sport

One school of thought holds that since there appears to be a percentage break-down between energy pathways in different sports, as shown in table 29, then training should be similarly divided. Another school of thought holds that the sport should be evaluated on its demands relative to short, medium and long-term endurance, as well as speed and strength endurance.

distance in m	aerobic	anaerobic
200	5%	95%
400	17%	83%
800	34%	66%
1500	50%	50%
5000	80%	20%
10,000	90%	10%
Marathon	98%	2%

TABLE 29 Aerobic v anaerobic contribution to energy requirement according to distance run.

Short-term endurance: the endurance required for covering efforts of 45 seconds to two minutes duration. Obviously, a high percentage of anaerobic involvement exists in such efforts. Speed endurance and strength endurance status is critical to short-term endurance.

Medium-term endurance: the endurance required for efforts of two minutes to eight minutes duration. Again, anaerobic processes are involved, but an apparent steady state has been achieved. Strength endurance and speed endurance determine medium-term endurance efficiency since a relatively high resistance, represented by the amount of force which the athlete must apply, must be expressed at a relatively high frequency over the whole period. Although present world times fall outside

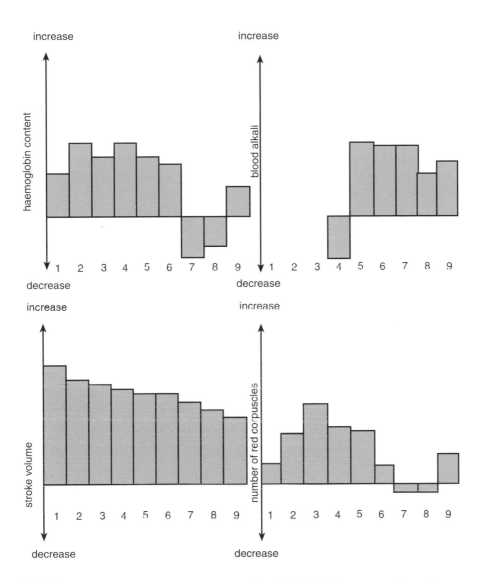

FIG. 76 Effects of certain training programmes on selected physiological parameters (adapted from work by Viru, Urgenstein and Pisuke, USSR, 1972). (1) Sets of 4–5 runs with 1½–2 mins recovery; 7–10 mins between sets. e.g. 3 x 4 x 150 m (75%); (2) Complex training involving various sessions; (3) Long steady distance; (4) Fartlek; (5) 2–5 flat out runs – full recovery; (6) Interval sprints (40–50 m sprint/jog); (7) Hill runs up 15° gradient; (8) Intensive interval runs 100–200 m at 80%–90% with 1–3 mins recovery until quality drops; (9) Extensive interval runs – such as slow/fast 200 m.

this range, steeplechase may be considered as having *very* high medium-term endurance demands.

Long-term endurance: the endurance required for efforts in excess of eight minutes duration and during which time there is no essential decrease in speed. The performance depends almost exclusively on aerobic efficiency. As the time increases, so the aerobic role becomes more exclusive. This type of endurance should be considered as virtually synonymous with aerobic endurance/heart endurance.

Speed endurance: the endurance required to resist fatigue due to loading at sub-maximum and maximum intensity (approx. 85–100% maximum intensity), and predominantly anaerobic production of energy. It is essential in sports demanding this type of endurance that speed is not reduced due to fatigue or innervation inhibition.

Strength endurance: the endurance required to continuously express relatively high strength efficiency when anaerobic by-products are accumulating. This is related not only to the alkali-acid imbalance in working muscle, the result of which painfully terminates activity, but also to the psychological aspects of willpower and the ability to tolerate pain.

The schematic relationship of these different endurance capacities is represented in figure 77.

Yet another school of thought holds that *all* endurance events are founded upon an extensive base of aerobic efficiency – so much so that approximately 67% of the training year is devoted to duration methods and their derivatives, and approximately 20% of the training year to the specific demands of a given endurance sport, as well as 13% to competition. Whatever basis is used for assessing endurance requirements, serious consideration must be given to such assessment because requirements vary for all sports.

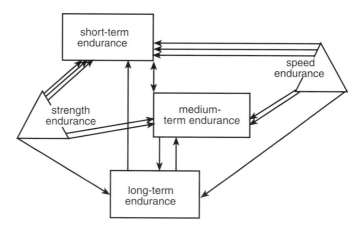

FIG. 77 Inter-relationship of various areas of endurance

The individual athlete's training status

This may be judged by bioprofiles, haematological analyses, VO2 maximum tests, etc., and by personal best performances at commencement of training, how long the athlete can run at a predetermined speed (e.g. 20 seconds/100 m), and standard training programme (e.g. the athlete runs 5 x 500 m at a speed of 90 seconds/500 m with a fixed recovery period). Before and after each repetition, and the total training programme, heart rate and lactate measures are taken.

The stage of development of the athlete

According to Williams (1974) (see also chapter 9) the exposure of pre-pubertal athletes to units consistent with anaerobic development is inadvisable. Also, training for general development of endurance must be stressed with emphasis on long stretches at a low intensity, rather than interval methods predominating. Methods which tax strength or strength/speed endurance in the young athlete are not recommended.

Long-/short-term objectives of training

The athlete will have some ultimate goal in mind as a supreme *raison d'être* for training. This may be an Olympic final, a world record, etc. However, he will also have landmarks that must be reached *en route*. This may be a particular level of performance, a victory at a National Championship, etc. Programmes will therefore be constructed to meet the various goals, each leading towards the ultimate and never being ends in themselves.

Limitations of the training environment

The proximity of hills, beaches, plough, surf, ideal stadia, basic stadia, gymnasia, sports halls, etc , must all be taken into account, together with their training value potential. Not every athlete has access to the ideal complex of training facilities so a programme may have to be created imaginatively in a situation that is not ideal.

Demands of the non-athletic environment

The problems of other commitments, e.g. to family, business, education, social scene, cultural pursuits, and so on, must be solved with the assistance of athlete, coach, and a carefully constructed plan.

The athlete's own personality

According to Harre (1973) (see also chapter 10), duration methods encourage development of buoyancy and elasticity of mind. Buoyant behaviour 'includes all those volitional controlling qualities of personality that help to overcome inward and external difficulties and problems, by a consistency in readiness to make an effort of will'. On the other hand, he suggested that interval training develops that form of control which he refers to as 'impetus of will'. By this he means a fluctuating, varying nature. He goes on to point out that only in consideration of specific demands can buoyancy and impetus of will have a positive or negative value, and that they can be present as integrated behaviour patterns in an athlete.

Working from strength v compensatory work

There are two poles of opinion when attending to the specific needs of an endurance athlete. The first looks to building a programme based on the athlete's strength, and by so doing gradually make ground on his weakness. The other looks to focusing on the weakness, and building a compensatory programme. This method is founded on the belief that the athlete's strengths need little work to maintain a high level, and the weaknesses can therefore be afforded more time – and brought up to the same level as the strengths. To give an example, if an athlete can run 200 m in 23.00 secs, and 800 m in two minutes, it is clear that endurance should be worked on. The 'working from strength' coach will build his programme around repetition work over 100 m, 200 m, and 300 m, gradually introducing longer repetitions and long runs. The 'compensatory' coach will look to longer endurance work and longer repetitions from the outset. Working from strength fits better into Harre's idea of building programmes according to the athlete's personality. Moreover, at a most fundamental level, it ensures that the athlete enjoys a positive motivational profile through a period of hard work.

Examples of endurance training plans

But what of the plan itself? It would appear that whatever it might be, it must fall into one of two categories: the Lydiard method or the Complex method. The former has now appeared in many forms and varieties, for example that used by Kari Sinkkonen with the Finnish distance athletes in 1975 (fig. 78), or any of the African systems. The latter has new varieties every day!

Every athlete and coach evolves a different interpretation of the complex method, but for the sake of illustration, figure 79 includes a variation on the model (referred to as 'the Oregon method') used by Bill Bowerman of the University of Oregon.

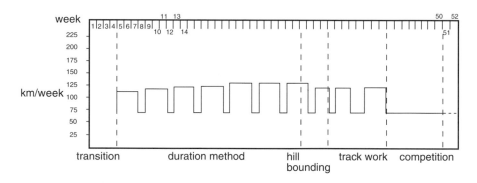

FIG. 78 Interpretation of Lydiard method of planning endurance training (from Sinkkonen, 1975)

Altitude training in practice

Training at altitude has become a regular feature in the annual cycle of preparing athletes for major championships. The following notes are a distillation of the experience of Bulgarian, Romanian, former Soviet Union and the former German Democratic Republic (GDR) coaches in using altitude training camps.

(1) Training at altitude for young athletes (17–19 years) is only recommended if these athletes have already achieved a very high level of training.

(2) Only athletes who can train with a full load should go to altitude. They must, therefore, be healthy. Altitude exacerbates infections and dental problems, so a complete health check is required before athletes can participate in an altitude camp.

(3) Athletes should have a trial period at altitude outside the competition season before using it as final preparation for a major championship. This affords the opportunity to learn what suits a given athlete.

(4) The minimum period for altitude training should be 21 days.

(5) Athletes should be tested under normal sea level conditions to establish different speeds for endurance training at altitude. For example, this will indicate the point at which activity changes from aerobic to aerobic/anaerobic. Once this information is recorded (in metres/sec), subtract 0.20–0.30 metres/sec and these are the speeds for use at altitude. For example: 4.70 metres/sec – sea level = 4.40–4.50 metres/sec – altitude.

(6) Young athletes should work primarily on:

- steady running at low-medium intensity, 30 mins-60 mins
- sprint training over distances which *do not* go into lactic anaerobic work
- general conditioning training.

(7) Because there is a feeling of euphoria after some days of training at altitude, athletes often feel motivated to push too hard in training. Coaches *must* apply a friendly discipline and carefully supervise all training to ensure that altitude will not have a negative effect. Interval work should permit recovery to midway between steady resting and maximum heart rate. Steady runs should be resting heart rate plus 65%–70% heart rate range.

(8) In the first three days at altitude, athletes should keep things at the intermittent walk/jog level to allow gentle adaptation. This is *essential* for first time trainers at altitude, but even established altitude trainers should have two days like this. At the end of the training period, days 19, 20 and 21 should be at a reduced training level.
   The pattern should be:

days 1–3/4   acclimatisation, e.g. instead of 2 x 60 m runs – 4 x 30 m runs.
days 3/4–18   hard training – normal programme but gentler progression; longer recoveries, etc. (bearing in mind note 5).
days 19–21   assimilation and recovery – lower intensity and extent.

(9) Athletes dehydrate readily at altitude so *must* take extra fluids (2.5 litres water per day minimum including electrolyte replacement). Athletes also require a higher intake of carbohydrate. Iron and water soluble vitamin supplementation is also advised, under medical supervision.

(10) After the end of altitude training athletes may feel unwell and, although tired, will have difficulty sleeping. For these first 2–3 days back at sea level, training loads should be lower. After this period the athlete will feel much better and performance capacity increases.

(11) Athletes may, however, record an exceptional performance within 3–4 days of returning to sea level (but this is an individual matter!). Then performance goes down for about seven days – to be followed by a return to high performance from the 10th, 11th, or 12th day which can continue for about four weeks. Around 85%–90% of all experienced altitude trainers produce their *best* results after 3–4 days and after 18–24 days.

(12) Ultraviolet radiation is more intense at altitude. Sun creams/blocks and sunglasses should be worn.

(13) Warm clothing should be taken for evenings and for immediate post-training.

(14) An extra 1–2 hours sleep should feature in the training period at altitude.

(15) The most used altitude facilities are as listed below in table 30; 2000–2200 metres is generally agreed as the best training altitude.

	venue	*country*	*altitude (m)*
1	Belmeken	Bulgaria	2000
2	Tzahkadzor	Armenia	1970
3	Font Romeau	France	1895
4	St. Moritz	Switzerland	1820
5	Sestriere	Italy	2035
6	Pyatra Arsa	Romania	1950
7	IssykKull	Kirgizia	1600
8	Zetersfeld (Linz)	Austria	1950
9	Addis Ababa	Ethiopia	2400
10	Nairobi	Kenya	1840
11	Ifran	Morocco	1820
12	Kunming	China	1895
13	Mexico City	Mexico	2200
14	Toluca	Mexico	2700
15	Colorado Springs	USA	2194
16	Keystone	USA	2835
17	Flagstaff	USA	2300
18	Bogota	Colombia	2500
19	Boulder	USA	2000
20	La Paz	Bolivia	3100

TABLE 30 Altitude training venues

	venue	country	altitude (m)
21	Quito	Ecuador	2218
22	Davos	Switzerland	1560
23	Pontresina	Switzerland	1900
24	Crans Montana	Switzerland	1500
25	Kaprun	Austria	1800
26	Zilvretsha	Austria	1800
27	Medeo	Kazakstan	1691
28	KesenoyAm	Russia	2000
29	Pzhevalsk	Kirgizia	1800
30	Tamga	Kirgizia	1700

TABLE 30 Continued

Endurance sports and the female athlete

Although strength and structural disadvantage are critical factors in the lower performance ability of women in endurance sports (compared with men), Wagner (1976) maintains that the most important factor is the poorer status of aerobic capacity. Keul (1973), in demonstrating that there is no difference between men and women in anaerobic capacity, appears to endorse this. Wagner (1976) further suggests that an increased emphasis on aerobic training, coupled with an increased number of training units per week, may explain the rapid improvements there have been since 1975 in women's middle distance events in track and field athletics.

Pace for the month   62 sec / 400 m   Next month 61 sec / 400 m

	Week 1	Week 2	Week 3	Week 4
Sunday	20 miles continuous			
Monday	8 x 400m: 62: jog 400 m	10 x 400 m: 62: jog 200 m	8 x 400 m· 62· jog 100 m	10 x 400 m: 62: jog 100 m
Tuesday	10 miles alternating 800 m jog between sets	as before	as before	as before
Wednesday	2 x 5 x 300 m: 46.5: jog 300 m	3 x 4 x 300 m: 46.5: jog 200 m	4 x 3 x 300 m: 46.5: jog 100 m	5 x 3 x 300 m: 46.5: jog 100 m
Thursday	Fartlek – 60 mins			
Friday	10 miles continuous			
Saturday	Competition-training / cross country / time trials / indoors / etc.			

FIG. 79 Interpretation of complex method of planning endurance training

SUMMARY

The preparation of endurance training plans and their progressive units (from the wide range of training practices) is a most interesting and rewarding exercise for the coach. Our well-documented knowledge of related physiology offers an excellent framework within which to apply training units consistent with the laws of specificity, overload and reversibility. Thus, with insight, the coach may accurately evaluate the endurance demands of sports (ranging from the marathon to ice hockey) and create a training programme geared to adapting the athlete's physiology to meet these demands.

The female athlete must have aerobic training emphasised in her training plan. Nevertheless, the coach should be aware that it is not sufficient to compensate for weaknesses and that he should build upon strengths when planning training.

17 THEORY AND PRACTICE OF MOBILITY DEVELOPMENT

MOBILITY CLASSIFICATION

Mobility is the capacity to perform joint actions through a wide range of movement. In sport, it should be considered in the light of an optimum application of strength throughout a range of movement appropriate to the demands of a given technique. Mobility is measured in degrees, radians or centimetres. Passive values are greater than active values and the reduction of the active-passive difference is often used as a criterion of achievement. There are three distinct varieties of mobility: active, passive and kinetic.

Active mobility: the capacity to effect movement by contraction of those muscles which naturally cause the movement. In figure 80, the athlete is flexing the femur on the pelvis by contraction of the hip flexors. In this instance, the neuromuscular pattern provides stimulation of the hip flexors (protagonists) to contract, and inhibition of the hip extensors (antagonists). The relaxed hip extensors are consequently 'stretched'. This represents the classical reciprocal inhibition.

Passive mobility: that movement which is effected by expression of external force on the joint action (e.g. apparatus, the weight of the body, a partner). In figure 81, the femur is being flexed on the pelvis by the combined effects of body weight and resistance of the wall bars. In this instance, the neuromuscular pattern stimulates neither the hip flexors nor hip extensors to contract. There is a variant of passive mobility which merits special mention here. This involves inhibition of reflex contraction in the antagonist muscles. This is referred to more in terms of training method than a sub-classification of mobility, as 'Proprioceptive Neuromuscular Facilitation' (PNF method).

Kinetic mobility: that movement which is effected due to momentum of one or other or both of the levers involved. In figure 82, the femur has been flexed on the pelvis by the momentum of its swing. In this instance, the neuromuscular pattern provides stimulation of the hip flexors (protagonists) to contract forcefully, and inhibition of the hip extensors (antagonists). However, as the movement reaches the limit of extensibility of the hip extensors, the muscle spindle reflex mechanism may initiate a reflex contraction of the 'overstretched' hip extensors. Consequently, this type of mobility presents the possibility of muscle damage, not only when it is applied as a means of developing mobility in general, but also when it is applied as an essential feature of technique. Kinetic mobility is also

FIG. 80 Examples of active mobility exercise

known as 'ballistic mobility' and 'bouncing mobility' and has also been covered by the umbrella title of 'dynamic mobility' (discussed below).

Factors influencing mobility

(1) The elasticity of muscle and tendon of those muscles being stretched (but note that increased strength of a muscle does not reduce its extension capacity).

(2) The elasticity of ligaments supporting the joint involved. This presents one of many coaching dilemmas. The ligaments provide joint stability but the characteristic to be developed is joint mobility. Ligaments do not display any apparent elasticity but, given extensive exposure to stretch, may be extended to a new length. This, while providing increased mobility, reduces the stability of the joint. Consequently, great care must be taken to ensure that those muscles which cross the joint are strong enough to provide some compensatory stability to protect it from injury.

FIG. 81 Examples of active mobility exercise

a.   b.   c.

FIG. 82 Examples of active mobility exercise

(3) The structural barriers of any muscle hypertrophy, or any skin and tissue folds which prevent freedom of joint range (e.g. 'spare tyres' – in hip flexion).
(4) Structural barriers of joint construction and bone.
(5) The strength of the protagonist in active and kinetic mobility.
(6) The capacity of the neuromuscular system to inhibit the antagonists (those muscles being stretched).
(7) The degree of technical mastery of the movement concerned, especially if the movement is one of several which comprise a sports technique.

conditions	time	result in mm
After night's sleep	8.00	−15
" "	12.00	+35
10 mins with body exposed at 10°C	12.00	−36
10 mins in warm bath at 40°C	12.00	+78
After 20 mins loosening up	12.00	+89
After tiring training	12.00	−35

TABLE 31 Alterations in mobility under different conditions from Osolin (1952).

(8) The athlete's internal and external environment (table 31).

(9) The effect of recent injury in the muscles or joints concerned, or of fibrous adhesion of an old injury which has caused the athlete to be restricted in a given movement for a considerable period.

(10) The restrictions of inappropriate clothing.

(11) The athlete's age and stage of development. After the age of approximately eight years, mobility will gradually reduce. Mobility training is therefore essential to the athlete.

(12) Structural adaptation to occupational postures (e.g. stooping over a machine, studying in a cramped position) or muscle habits may reduce free movement in certain joints.

Role of mobility

Mobility is fundamental to the efficient performance of any action, both in nature and degree. Poor mobility development will present the athlete with several problems.

(1) The learning of sports techniques is difficult and in some cases impossible. This prevents the athlete from successful participation in certain sports. Moreover, the coach may believe an athlete's inability to perform a given technique is due to poor motor learning, lack of strength, etc., when in fact the problem may be quite simply that the athlete has insufficient mobility to assume a requested position.

(2) There exists the very real problem of injury due to muscle, tendon or ligament strain. For instance, when the athlete attempts to exceed his mobility range, there can be strain of other muscles and tendons which are employed to compensate for poor mobility in a given range, or strain of ligaments which become excessively loaded when restricted range of movement demands extraneous compensatory and balance adjustments.

(3) The development of other characteristics (e.g. strength and speed), or their effective application in technique, may be retarded. Ultimately, in terms of results and execution, this will lead to poor technical performance.

(4) The range of movement through which force may be applied (e.g. throws, golf swing, tennis strokes, stride length, etc.) is reduced and consequently the total performance is impaired.

(5) If the quality of a given movement is reduced due to lack of mobility, that movement cannot contribute fully as a component of more complex or similar movements. Thus the total movement potential of the athlete is reduced.

(6) A lack of mobility in any joint action imposes an extra workload and tension on those muscles compensating for this deficiency. The result is more rapid tiring and a reduction of performance capacity.

(7) Before performing in speed or elastic/fast/strength training or competition, kinetic mobility should predominate in warm-up. This supports the energy resource and neuromuscular dynamics of the activity to follow. Sustained slow stretching, whether as active or passive mobility, inhibits both resource and dynamics.

The net result of all of the above is that a lack of appropriate mobility reduces the athlete's 'sphere of influence' in game situations, and his adaptability and technical efficiency of sports performance. Moreover, it increases the athlete's risk of sudden injury and unnecessary cumulative strain of muscle, tendon and ligament. A lack of mobility, then, has far reaching effects. The athlete must develop and maintain a level of general mobility to gain maximum advantage from training, freedom from the risk of injury, and attainment of a certain level of specific mobility, in order to meet the demands of technique.

MOBILITY TRAINING

Training to develop mobility must also obey the laws of specificity, overload and reversibility.

Specificity: training must focus on a particular joint action and the active, passive or kinetic nature of the mobility required in that joint action. 'Specific', here, refers to athlete, joint action and technical demand.

Overload: the range of movement will not be maintained unless the existing limit is reached regularly, nor will it be improved unless that limit is exceeded. For instance:

- active mobility exercise is acceptable for maintaining a range of movement, provided strength of the protagonists is not lost. It has only limited value for developing mobility and implies increased strength of the protagonists and work in the end position, i.e. at the existing limit of the range of movement
- passive mobility exercise, given appropriate external force, will maintain or increase the range of movement
- kinetic mobility exercise makes its greatest contribution by relating mobility which is achieved through active or passive exercise, to the dynamics of a sports technique. However, as a carefully supervised type of exercise, it may also improve mobility.

Reversibility: mobility status is lost more slowly on cessation of regular specific training than other characteristics. Nevertheless it is gradually lost so the athlete should include mobility training either as an introduction to a unit, or as a unit in its own right.

Mobility unit construction

There are virtually thousands of mobility exercises to choose from but, for the guidance of coaches, a summary of points relative to mobility unit construction is included here. Obviously, the coach must understand the specific joint actions to be mastered by the athlete and, as always before selecting training units, the laws of specificity, overload, and reversibility must be obeyed. The following order of events should also be observed.

(1) Raise body temperature by jogging, striding, and gentle warm-up activity in natural fibre sweat suit (if air temperature is 22 degrees or higher) or in a natural fibre sweat suit plus wet suit (if the temperature is 21 degrees or lower). The purpose of this warm-up is to settle the body temperature at 37.5–38.5 degrees.
(2) Active and slow, sustained exercises for each joint action.
(3) Passive exercises with partner, apparatus, body weight, etc.
(4) Kinetic exercises and combined elastic strength/mobility exercises (experienced athletes only).
(5) Specific exercises related to the whole technique(s), and whole techniques up to competition or training performance speed.

When the activity to follow is not speed or elastic strength dependent, the priority of each item is approximately: (1) 25%, (2) 20%, (3) 20%, (4) 10%, (5) 25%.

If the following activity is speed or elastic strength dependent, the priority is: (1) 25%, (2) 10%, (3) 15%, (4) 25%, (5) 25%.

Mobility work should *always* precede other training and *never* be practised in a state of fatigue (following strength or endurance training, etc.) unless gentle active mobility is used. Like all training, mobility must be carefully supervised while the athlete learns training discipline (e.g. no experimentation, no interference with other athletes, no lazy 'compromised' movements, etc.).

Especially with the young athlete, *all* joint actions must be afforded mobility training as the basis upon which specific mobility training will develop. With the advanced athlete, general mobility training holds high priority in mesocycle 1 of the annual cycle and should be included (possibly in warm-up for other training units) throughout the year. Highly specific mobility is for advanced athletes only. However, all levels of athlete require a complementary development of strength, but in separate training units. The advanced athlete may combine mobility and strength work in kinetic mobility exercises, but this work should be supervised and never taken to the point of fatigue.

Sets of exercises should comprise 10–15 repetitions, since only after several repetitions is there any visible increase in range of movement. The recovery period between sets must not be long enough to permit temperature reduction. It may also be active (walking, jogging, general stretching) or passive (relaxing in warmth). When active or passive mobility exercise is used in training units, the end position of stretch should be maintained for 6–10 secs in each repetition. Several authorities recommend daily or twice-daily units of mobility training. Personal experience suggests that general and/or specific mobility work as part of warm-up for daily training units, supplemented by separate units within the microcycle where mobility is trained exclusively, is sufficient for athletes in the majority of sports. Exceptions are sports such as gymnastics, where daily mobility units are essential.

PNF method would be used at stage four in the training unit. It must be used with care, and partners should be mature, responsible persons, trained in application of the method. The athlete's partner slowly forces the relevant limb to the existing comfort limit of a range of movement. When the athlete feels discomfort, the movement stops and the partner then offers a resistance so that the athlete can perform an isometric contraction against the original direction of movement. This is held for 6–10 seconds. Athlete and partner rest for 30 seconds then repeat the exercise 3–6 times. An extension of this method, referred to as 3 PIC requires the athlete to contract the protagonist muscles for 3–6 seconds immediately following the isometric contraction. The partner then recommences the cycle of forced stretch, isometric contraction against the direction of stretch, and active contraction *with* the direction of stretch. The cycle is repeated 3–4 times before resting for 30 seconds and going through the exercise again. The total number of repetitions of the exercise is 3–6.

Mobility derivatives

Fleishman (1964) distinguishes between 'extent flexibility', which is defined here as mobility, and 'dynamic flexibility' which is an ability to perform repeated contraction and stretching of muscle. This derivative of mobility appears to embrace innervation, as previously discussed, and kinetic mobility. Thus, dynamic flexibility may be more accurately thought of as a specific 'functional' or 'applied' mobility. This moves close to the areas of 'agility' and 'quickness' which links technique, speed and mobility. These complex characteristics are derivatives of the basic fitness characteristics. Listing and explaining all of them is impossible due to lack of standard definitions.

SUMMARY

Basic to a development of the technical model, or models demanded of a sport, is a wide range of movement in all joint actions. A limited range of joint action compromises movement potential for the interpretation of technique, and the range through which force is applied is a critical factor in determining the nature and degree of force expression. The structure of joints, elasticity of soft tissues, and neuromuscular coordination are significant. The most important factors determining active, passive or kinetic mobility are specific exercise, joint structure, elasticity of soft tissue surrounding joints, neuromuscular coordination, and temperature.

18 EVALUATION IN SPORT

Training programmes must be planned to meet the stressors of the athlete's lifestyle and chosen sport in pursuit of agreed development and/or performance goals. The coach and athlete(s) must first agree the goal and conditions which must be met to achieve it. They must also know where they are now relative to those conditions to establish what developmental process is required against a background of evaluating the demands of the sport and the athlete's capacity to adapt to process and demands. The coach may then plan the appropriate programme for the athlete(s) to achieve the goal.

It is beyond the scope of this book to deal with the complex subject of evaluation in detail. However, a general guide to evaluation in sport may be helpful and it should be emphasised that evaluation is essential to the athlete's progress, as the coach applies the cycle: TARGET–PLAN–DO–REVIEW.

STATUS CLASSIFICATION

The primary objective of applying testing procedures is to establish the athlete's status in the parameters which are being measured. The classification of possible parameters is as follows:

GENERAL PARAMETERS	EXAMPLE
Anthropometric measures	Height, somatotype, lean body mass
Physical capacities	Strength, (e.g. leg press), power (Abalakov test), mobility (e.g. ankle flexion – extension)
Physiological capacities	VO2 maximum, blood pressure, resting heart rate
Psychological capacities	Self-regulation strategies
Technical abilities (neuromotor)	McCloy's general motor ability
SPECIFIC PARAMETERS	
Sports performance	Personal bests, development norms
Tactical performance	Decision-making, problem-solving
Technical performance	Shooting accuracy, correct response selection
Functional performance	ECG during training or competition
SPORT SPECIFIC GENERAL PARAMETERS	
Jumping strength	Bosco test

Due to the 'chicken and egg' relationship of athlete and environment, factors known to influence athletic performance must also be evaluated. Classification of environmental factors might be:

- finance – financial assistance for sports equipment
- nutrition – dietary supplements, calorie intake, smoking
- occupation – student, labourer, mother
- social – family, institution, religion
- training – equipment, facilities
- support – physiotherapy, sport science, lifestyle management.

Mass longitudinal screening techniques, or bioprofiles, assess the athlete's status in all quantifiable parameters and environmental factors relevant to athletic performance. Such information, married to the athlete's training programme over many years, may benefit the athlete if an exchange of information can be established between coach and researchers.

The measurement of status is a simple statement of fact. The next step is to evaluate these facts by comparing current results of a given test with the athlete's previous performance, with relevant norms or standards, and with other athletes. Thus, a girl athlete's VO2 maximum, say on 15th March 1989, may be 59 ml/kg/m, while on 15th September it was 55 ml/kg/m, and on 15th March it was 56 ml/kg/m. She runs 800 m and 1500 m for which the Swedish norms are 52–58 ml/kg/m. Her team-mate training for the same event recorded 57.5 ml/kg/m on 15th March and 56 ml/kg/m on 15th September. The coach, equipped with this information, can make any of the above three comparisons.

Having done this, the evaluation may help the coach reach important conclusions or decisions in several areas. Measurement and evaluation may be used as detailed below.

(1) To assess the athlete's aptitude for a given sport: testing procedures are not yet sufficiently sophisticated to assess this quality with scientific precision. However, indices of aptitude may be derived from the collective evaluation of the following:

- the status of the athlete's performance of the given technique/sport, with respect to existing norms according to age, gender, etc.
- the athlete's status in those capacities characteristic of the given sport (physiological, physical, anthropometric, etc.)
- the speed at which the athlete improves performance during the period of instruction
- the ability to reproduce consistently good performance (stability).

Clearly, the most important condition for diagnosing aptitude is regular participation in the sport concerned.

(2) To plan the athlete's developmental programme: only by exposing the athlete to a comprehensive battery of tests and comparing the athlete's status with norms according to chronological age, developmental age, gender, etc., in a given sport, will the coach be fully equipped to set out a plan for the athlete's development. The general scanning concept represented by the bioprofile system just discussed should be applied here.

(3) To assess the effect of training systems on performance: here, the athlete's status in those parameters which are to be developed by the training system (e.g. strength, aerobic endurance) is compared with performance in the sport. The results are also compared with previous results in the same testing situation. The contribution of the athlete's status in each parameter to the performance is thereby assessed.

(4) To assess the efficacy of training systems in developing specific parameters: as the athlete works to develop strength, speed, etc., via various specific training units, the athlete's status in these parameters must be constantly monitored. Evaluation of results will allow any necessary adjustment of loading within each training unit.

(5) To establish homogeneous groupings for training: it is reasonable to group athletes according to physical capacities such as speed, strength, endurance, and so on. Evaluation will enable the coach to form those groups to the best advantage of their members.

(6) To access knowledge of a given sport: the athlete must understand tactics, rules, training principles, and so on. Although it is not commonplace to test the athlete's command of this knowledge, it is important and may be seen as part of the training process.

(7) To establish the characteristics demanded of a given sport: a detailed study of biomechanics, physiology, psychology, etc., provides some insight into the demands of a given sport. However, by evaluating the status of successful athletes in physical, physiological, and other parameters, a more substantial link between athlete and sport can be established.

Tests are not ends in themselves, but a means of evaluating an athlete's status. In short, testing procedures assist the coach in understanding the athlete's training status and its development, and in making training programmes more efficient.

Notes on tests and testing

The coach must conduct testing sessions with care. Every testing procedure must be valid (testing what it purports to test), reliable (consistency of reproduction), and objective (consistency of result, irrespective of tester). The following points may help to achieve these aims.

(1) A test should measure only one capacity/ability/factor.

(2) Unless technique is being assessed, the tests should not require technical competence on the part of the athlete.

(3) There is little purpose in duplicating tests within the same unit (i.e. testing the same parameter with different tests) unless the purpose of the session is to validate new methods of testing.

(4) Each athlete in the test situation must understand exactly what is required, what is to be measured, and why. At conclusion, the results should be interpreted for the athlete.

(5) The method of conducting the test (e.g. administration, organisation, environmental requirements) should be standardised. (A set of simple instructions will help to standardise procedure on subsequent sessions. For example, in strength tests, starting and finishing joint angles must be specified and adhered to.) The standardisation of procedure should be as strict as possible (e.g. constant venue, temperature, time of day, day of menstrual cycle for girls, degree of motivation, tester, previous nutrition, time allowed for warm-up, nature of the equipment, etc.).

(6) The venue, score cards, equipment, etc., should be prepared in advance of carrying out the tests.

(7) The coach will find knowledge of statistics, mathematics, and presentation of data (e.g. graphs) very useful.

(8) The complete evaluation process involves physiologists, physiotherapists, general practitioners, psychologists, the coach and, in some cases, parents, other coaches and athletes. The sum evaluation by this 'team' should be documented and filed, but a record of tests conducted by the coach may also be kept in the athlete's training diary.

(9) Technological advances are enhancing the efficiency of evaluation techniques, e.g. photoelectric systems, laser, radar, high speed digitised video, EMG, force sensors, notational analysis etc.

The basis of evaluation and review are built into training units as target times, weights, repetitions, and so on. So whether or not an athlete or athletes are achieving the agreed challenges of units, microcycles and mesocycles are part of the review. This approach applies on a day-to-day basis and is summarised at six weekly intervals throughout the year, or 1-12-week intervals during periods such as rehabilitation or critical pre-competition preparation. The training process is clearly dynamic, with multiple variables impacting on its smooth running. The key for coach and athlete(s) is to 'read the game' fast; to learn from how it is 'read' through agreed evaluation procedure; then to adapt and move on in a different direction as suggested by the evaluation and review.

Ideally, the athlete takes ownership of at least part of the continuous monitoring process. General wellbeing or wellness self-assessment instruments are being developed and are available on the internet. They focus on creating a broad picture of the user's personal status across a range of performance related areas. For example, www.wellgoal.com covers the areas set out in table 32. Such instruments afford a basic valuable, user-friendly resource in assessing the user's overall stressor profile. More sport specific and elite performer specific variants will undoubtedly become the norm.

AM	Resting heart rate	Weight factor	Sleep	Hydration	Attitude	Perceived stress	Health
PM	Nutrition categories A, B, C, D, E	Activity	Smoking	Pursuit of purpose	Alcohol	Caffeine	RufStuff

TABLE 32 Areas for assessing the user's overall stressor profile, covered on www.wellgoal.com

SUMMARY

Evaluation is an essential ingredient of modern coaching methods. By assessing the demands of each sport, and the status of the athlete relative to these demands, a specific progressive programme of training may be constructed for that athlete. This is achieved by applying knowledge gained from an ongoing system of evaluation. The well-designed system aids in selection of sports most suited to the athlete's abilities, in planning training most suited to his needs, and in monitoring the contribution of training to the progression of fitness for a specific sport. Evaluation is part of a regular monitoring and review system. As such it is the keystone of learning.

SUMMARY OF PART 4

The interpretation of fitness for an individual is unique to his lifestyle. For athlete and non-athlete it should be understood that lifestyle in the teens influences that in the 20s and this, in turn, influences that in the 30s, and so on. A well-balanced daily routine which includes physical activity might be seen as a basis for a healthy life and should be established early on. Physical activity will range from walking and jogging, each of which requires little or no equipment, to those aspects of physical recreation which are practised in recreation or sports centres or which require specialist facilities, as in skiing and sailing.

For the athlete, part of his lifestyle is pursuit of competitive advantage and fitness must be developed accordingly. On the sound basis of general strength, endurance, and mobility, technical efficiency is developed and progressed towards the specific requirements of physical and physiological status demanded of a given sport. The broad direction of development is from general to specific, as well as from a basic technical model (or models) towards expressing that model with greater strength and speed, sometimes in the climate of endurance factors where there are such facets of a particular sport. Against the constant backcloth of a well-managed training and non-training environment, the final sophistication of development is a mature competitive attitude which permits sound performance in progressively variable situations.

Perhaps the most demanding problem for the coach is arriving at the most appropriate training plan for the development of physical and physiological status. The relative contributions of strength, speed, mobility, endurance (and their derivatives) may, in most instances, be established with the intelligent use of evaluation procedures. Nevertheless, the coach requires the full measure of his artistry to create an individually orientated programme from the expanding areas of related theory and practice.

REFERENCES FOR PART 4

Arbeit, G. (1998) Practical training emphasis in the first and second decades of development, HAS, 13–20

Astrand, P. O. & Rodahl, K. (1970) *Textbook of Work Physiology.* McGraw Hill, Toronto Ballreich, R. (1975) *A Model for Estimating the Influence of Stride Length and Stride Frequency on the Time in Sprinting Events.* Proceedings of the VIth International Congress of Biomechanics, Jyväskylä, Finland

Brunner, J. A. (1967) Untersuchungen über Statisches (Isometrisches) und Dynamisches (Isotonisches) Muskelwaining. *Körperererziehung* No. 5, Switzerland

Bührle, M. (Jan 1971) Prinzipen des Krafttrainings. Die Lehre Der Leichtathletik Dyatchkov, V. M. (1969) High jumping. *Track Technique*, No. 36 Endemann, F. (1975) *Learning Practices in Throws.* VIth Coaches' Convention Report

Fleishman, I. E. (1964) *The Structure and Measurement of Physical Fitness.* PrenticeHall, New Jersey

Gundlach, H. (1968) Zur Trainierberkeit Der Kraft–Und Schnellkeitsfahigkeiten Im Prozess Der Korperlichen Vervollkommnug. In *Theorie Und Praxis Der Korperkultur* 17, Beiheft, Teil 11, S., 167

Harre, D. (1973) *Trainingslehre.* Sportverlag, Berlin

Hettinger, T. & Muller, E. A. (1953) Muskelleistung Und Muskeltraining. *Arbeitsphysiologie,* 15, 111–126

Ivanova, L. S. (1967) *u.a.: Die Korperliche Vorbereitung Der Sportler Hoherer Leistungsklassen.* Entwicklung Der Kraft. (Fiziceskaja Podgotovka Sportsmenok Wyssych Razrjadov. Razvitie Silyl), Fiskultura i Sport, Moscow, Ubersetzung An Der DHfK Unveroffenlicht

Jäger, K. & Oelschlägel, G. (1974) *Kleine Trainingslehre.* 2nd Edn. Sportverlag, Berlin

Karvonen, M. J., Kentala, E. & Mustala, O. (1957) The effect of training on heart rate. *Annales Medicinae Experimentalis et Biologae Fenniae, Vol 35*

Keul, J. (1973) *Limiting Factors of Physical Performance.* Thieme, Stuttgart

Kusnetov, V. V. (1975) *Kraftvorbereitung–Theoretische Grundlagen Der Muskelkraftenwicklung.* 2nd Edn. Sportverlag, Berlin

Lay, P. Fundamentals of weight training. *Athletics Weekly* (13th Dec 1969, 10th Jan, 7th Feb, 28th Feb, 11th Apr, 16th May 1970)

Murase, Y., Hoshikawa, T., Yasuda, N., Ikegami, Y. & Matsui, H. (1975) *A Study of Analysis of the Changes in Progressive Speed of 100m from the Points of View of Anaerobic Energy Output and Running Patterns.* Proceedings of Vth International Congress of Biomechanics, Jyväskylä, Finland

Osolin, N. G. (1952) *Das Training Des Leichtathleten.* Sportverlag, Berlin

Osolin, N. G. (Jan 1973) Speed endurance. *Modern Athlete and Coach, Vol 11,* No 1

Pahud, J. P. & Gobbeler, C. (1986) *Training at Altitude: General Principles and Personal Experience.* New Studies in Athletics, September 1986, Rome

Pohlitz, L. (1986) *Practical experiences of altitude training with female middle distance runners.* Leichtathletik. Berlin 25, vol. 3

Saziorski, W. M. (1971) Die Korperlichen Eigenschaften Des Sportlers. In *Theorie Und Praxis Der Korperkultur.* Beiheft 2

Sinkkonen, K. (1975) *The Programming of Distance Running.* Paper to E.L.L.V., Congress, Budapest

Teglbur, U., Bussg, N. and Braumann, K. M. (1993) Estimation of an individual equilibrium between lactate production and catabolism during exercise, *Medicine and Science in Sports and Exercise*, 25, 620–627

Upton, A. R. M. & Radford, P. F. (1975) *Trends in Speed of Alternated Limb Movement During Development and Amongst Elite Sprinters.* Proceedings of Vth International Congress of Biomechanics, Jyväskylä, Finland

Van der Woude, L. H. V., Veeger, H. E. J. and Dallmeijer, A. J, (1995) The ergonomics of wheelchair sports – *Sport, Leisure and Ergonomics* (Eds Atkinson, G. and Reilly, J.), pp. 3–12, E. and F. M. Spon, London

Verhoshansky, J. W. (1971) Grundlagen Des Speziellen Krafttrainings Im Sport. In *Theorie Und Praxis Der Korperkultur*

Viru, A. A., Urgenstein, Y. U. & Pisuke, A. P. (1972) Influence of training methods on endurance. *Track Technique*, No 47

Wagner, P. (1976) *MaleFemale Differences in Middle Distance Training and Competitions.* VIIth Coaches' Convention Technical Report

Wasserman, K. (1986) The anaerobic threshold: definition physiological significance and identification, *Advances in Cardiology*, 35, 1–23

Williams, C. (1974) *Special Forms and Effects of Endurance Training.* Vth Coaches' Convention Report

BIBLIOGRAPHY

Arthur, R. (May 1973) What swimmers can teach to runners. *Modern Athlete and Coach*, Vol 1, No 3

Clarke, H. H. (1967) *Application of Measurement to Health and Physical Education.* 4th Edn. PrenticeHall, New Jersey

Counsilman, J. G. (1970) *The Science of Swimming.* Pelham Books Ltd., London

Elliott, B. (1999) *Training in Sport,* Wilgy, Chichester, UK

Hettinger, T. H. (July 1975) Muscle trainability of men and women. *Modern Athlete and Coach, Vol 13*, No 4

Hogg, J. M. (1972) *Land Conditioning for Competitive Swimming.* E. P. Publishing Ltd, Wakefield

Jensen, C. R. & Fisher, A. G. (1972) *Scientific Basis of Athletic Conditioning.* Lea & Febiger, Philadelphia

Jesse, J. P. (July 1976) Young athletes and weight training. *Modern Athlete and Coach, Vol 14*, No 1

Kendrick, D. (May 1975) Activity and ageing. *New Behaviour, Vol 1*, No 6

Koslov, V. (July 1970) Application of maximum power in throwing. *Modern Athlete and Coach, Vol 8*, No 4

Margaria, R. (1976) *Biomechanics and Energetics of Muscular Exercise.* Clarendon Press, Oxford

Petrovski, V. & Verhoshansky, J. (1975) Aspects of sprint training. *Modern Athlete and Coach, Vol 13*, No 4

Pickering, R. J. (1968) *Strength Training for Athletics*. 2nd Edn. B.A.A.B. Instructional Booklet, London

Polunin, A. (1994) *Training in Middle and High Mountains*. EACA Workshop Paper, Belmekan

Schmolinsky, G. (1974) *Leichtathletik*. 7th Edn. Sportverlag, Berlin

Schon, R. (1994) *Recommendations Based on Experience of Altitude Training with Young Athletes*. EACA Workshop Paper, Belmekan

Shephard, R. J. (1969) *Endurance Training*. University of Toronto Press

Skaset, H. B. (1970) *Trainingslaere*. Norges Idrettsforbund, Oslo

Taylor, A. W. (1972) *Training–Scientific Basis and Application*. Charles C. Thomas, Illinois

Whitehead, N. (1988) *Conditioning for Sport*. A & C Black, London

Young, W. (1995) Laboratory strength assessment of athletes, *H.S.A.* 10–1, 89–96

PART 5

PLANNING THE PROGRAMME

Without knowing our destination, we cannot plan our journey. Our destination in sport is the competition objective or goal. It might be to win a league competition, a cup tournament, an Olympic medal, a place in the National Championships, a qualifying performance for team selection, or a lifetime best performance in a particular competition. It must be 'beyond the probable' yet is realistically believed in, as agreed by coach and athlete. Our journey is the preparation programme planned to help reach the objective or goal; it is quantifiable and has a timescale.

The structure of that plan and its details must, however, be sufficiently flexible to move and adapt to the dynamics of athlete, coach and situation. The destination is not a terminus, but a milestone. The programme must be capable of adjustment on the way to that milestone, and for progressing beyond it.

We must, however, start with some kind of 'route map'. The division of the training year into periods of varying duration, characterised by their progressive contribution to reaching the 'destination', is such a 'route map'.

For athletics, it grew from such origins as:

Period 1	Autumn and winter	Training for and compet-ing in winter field games
Period 2	Spring	Training for athletics
Period 3	Summer	Lighter training and competing in athletics

to:

Period 1	Winter training
Period 2	Pre-competition training
Period 3	Competition training

to current systems of periodisation.

This evolution of how the year is planned might be thought of as a progressive shift towards considering training as a cyclical year-round process, which is part of a total development of training and performance over several years.

In part 5, in order to explain the underlying principles of designing a year-round programme, it is expedient to illustrate the process with reference mainly to a summer season sport – athletics. Here, the preparation portion of the year is long – and the competition portion(s) short. This makes things very simple. However, in long competition season sports such as winter games (e.g. soccer, rugby, hockey, lacrosse, basketball), or year-round racquet games (i.e. tennis, squash), life is rather more complicated and both preparation/conditioning and competition objectives must be pursued simultaneously on the foundation of a very brief (1–2 month) preparation/conditioning base.

Part 5 sets out the athletics training year and, where relevant, reference is made to the application of training principles in practice in long season/year-round sports.

19 PERIODISING THE YEAR

Periodisation may be described as an organised division of the training year in pursuit of three basic objectives:

* to prepare the athlete for the achievement of an optimal improvement in their performance
* to prepare the athlete for a definite climax to the competition season
* to prepare the athlete for the main competitions associated with that climax.

Occasionally, annual objectives are not embraced by the three stated. These may be considered under two separate headings:

* to aid recovery from injury, illness or a particularly stressful training year
* to prepare the athlete for meeting the above objectives in subsequent years, by increasing special training status, stabilising technique or performance, and so on, over the period of one or more years.

Special programmes are required to meet the last two objectives and, although they are not dealt with in detail here, the terminology and broad principles of programme construction still apply.

Modern theory of periodisation was originally advanced by L. P. Matveyev (USSR), in 1965, as an updating of work which he first introduced in 1962.

month	Oct	Nov	Dec	Jan	Feb	Mar	Apr	May	Jun	Jul	Aug	September
macro	← preparation ———————————————→							← competition ——→				← transition →
meso	I				II	III				IV	V	VI

FIG. 83 The division of the training year will obviously be influenced by the 'competition calendar'. The division shown here was used by USSR in preparation for Munich*YY*where athletes used a 'single periodised year' (from Osolin and Markov, 1972).

double		I		II		III_1		I		II			III_2	IV	V		VI
single				I				II	III				IV	V			VI
month	Nov	Dec	Jan	Feb	Mar	Apr	May	Jun	Jul	Aug	Sep	Oct

FIG. 84 Single and double periodised years

From early ideas of preparing an athlete for a competitive programme distributed throughout a season, he looked towards a specific competition climax or peak (e.g. National Championships, Olympic Games, etc.), for which not only training periods, but also a selected competition programme was a totality of preparation. Matveyev suggested that the year be divided into three periods: preparation, competition, and transition. These are referred to here as *macrocycles*, and they describe the cyclic performance development model of PREPARATION (ADAPTATION) – COMPETITION (APPLICATION) – TRANSITION (REGENERATION). He sub-divided these into shorter training phases, which are referred to here as *mesocycles* (fig. 83). A closer look at these mesocycles will help identify their individual character.

PREPARATION MACROCYCLE

Mesocycle 1

This is the longest phase in the annual cycle and should occupy one third of that cycle. Thus, in the single periodised year (fig. 84), it occupies four months (3 x 6 weeks) while in the double periodised year (fig. 84 and text) it occupies 8–10 weeks, to be reintroduced after the first competition macrocycle (3_1) for a further 6–8 weeks.

The main aim is to increase the athlete's ability to accept a high intensity (quality) of loading in mesocycle 2 by increasing the extent (quantity) of loading during mesocycle 1. The high volume of work involved necessitates a very gradual increase in intensity during this mesocycle, but this increase is essential to progress in mesocycle 2 and to the stabilisation of performance in the competition macrocycle. Training is more general in nature, and during this mesocycle the athlete is working at the endurance end of his event development. However, in the interest of continuous development of performance, it is also necessary to pursue related training and specific training. A mixed programme is required, which must take into account the particular event and the athlete's stage of development when establishing a ratio of general:related:specific training. It may be useful to describe these broad areas of training.

General training: this is training for the whole organism. A basic all-round programme is usual and, above all, the establishment of a sound basis of aerobic fitness, and a certain minimum status in the foundation of fitness for a specific sport (e.g. mobility and strength for jumps, goalkeeping, diving, etc.).

Related training: this is training to perfect the individual components of sports techniques and specific fitness, e.g. work with heavier implements (throws), technique work with resistances (gymnastics, swimming), drills (games), bounding, hill running, under/over distance work (endurance sprints/middle distance).

Specific training: this is training where technique is completely rehearsed and, more specifically, in the competition situation. This area varies from a shade of special training to actual competitions, embracing technique, tactics, etc. It plays a much smaller part in the total extent of training than the other two.

At the risk of being over repetitive, *all three areas* are covered throughout the year, but their contribution will vary from mesocycle to mesocycle. At the end of mesocycle 1, the basic components of fitness for a specific event must have reached the level necessary to ensure a planned increase in performance. Tests may be used to check this. For example, a long jumper working towards 8.00 m from a 20-stride approach should jump 7.00 m from 10 strides.

This mesocycle might be viewed as 'training to train', and is normally subdivided into Mesocycles 1_1, 1_2 etc. of up to six weeks duration.

Mesocycle 2

This mesocycle, according to Matveyev (1965), lasts eight weeks when single periodisation is used and six weeks in double periodisation. However, it is possible to stretch this to eight or 12 weeks, and four weeks plus four weeks respectively, if the annual cycle is extended slightly beyond 52 weeks. There are many advantages to such stretching, but most important is that the increase of load intensity will be gentler. There is no doubt, however, that this is the hardest working mesocycle in the year.

Mesocycle 2 runs directly into the competition period. Its aims are to unite the component parts or foundations of training into a harmonious whole (e.g. training moves from workshop to assembly line). While the character of this mesocycle is that of specialisation, the areas of training in the first mesocycle are continued. The training ratio decreases in the general area and, while the total extent of work remains the same or is gently reduced, the intensity of loading in related and specific training increases sharply. Technique must be schooled and stabilised as the athlete learns to use increased strength, speed, etc. It is absolutely essential that technical development and development of strength, speed, and so forth, are advanced together. A season can be completely lost if they are 'out of step'.

Towards the end of this mesocycle, the athlete must be exposed to more open competition situations such as wind, rain, noise, morning, floodlights, etc. Should training progress successfully, the young athlete will (according to Harre (1973)) improve on previous best performance after three competitions. The experienced athlete should at least equal his previous best. It would appear from personal observation that if the young athlete is within 2.5% of his best performance in a technical event after three competitions (spaced over 2–4 weeks), it is reasonable to assume that progress is 'on schedule'. By increasing load intensity, particularly via competitions, he will improve performance still further. If no improvements follow, it is frequently a result of the intensity having been raised too rapidly in the second mesocycle, or the extent of competition loading being too great, or the total extent of loading at the end of the preparation macrocycle having been excessively reduced.

This mesocycle might be viewed as 'training to compete'.

COMPETITION MACROCYCLE

Mesocycle 3

The main task of this mesocycle of the competition macrocycle is to develop and stabilise competition performance as fully as possible (see also chapter 24). The athlete will then be able to produce optimal performance in key competitions. The blending of new levels of specific sport or event fitness, which has been developed throughout the preparation macrocycle, must be continued in order to produce high-level performance. Moreover, these new levels of fitness must be maintained via specific loadings and competitions themselves. Consequently, the loadings in this area are increased, while those in the general and related areas are reduced. The total extent of training is therefore decreased as the intensity rises. The reduction of extent is very steep where sports demand maximum or elastic strength or speed (e.g. jumps, throws, weight lifting, games), but only slight in endurance sports in the interest of maintaining aerobic fitness. General training should be seen primarily as a means of active recovery in the non-endurance sports.

It is important not to neglect the status of basic fitness components such as strength, speed, mobility, etc., in favour of technical development. Strength losses, for example, can be considerable, even over 2–3 weeks and such losses, if continued, will be reflected in performance. Consequently, the strength programme has its place in the competition macrocycle (fig. 85).

The frequency of competitions depends on the individual athlete's capacity for

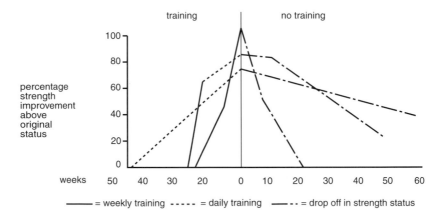

FIG. 85 An outline of work conducted by Hettinger, illustrating not only different effects of daily and weekly training, but how strength training loses its effect once stopped (from Hettinger, 1968).

the emotional and physical stress of competition loading. It is very difficult to establish ideal numbers of competitions and this topic is discussed more fully below. At one end of the scale, an elite athlete might feel that two major marathons in one year is acceptable but, at the other, a 13-year-old may be happy to spend all year competing twice a week in several sports.

Competition frequency and the amount of specific loading determine development of performance in the competition macrocycle. An optimal balance can only be arrived at individually, but, once known, the athlete can expect to record best performances 6–8 weeks from the start of this mesocycle (i.e. mesocycle 3 single periodisation, and mesocycles 3_1 and 3_2 double periodisation). Thus, after three competitions (4–6 weeks from start of mesocycle 3), the athlete will be within 2.5% of lifetime best and by 6–8 weeks will have improved upon lifetime best. Trials and qualifying competitions, and most of the main contests for young athletes, should therefore fall within mesocycle 3 (single) and mesocycle 3_2 (double).

This mesocycle might be viewed as 'competing to learn'.

Mesocycle 4

If competition is to continue beyond mesocycles 3 and 3_2, it is advisable to introduce a mesocycle of 4–6 weeks in which the proportion of specific training is reduced, competitions are eliminated, and general and related training are increased. The value of general training should be noted here, as it serves an important role in active recovery from the emotional and physical stresses of competition.

If the athlete has not been brought to peak performance in the previous 6–8 weeks, a longer period may be necessary, and mesocycle 4 may be omitted and the training ratio left unchanged. If the athlete has achieved peak performance, mesocycle 4 aids recovery, protects from injury, and prepares for mesocycle 5. The latter is most important in a major season (e.g. Olympic Games) as this mesocycle will be seen as a special preparation macrocycle. This mesocycle might be viewed as 'training to win'.

Mesocycle 5

Again, by evolving an optimal blend of competitions and specific training, further improvement in performance may be expected within 3–4 weeks. Ideally, the major event of the athletic calendar will fall within this mesocycle (Olympic Games, National Championships, etc.).

This mesocycle might be viewed as 'competing to win'.

TRANSITION MACROCYCLE

Mesocycle 6

Just as restful sleep must follow a hard day's work, so a period of regeneration must follow a hard year's training and competition. This period of regeneration must bring the athlete to commencement of the next training year totally prepared for training; from positive motivational profile through to fully 'recharged energy batteries'.

If the season has been 'low key', little wear and tear on the organism might be expected and, following a medical and physiotherapy check-up, the athlete will go straight into general activity for basic strength, mobility and aerobic endurance after mesocycle 5. In effect, it is a build into Preparation mesocycle 1. This would mean a rapid increase in the extent of training, and a drop in intensity. If, on the other hand, the season has been 'high key', 3–6 weeks active recovery must precede the next preparation macrocycle. The athlete should not start the new preparation macrocycle without a full recovery from the previous competition season, otherwise the effect of future loading will be extremely limited, adaptation problems will quickly arise, a risk of injury will occur, and the disappointment of poor progress in training may have effects reaching into the next competition macrocycle.

The transition macrocycle sees the gentle reduction of all loadings, with general training assuming the leading role in the training ratio. While technical schooling may now be introduced, the emphasis should be on physical, and emotional and intellectual regeneration involving leisure pursuits. On no account should this macrocycle be passive.

This mesocycle might be viewed as 'recharging to train'.

YEAR-ROUND ADAPTATIONS

In broad terms, it is possible to establish a 'competition' macrocycle which constitutes priority competitions, and another 'preparation' macrocycle where there are no competitions or very low priority ones. For example, soccer's competition macrocycle in the UK commences mid-August and concludes mid-May. This leaves approximately 12 weeks for the preparation macrocycle during which the regeneration objectives of mesocycle 6 and the objectives of mesocycles 2 and 4 are pursued. The loose guide to training unit distribution here is general:related:specific – 50%:30%:20%. Through the competition season it is a matter of ensuring that microcycles of seven days, variously having one or two or even three competitions, are designed to regenerate; to produce competition sharpness; and to maintain general:related:specific conditioning status. A possible unit distribution to achieve this would be 20%:30%:50%, bearing in mind that competitions themselves are included in the 50% specific.

This said, the programme should be sufficiently flexible to return to the preparation macrocycle distribution should the opportunity arise. In rugby union in the UK, such an opportunity is afforded by the midwinter league break. In international tennis, players must create blocks of time to regenerate and build a conditioning base by prioritising their tournaments through what can amount to a 12 month 'season'!

SUMMARY

Periodisation is an organised division of the training year in pursuit of basic objectives of training. The divisions are, in the first instance, those of preparation, competition and transition. These are referred to as *macrocycles*, which are further subdivided into *mesocycles*. Mesocycles 1, 2 and 4 are planned according to specific objectives of preparation, while mesocycles 3 and 5 are planned in pursuit of specific objectives of competition. Mesocycle 6 coincides with the transition macrocycle.

20 VARIATIONS IN PERIODISATION

Preparation for achieving an athlete's lifetime competitive goal of the Olympic Games or gaining a World Title etc., commences with his earliest experience of sport and is brought to fruition sometime during the athlete's peak performance years in his chosen sport; hence the timetable of the development process set out in table 33. Management of this process through the several years should be considered a shared 'partnership' responsibility and might take the shape of fig. 86.

Each year of development must be carefully structured to build on previous years' development and as preparation for those to follow. They are each quite different. Here, a close examination is made of the 12-month cycle of an athlete committed to high-level achievement in sport.

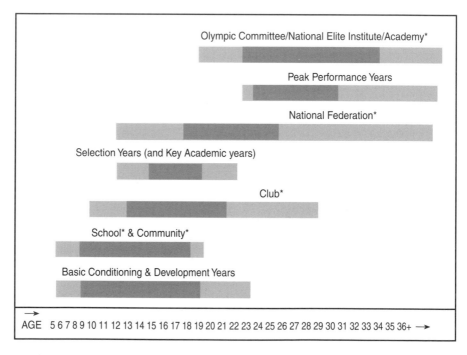

FIG. 86 Management of the athlete's development progress requires a commitment to partnership as the athlete moves through the process. Possible 'partners' are indicated*.

approximate age range	development emphases
4–11/12 years	• General all-joint mobility • General all-round strength • Basic health • Positive attitude to exercise and sport • Wide range of sound basic technical models and complex model components • Competitive attitude – challenge/ performance
12/13–18/19 years	• General/related/specific strength • General/related/specific endurance • Specific technical models • Participation/competition opportunity in range of sports • Speed of technical execution • Competitive attitude – performance/results
19/20–22/23 years	• Progressive competition experience • Performance goals acceleration • Dedicated specific training programmes • Long-/medium-/short-term goals preparation • Competitive attitude – results performance
22/23–35+ years	• Pursuit of critical career best performance • Refinements of specific training programmes • Long-/medium-/short-term goals delivery • 'Full-time' approach • Competitive attitude – results
35+ – Life	• 'Detraining' = fitness programme for life wellness

TABLE 33 An athlete's development from the earliest years of exercise/sport involvement through the post-competition years requires a strategic approach to addressing development objectives/emphases.

SETTING OUT THE TIMESCALE

The start of the competition macrocycle(s) is dictated by (1) the number of competitions necessary for the athlete to reach and stabilise best performance, (2) the dates of the major competition and main competitions, (3) the recovery period required by the athlete between competitions, and (4) the period required for preparation for the major competition (this period must take into account possible acclimatisation to a new environment – time adjustment in East/West shift, altitude adjustment, etc.). These conditions are worth further explanation.

(1) **Number of necessary competitions.** Although Harre (1973) suggested 6–8 weeks, other authorities have advanced 6–10 weeks as a reasonable range of time

for athletes to reach and stabilise their best performances in mesocycle 3. Harre's (1973) suggestion is more acceptable for mesocycle 3_2 if double periodised. Some athletes commence the competition macrocycle with low-key, non-pressure competitions which are virtually an extension of training time trials. These constitute a type of 'competition control', reintroducing the disciplines of competition warm-up and reporting procedures. Moreover, irrespective of the athlete's level of performance, he has an opportunity to 'get the adrenaline moving' without the stressors of pressure which will come later in the season. Once this stage is completed, the athlete then decides with his coach the venues, levels of competition, and frequency of competition which are required to produce his best performance, his springboard for the main business of the season.

The coach should be aware of the influence which early good performances by opponents have on an athlete. The season's objectives *and* the week by week objectives must be understood by athlete and coach. The athlete's early season performances should not be so far adrift from those of the opposition that the athlete feels pressure. Consequently, coaches should introduce the athlete to competitions *only* when the athlete is ready and only when the objective is understood and attainable.

(2) **Dates of competitions.** The important qualifying rounds should be found in the latter 2–4 weeks of the suggested range, thus giving up to six weeks of preparatory contests and up to four weeks of main contests. The major competitions will be, as it were, the 'fixed point' of the season. Thus, if the athlete views the National Championships as the major competition, mesocycles 3 or 3_2 and 4 are worked from that date. The coach has the problem of providing the relevant mesocycle 3 (3_2) levels of competition for the athlete over the time-span dictated by the National Championships date. On the other hand, the major competition may be an Olympic Games. It would then be in the interest of the Olympic athletes for trials and competitions, designed to produce qualifying marks, to be timetabled for a relevant mesocycle 3 or 3_2. Moreover, as Olympic Games and other major championships constitute a tournament rather than one-off competitions, the athlete must be afforded the opportunity to rehearse the sequence of qualifying rounds/heats and finals in the period leading up to the final selection dates or in the course of the final selection dates.

(3) **Recovery period.** This will vary from athlete to athlete according to event, age, experience and standard of competitions. The young athlete, whose ability to produce performances near the limit of his capacity is as yet undeveloped, will compete very regularly – as often as twice to three times per week in interclub, intra-club, league or open meetings, etc. Although competitions are meaningful to such an athlete, times, distances and heights are a long way from being an ultimate expression of ability. On mounting the club/district/regional/national/ international record ladder, however, the athlete begins to take a more serious view of success and failure. With this change of approach from 'playing' to commitment, both physical *and* psychological stressors mean more time to prepare for and recover from competitions. It is not unusual, then, to find an athlete at this

stage competing only once a week, or every other week. Again, the idea might be extended so that there are only two or three competitions in the season (specific competition climaxes or peaks), while a few other competitions are entered to test fitness or for practice.

Matveyev (1965) suggests that in explosive sports, where the technical component is high (e.g. field events, tennis, gymnastics, team games), several peaks may be pursued. However, where the technical component is lower (e.g. sprints, hurdles), three peaks per season at most can be worked for. This argument can only be defended if, by 'peak', we consider a block of time rather than a particular time on a particular day. On this basis, it is suggested that most athletes cannot sustain maximum performance levels beyond 21 days, and even then such performances are not being repeated at high frequency within these 21 days. The main problem here is as much a psychological/emotional one as it is physiological/physical. Clear understanding and application of the concept of regeneration is essential to ensuring that peak 'blocks of time' can be repeated not only within a given season, but also over several seasons.

In endurance events, where complex training has been used, only two peaks can be expected. The first of these peaks might be considered a 'performance peak' where the athlete pursues a performance objective such as a record, or a performance control on which to base achievement targets for the main competition focus. The second is a 'competition peak' where the athlete builds on what has been achieved in pursuit of the first peak through tournament planning and tactics, to reach for success in the season's major championships. Endurance athletes using the Lydiard method normally aim for one peak in the season. This peak embraces pursuit both of performance and competition objectives and is sustained over a period of up to six weeks during which time competitions are judiciously spaced to have both objectives coincide with the major championships.

It is clear that the process of planning an athlete's season up to a selection date is unique to a given athlete. Ideally, the programme of local, area, national and international competitions made available to athletes is such that the athlete can select those competitions which best suit his programme of preparation. This means that athletes must occasionally make value judgements on whether or not to compete on occasions which have high priority for those organising the competitions, but low priority for the athlete. The objectives of periodising the year were set out at the start of chapter 19. The athlete's value judgements must be made within the framework of these objectives if he is to produce optimal performance at the major championships.

(4) Preparation period. This period is really mesocycles 4 and 5 looked upon as a whole, with mesocycle 4 lasting 4–6 weeks and mesocycle 5 lasting 3–4 weeks. The content of mesocycle 4 will, of course, be altered considerably from that just described in that it represents a specific programme of preparation for a specific competition. For the young and developing athlete, there seems little justification for imposing a rigid structure of competition in the competition macrocycle. For the mature national and international athlete, however, it is essential.

Top-level athletes cannot be expected to produce maximum performance on every outing. To avoid pressure to do so they may choose not to compete against key opposition. In commercially orientated sport, the pressure is great to meet various contractual obligations. Decisions must be made early when planning the year's programme to strike a balance which will avoid compromise to the pursuit of performance and competition objectives, yet will satisfy the sport's commercial sector. When an athlete is preparing to meet the best in the world, both preparation and competition represent intense mental, emotional and physical efforts and cannot be entered into at short intervals. Failure to accept this will lead to an athlete 'burning himself out', and can set the scene for falling short at the major championships. In long, persistent season sports like soccer, managers must rotate players over approximately 6–8-week cycles to avoid similar burn-out. This ensures a generally consistent high quality team output while allowing regeneration and learning opportunity across the squad of players.

According to Harre (1973) the total process of the main competition period spans 12 weeks. Personal experience suggests that this can be 16 weeks in a single periodised year. Young and developing athletes should not go beyond 12 weeks; developing athletes may reach 16 weeks due to the more general nature of their training; and top-level athletes will operate between 10 and 16 according to how they have periodised the year, and how they may have organised the progression of competitions and the competition peaks within the season. Several countries arrange their fixture lists in such a way that a periodised competition season may be followed, e.g. the German soccer season.

Before leaving this general look at the phasing of the competition period, comparative study of Olympic performances in Mexico and Munich is worth comment. Kruger (1973) found that those following Matveyev periodisation of the summer improved significantly (0.5 level), compared with nations who did not. If the Belgians and Finns were excluded, significance was at the 0.1 level! This study had one or two limitations in that it had information on the athlete's main event alone, and on competition results only, but no knowledge of competition conditions. Moreover, Matveyev periodisation *should* show Matveyev results! Nevertheless, within these limitations, the value of this approach to periodisation seems considerable. The ability of an athlete to peak at the right time must be considered a possible cause of such significant results.

SINGLE AND DOUBLE PERIODISATION

Several attempts have been made to accelerate performance improvement by establishing two competition seasons. The concept of two competition seasons is referred to as double periodisation, while one competition season is single periodisation. The double periodised year has been successfully applied to swimming and track and field. Matveyev (1965) has demonstrated that by this method it is possible to achieve a greater increase per year in those events where maximum and elastic strength are key characteristics (table 34).

event	double periodisation	single periodisation
100 m	1.55%	0.96%
Long jump	1.46%	1.35%
High jump	5.05%	2.40%
Shot	3.85%	2.58%

TABLE 34 Percentage annual improvement in performance comparing double and single periodisation from Matveyev, 1965 Die Periodisierung, Des Sportlicher Trainings—Fiskultura i Sport—Moscow Discus (3.87% 3.11%)

Matveyev's explanation is that the more rapid sequence of competition periods prevents an undue fall-off of competition performance and contributes to the stabilisation of technical performance. By stabilisation it is presumed he is referring to the continued integration of technique and conditioning of one keeping in step with the other. However, this implies a certain status in technical development. It should be emphasised, then, that where long periods of consolidation and development are needed (e.g. basic strength, speed, etc.), and in technique as in the young and developing athlete, double periodisation does not have a strong case. To sub-divide the year into short periods of preparation will only result in incomplete mastery of technique, unstable performance, and a reduced rate of development in the foundations of fitness. The stressor of competition in these circumstances will exaggerate those faults which accompany the pursuit of immediate wins, as opposed to an ultimate optimal improvement in performance. This said, any discussion of single or double periodised years should assume that the athlete has a training maturity of several seasons. The young and developing athlete should therefore use any second season as an adjunct to training rather than a deliberate competition climax (e.g. other games, cross-country, etc.).

Since this discussion implies mature athletes, the main competition period is long both for single and double periodisation. This period is subdivided for both systems into mesocycles 3, 4, 5 or 3$_2$, 4, 5. So the fundamental difference between single and double periodisation, then, is the existence of a second season. Despite Matveyev's evidence to support the double season, it is not without its antagonists. Although, their criticisms are more requests for caution than rejections, and should be noted, it was always made clear by Matveyev and interpreters of his work that the notion of double periodisation was not generally suited to endurance sports. Of course there are exceptions where athletes have won world indoors or cross-country titles, then achieved World or Olympic titles in the summer season. However, the breaking up of the preparation period necessary for endurance excellence does not lend itself to continuing endurance sport competition achievement.

Implications for the long season sports

Simply playing a team game, as opposed to an individual sport, does not make players different in their capacity to produce peak performance. It becomes essential, then, for team managers in sports such as rugby, ice hockey, basketball, etc. to establish some form of rotation of players as suggested. Of course the first team will be critical to achieving success in big competitions, but these must be prioritised and individual player preparation plans should be woven round the prioritised competition dates. If players are also to be able to peak for international team duties, these dates must be included in the prioritised list. If international tournaments such as World or European cups extend the season to the point where the transition cycle is substantially eroded, it is essential to the players' wellbeing that additional weeks are made available for regeneration.

So many peaks, by definition, means a well-planned regeneration programme and the cyclic reintroduction of general and related training units. In those sports with high and multiple technical demands and conditioning demands, there is a year-round requirement for technical and conditioning work. Cycles of general:related:specific work cannot be compromised to meet the demands of ranking systems. Short-term objectives *must* be consistent with long-term objectives, and not ends in themselves. The key is to ensure the unbroken competition period is not so long as to erode the general/related conditioning base.

SUMMARY

A double competition season provides a greater potential for increase in annual performance in most disciplines, but probably not endurance. The advantage gained by expanding the time available for competition opportunity must be weighed against the loss to preparation time. Consequently, when applying double periodisation, careful thought must be given to the phasing of the preparation period within the annual cycle. Moreover, in the athlete's competitive 'life', sound judgement is required in the distribution of double periodised years.

21 UNITS, MICROCYCLES, MESOCYCLES AND MACROCYCLES

The world of 'schedules and sessions' is now examined, although these expressions are losing their popularity. Consequently some of the expressions used here may be new and it may therefore be useful to define them.

THE TRAINING UNIT

The training unit is a single practice session in pursuit of a training objective. For example, the objective may be to develop sprinting speed so the unit might then be 3 x 4 x 30 m rolling start sprints, four minutes between repetitions, 7–10 minutes between sets. The objective may be development of aerobic endurance so the unit might be a 20 km steady run, or the objective might be active recovery so the unit could be 20–30 minutes squash, and so on.

An athlete's visit to a training venue may, in fact, allow him to work on one or several training units. For instance, a female basketball player may work through three units in one visit to the gym. At 13.00 hours she begins the first unit (mobility exercises) to develop mobility. At 14.00 hours she practises shooting drills to develop accuracy. At 15.00 hours she begins the third unit of 3 x 3 x 3 lengths turnabout court sprints in 15 seconds, with 60 seconds easy run between reps and two minutes between sets, to develop running speed endurance. On the other hand, an evening or lunchtime session may only allow time for one unit. So, simply referring to both situations (i.e. three units in one day, and one unit in one day) as two 'sessions' might cause confusion. This would certainly be the case if one were discussing the number of units per week. To say 'six sessions per week' might mean anything from six to 18 units!

THE MICROCYCLE

The microcycle is a group of units organised in such a way that optimal training value can be obtained from each unit. Moreover, the microcycle may be repeated several times in pursuit of the overall objectives of a mesocycle or macrocycle.

It is expedient to plan microcycles for a period of one week (table 35) as this helps to fit training units into the general framework of social routine. However, it is clear that for many younger athletes the unit ratio of work to rest, even on a one unit per day basis, can lose its training value at 6:1.

day	objective	unit	*demand
Sunday	general conditioning and mobility	Fartlek and woodland conditioning circuit	medium
Monday	elastic and maximum strength	maximum and sub-maximum weights	high
Tuesday	special development	throws in weighted jacket with heavy implements	medium-high
Wednesday	elastic strength	combined submaximum weights and jumps	high
Thursday	maximum strength	maximum weights	very high
Friday	general throwing	other throws, jumps, hurdles, special exercises	medium
Saturday	technique development and strength testing	throws and tests	high

*Note varying demands of each unit. Classification was made according to athlete's own impressions in working through programme.

TABLE 35 Mesocycle 1 microcycle of a male discus thrower

A regular cycle of 3:1 may suit this athlete's development better, but the training cycle will fall out of synchronisation with the calendar cycle of one week. If this caused problems, the units might be rearranged. For example, one unit on Saturday, two on Sunday, none Monday, one each on Tuesday, Wednesday and Thursday, and none on Friday. Naturally, the units on Sunday would require careful selection. The ratio of the number of training units to the number of recovery units within a microcycle is the inter-unit *training ratio*.

Several points are worth noting on the construction of a microcycle.

(1) The profile of extent of loading and intensity of loading must be given careful consideration (fig. 87). This profile is often referred to as 'the *structure of loading*'. Both extent and intensity of loading will be dealt with in greater detail in chapter 22.

(2) The demands made on the athlete vary in individual training units in terms of the intra-unit training ratio. This is the relationship of stimulus:recovery within a unit. Thus, the training load represented by each unit has anything from a very high to a slight demand upon the athlete. The athlete must not be exposed to very high demands upon his system in successive units (table 35). Although assessments of demand are mainly subjective on the part of the athlete, the observant coach should read the effect of units upon the athlete with whom he is working. Athlete and coach share responsibility for value judgements on the effect of training, and apply their collective input to programme planning as a consequence.

(3) Each unit is in pursuit of a specific objective and should vary within a day, and from day to day. Programme planning should then have not only an inbuilt variety of general, related and specific units according to athlete, sport and place of training, but also variations in unit detail in pursuit of a specific objective. Notwithstanding the need for variety, athletes also require a sense of routine in the programme. The values here range from a basis for comparison to monitor progress, through to the 'comfort' of an established microcycle design. Part of the coach's art is to arrange microcycles in such a way that variety is a key feature within a flexible framework of routine.

(4) In order to avoid over-exertion, the interval between two training units should be long enough to allow the athlete to recover sufficiently to gain maximum training effect from the next unit.

(5) Recovery is accelerated if units of active recovery, or 'regeneration' units are introduced into the microcycle (see chapter 23).

(6) When training units with different objectives and varying demands follow each other, it may not be necessary to await complete recovery. This is the case when different systems are being stressed. According to Craig (1973), this also protects the athlete from 'overuse' types of injury.

(7) Microcycles also permit concentration on one particular objective in individual units, allowing some optimal period of time when the athlete can be exposed

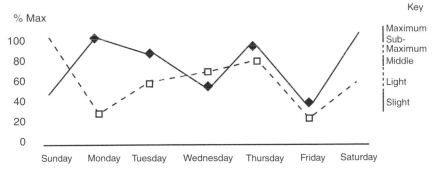

FIG. 87 Alterations in intensity:extent ratio in the course of a microcycle in Mesocycle II. The subject is a female long jumper, and the scale of intensity (maximum, submaximum, etc.) is read against percentage of maximum (vertical scale). The scale of intensity is as suggested by Carl when he advanced the concept as 'spheres of intensity' for weight lifting (from Carl, 1967).

to the desired stimulus. This helps adaptation to develop in a particular area. Poor organisation may bring conflicting objectives into badly grouped units (e.g. when speed loading and endurance loading are brought together *some* contribution is made to speed and endurance, but the maximal development of either is impossible). Similarly, when an athlete rushes intervals between repetitions of set pieces in games, development of technique is impaired and very little contribution to speed or endurance is made.

(8) Microcycles reduce monotony in training despite high frequency of training units. Failure to use these cycles may mean a standard unit or variation on a unit being used *ad nauseam*, the result of which would be a stereotyped reaction to the exercise stimulus and an ultimate stagnation of performance, as there is no adaptation challenge.

(9) Demands on speed or elastic strength or maximum strength should be carried out on days of optimal capacity and never following days of high demand, especially if this involves lactic-anaerobic endurance training. A similar rule will apply when several units are being worked in the course of one day. So the following order of events should be pursued:

Several units in one day:

- warm-up and/or mobility
- neuromuscular work (e.g. technique, speed, elastic strength, maximum strength)
- energy systems work (all endurance – heart, speed, strength)
- aerobic warm-down.

From day to day:

- aerobic/general/recovery
- neuromuscular
- anaerobic endurance.

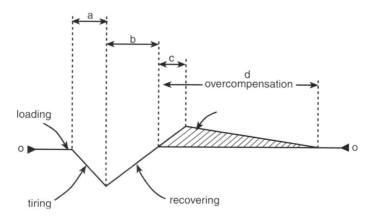

FIG. 88 Cycle of over-compensation (from Yakovlev, 1967). a–d represent periods of time; o represents original status of capacity being trained. a = catabolic effect of training; c = anabolic effect of training.

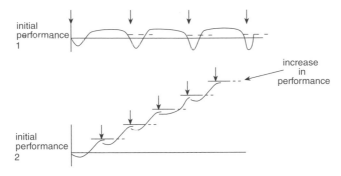

FIG. 89 This illustrates the cumulative effects of training. Since the period of overcompensation, or improved performance, gradually diminishes, there is less increase in performance with longer intervals (1) than with shorter intervals (2). The optimal improvement in performance is achieved when the new loading is presented at the highest point in the overcompensation phase (from Harre, 1973).

In the events carried out for maximum strength training the day-to-day pattern alters by intensity and/or exercises.

(10) As a rule, 48 hours minimum are required to recover from maximum loadings which will, of course, include competitions. Consequently the loading in the competition period must be so placed that the competition can be carried out in the phase of accentuated capacity (or overcompensation) brought about by optimal loading two to three days beforehand (figs 88 and 89).

Adaptable microcycles

For some sports, there are occasions where microcycle design cannot be fixed for any length of time. For example, where players are 'on the road' in constant national or international travel, changing time zones, training and competition venues; or where what happens in terms of tournament progression dictates subsequent training time, availability and location. This is very much the situation for the full-time professional athlete or player.

In these cases, against the background of the foregoing points on microcycle construction, and on the understanding that there is a sound conditioning base, the following notes may help meet the player's or athlete's training needs.

(1) In the main, try to follow a cyclic pattern of adaptation; application; regeneration; through training units, with full recovery between units. Extent and intensity of loading in adaptation units should be low to medium, while loading in application units should be low to medium in extent, but high to very high in intensity.
(2) Create for the athlete/player a selection of those microcycle structures which may be called for, given certain situations. For example there should be a structure provided for one, two, three, four, or five days training opportunity. Where there

are more days, either the basic microcycle for that mesocycle in the year, or a special training camp microcycle will apply.

(3) Provide a selection of training units from which the athlete will choose the best suited to a given training situation. For example, a player's training microcycle has 'aerobic run' as a unit. The selection on the programme is either 45 minutes easy run (heart rate 155–165) **or** 30 minutes hard Fartlek on undulating terrain (heart rate should vary between 140 and 180) **or** 30 minutes steady aqua jogging (heart rate 155–165) **or** steady mountain bike ride for 75 minutes (heart rate 150–160) **or** 20 x interval runs using the diagonal of a soccer pitch for the fast run (heart rate 180), jogging the length of the sideline as recovery (heart rate 135–145 in 60 seconds).

If the player is in a hotel in the centre of a city which has a swimming pool, the player is able to aqua jog. The next day, the player may travel at midday and will not arrive at his destination until late at night. The training unit for that day is 'general strength' for which the selection on the programme is either personal weight training programme (60 minutes) **or** personal strength machine programme (45 minutes) **or** personal body circuit (30 minutes).

Time and limited equipment suggest the latter programme. In other words, the coach must prepare a series of options in advance.

(4) Encourage the player/athlete to keep a record of what is done so that this information can be considered in designing the next basic microcycle.

(5) Regeneration units should also be on the basis of a selection to choose from. The player/athlete will, then, develop an involvement in establishing his area of training as part of a lifestyle which can become stressful. Regeneration units are very important inclusions in the 'adaptable microcycle' as a contribution to stress management.

MACROCYCLES AND MESOCYCLES

The macrocycle, and smaller mesocycle, is the sum of all units required to bring the status of training to that level required to meet the macrocycle objectives which relate to Preparation (Adaptation), Competition (Application) and Transition (Regeneration) within the annual cycle. To achieve those objectives, the coach designs and manages the content and duration of *mesocycles*. The mesocycle then becomes the vehicle for adjusting and adapting *macrocyles* to address the variance of annual objective within the overall purpose of Olympic or longer cycles. The mesocycle affords capacity for a quick and flexible response in the continuous process of reviewing, learning and changing to make macrocycles effective in their function.

A mesocycle is the sum of all units required to bring the status of training to that level required to meet its objectives. They exist to characterise progress of intensity and extent of loading, and are required to make the rhythmic changes from periods of high average loading to shorter periods of reducing loading.

Clearly they are regulated by the competition macrocycle(s). Although some mesocycles may be stretched to eight weeks, extending beyond six weeks can dull the athlete's motivation and capacity to work beyond the limits of present adaptation levels.

The shape of loading in the preparation macrocycle arises from the basic principle that within each macrocycle one establishes an optimal intensity consistent with a sound technical model, an increase in extent of loading is achieved, then the intensity in each unit is raised. The Oregon (Bowerman) method of endurance training classically illustrates this principle. Ter Ovanesyan (1965) describes extension of the principle to competition preparation, where, over a five week mesocycle, the total extent of loadings were increased over weeks 1–3, and then reduced, while intensity continued to increase to the competition itself.

In meeting macrocycle objectives, the coach must have collected the following information:

- the number of units of training available in the mesocycle(s). For example, in the months of November/December, the athlete may be able to programme nine units per week – approximately 70 units in total
- the % distribution of general, related and specific training
- the inter-unit training ratio
- the structure of loading for the mesocycle
- the structure of loading and intra-unit training ratio relevant to each type of training in microcycles
- the manner of increasing extent and intensity within the macrocycle
- the athlete's evaluation of the effects of training at unit, microcycle, mesocycle and macrocycle levels.

training area	classification	% units
aerobic endurance	general	11
speed endurance	special	11
strength endurance	general	11
speed	competition specific	5.5
elastic strength	special	11
maximum strength	special	5.5
mobility	general	11
sprint technique	competition specific	11
active recovery	general	23

TABLE 36 Possible breakdown of units for a 17-year-old girl sprinter – mesocycle 1

For example, in table 36 we have a suggested breakdown of units for a 17-year-old girl sprinter in mesocycle 1. This represents 10 units per week for five weeks. In each microcycle of one week, the athlete has a programme which is set out below:

Saturday   2   Wednesday   1
Sunday   2   Thursday   2
Monday   1   Friday   0
Tuesday   2

The next step will be to detail the objective of each unit indicated on the weekly microcycle, over all five weeks of the mesocycle. This might be done as shown in table 37. Obviously, the final interpretation of the percentages is flexible, but they have been kept, in the main, close to the original suggestion.

day		week 1	week 2	week 3	week 4	week 5
Saturday	A	sprint tech	sprint tech	sprint tech	sprint tech	sprint tech
	B	aerobic	aerobic	aerobic	aerobic	aerobic
Sunday	A	max strength	elastic strength	max strength	elastic strength	max strength
	B	speed/ endur	speed/ endur	speed/ endur	speed/ endur	speed/ endur
Monday	A	active recov	active recov	active recov	active recov	active recov
Tuesday	A	speed	sprint tech	speed	sprint tech	speed
	B	mobility	mobility	mobility	mobility	mobility
Wednesday	A	active recov	active recov	active recov	active recov	active recov
Thursday	A	elastic strength	elastic strength	elastic strength	elastic strength	elastic strength
	B	strength end	strength end	strength end	strength end	strength end
Friday	A	0	0	0	0	0

TABLE 37 Approximate distribution of training objectives against the suggested percentages

When working with an experienced athlete, the coach weighs all such considerations in setting out mesocycles as building blocks through the 52 weeks of the annual cycle.

The following is an example of a mesocycle breakdown for an experienced sprint athlete over the year.

Mesocycle 1₁   2 weeks   General training – strength, endurance, mobility (if required, some compensatory focus for reinforcing rehabilitation, etc., post previous season).

Mesocycle 1_2	6 weeks	Core training to provide very strong foundation for the more specific work to follow.
Mesocycle 1_3	5 weeks	Discipline – specific training focus.
Mesocycle 2_1	4 weeks	Competition preparation including training competitions.
Mesocycle 3_1	4 weeks	Competition (indoor athletics season).
Mesocycle 4_1	1 week	Regeneration, review, refocus.
Mesocycle 1_4	4 weeks	Core training 'top-up'.
Mesocycle 1_5	6 weeks	High-intensity discipline – specific training.
Mesocycle 2_2	4 weeks	Competition preparation including training competitions.
Mesocycle 3_2	6 weeks	Main competition season including key championships qualifying competitions.
Mesocycle 4_2	2 weeks	Regeneration, review, refocus (including competition preparation units).
Mesocycle 5	4 weeks	Major Championships goal.
Mesocycle 6	4 weeks	Regeneration.

Fitness and medical controls relate to key performance development milestones throughout the annual cycle.

Next, the detail of each training unit in terms of number of repetitions, sets, distances, intervals, kilos, exercises, etc., would be listed. Finally, the progression of extent and intensity would be established. For example, numbers of repetitions and/or sets will be increased in weeks 1–3, while in weeks 4–5 repetitions and sets will return to those of week one, but runs will be faster, loads heavier, or intervals shorter.

As a guide to training ratios, table 37 is offered as suggested percentages on which to work for track and field. It will be noted that columns are headed G (general), R (related) and S (specific). Osolin and Markov (1972) suggest statistics for the three periods and their figures have been used in compiling the percentages listed here.

	Percentage of training units					
beginners and developing athletes	I	II	III	IV	V	VI
	G R S	G R S	G R S	G R S	G R S	G R S
10–14 yrs	70 10 20	60 20 20	50 20 30	60 20 20	50 20 30	80 10 10
15–17 yrs	60 20 20	50 25 25	50 20 30	50 25 25	50 20 30	70 20 10

TABLE 38 Percentage distribution of general (G), related (R), and specific (S) training units according to the phase of the periodised year

	Percentage of training units					
beginners and developing athletes	*I*	*II*	*III*	*IV*	*V*	*VI*
18–19 yrs	50 25 25	40 25 35	25 25 50	45 30 25	15 25 60	75 15 10
novice seniors	50 25 25	40 25 35	25 25 50	45 30 25	25 25 50	75 15 10
experienced athletes						
sprints, long and triple	25 55 20	15 60 25	10 55 35	25 55 20	10 60 30	80 10 10
middle distance and walkers	20 75 5	20 70 10	10 70 20	10 85 5	10 80 10	55 40 5
long distance and marathon	10 85 5	10 85 5	5 90 5	10 85 5	5 90 5	45 50 5
hurdles, high, pole vault	35 35 30	25 35 40	10 40 50	20 40 40	10 40 50	80 10 10
throws	25 35 40	15 45 40	10 40 50	20 40 40	10 40 50	80 10 10

TABLE 38 Continued

SUMMARY

The pattern of the training plan should be seen in relation to that of all other natural phenomena. Just as the seasons follow a cycle, and our various physiological systems follow the laws of chronobiology, so training must follow a cyclical pattern. The broad areas of the cycle may be summarised as preparation (adaptation), competition (application), and transition (regeneration). These are the macrocycles of the annual cycle. The areas are reflected at all levels from unit to annual cycle to the athlete's competitive 'life'. To progress the athlete's pursuit of competitive advantage, training units that represent specific structures of loadings are organised for optimal effect by applying correct training ratios into microcycles. These are repeated with progressions to form mesocycles, which are designed to achieve the purpose of the macrocycle to which they belong. By careful emphasis on distribution of general, related and specific training, the phases are structured to meet objectives relative to progression through the periods of the annual cycle. Finally, each annual cycle has a unique character in terms of its contribution to the athlete's ultimate sporting objective.

22 ADAPTATION TO LOADING

Adaptation is the raising of the athlete's functioning capacity due to external loading and/or adjustment to specific environmental conditions. Physical, intellectual and emotional adaptation must be seen as one process.

We adapt to a stressor by 'learning' to cope with it. The 'learning' follows a stress response where adaptation energy is applied to accommodate the threat to normal functions capacity represented by the stressor. Whether the stressor is physical, intellectual or emotional, it's the same general adaptation energy source which is accessed. We seldom have single stressors to cope with. Rather, they are multiple and their energy requirement cumulative (fig. 68, p. 223). So, although the adaptation focus may be, say, strength in a training unit, other stressors vie for adaptation energy. Because the total amount of adaptation energy is finite, the total stressor picture must be understood to ensure a positive, rather than negative, effect of training.

DEFINITION

Training offers the athlete external loading and it is quite obvious that there is a relationship between loading and adaptation. The three laws of training (specificity, overload and reversibility) qualify and quantify loading. However, while these laws are fairly explicit, there are some points which should be emphasised.

(1) A high extent of load without the necessary minimum intensity fails to produce adaptation just as much as high intensity with too little extent.
(2) The more the amounts of loading approach an optimal value relative to the athlete's capacity *at the moment of loading*, the more rapidly adaptation takes place. Conversely, the greater the departure from that value (either over or underloading) the less the adaptation.
(3) If the demands of loading exceed the athlete's capacity, or if the structure of loading is wrong, then the athlete's capacity to adapt is compromised and performance will stagnate or even be reduced.
(4) The relationship between loading and recovery is critical and they should be seen as a whole (fig. 88, p. 322). This will be discussed in greater detail in Chapter 23.
(5) While 'overcompensation' is quickly transformed to a higher level of performance in the young and developing athlete, this process takes weeks or months with the mature athlete. Each loading close to the optimum will leave behind it a trace of overcompensation, but for the mature athlete it is only due to the cumulative effect of

training that improvements come at intervals, and not necessarily regular intervals. Matveyev (1965) refers to this as 'delayed transformation': '(it) prevents the continuous flow of information on the effect of loading on training that is necessary for the optimal regulation of the training process'. Progressive adaptation is not therefore easily apparent and only the results of competition or tests at the end of mesocycle 2 or at the start of mesocycle 3 show whether or not loading has been effective. Periodic checks and test procedures geared to accurate prediction are therefore vital throughout mesocycles 1 and 2. It is feasible that the introduction of mesocycle 3_2, in double periodisation, may provide a most relevant testing procedure.

(**6**) Loading must be systematically and progressively increased. Loadings that remain unchanged are more easily overcome in time and cause less disruption of the body's systems, but their effect diminishes until they simply maintain a stationary state of adaptation. The organism will adapt only if it is challenged to do so. The challenge of a well-designed mesocycle is optimal between six and eight weeks.

(**7**) The rate at which capacity reduces on reduction or cessation of loading is critical to the athlete. Illness, travel during the competition season, examinations, injury, etc., all imply disruption of the systematic increase of loadings. Moreover, during the competition season, loadings are frequently reduced in extent (and even intensity by some coaches). Again, this represents a break in continuity of the adaptation process. The more recent the level of adaptation, the more quickly it will be affected by reduced loading. Long periods of gradual development are therefore indicated. Lengthy transitional periods without training loading are to be avoided and, if the interval between training units is too long, the effect of loadings is lost. Finally, attention is drawn again to the relevance of a 'polyvalent' or mixed approach and to pursuing a changing training ratio throughout the year.

(**8**) The rate of return from the catabolic through to the anabolic/overcompensation peak in fig. 88 (see p. 322) is also critical to the athlete. The shorter the time interval, the more training can be performed per unit of time. Strategies within the laws of sport, to keep the interval short, should be applied in countering the energy-sapping effect of cumulative stressors.

(**9**) Loadings of great extent and slight to medium intensity primarily develop endurance capacity. Those of less extent, but sub-maximum to maximum intensity, mainly develop maximum strength, elastic strength and speed. While this may be accurate for the mature athlete, the young and developing athlete is affected by loadings in a far more complex way. Consequently, as Harre has noted (1973), the bulk of his work which is low to middle intensity, also develops strength and speed, to a certain extent. But what exactly do expressions like 'middle intensity' mean? To arrive at an explanation, one must first examine the expression 'intensity'.

Intensity of loading

The intensity of loading is characterised by the strength of the stimulus, or by the concentration of work executed per unit of time within a series of stimuli. Intensity for endurance or speed is calculated according to the speed in m/second or the frequency of movement, e.g. cadence in sprinting. For strength exercises the amount of resistance is measured, and for jumping or throwing, the height or distance (loaded and/or unloaded) is used. Since intensity varies in exercise it is useful to distinguish between 'spheres of intensity', as Carl (1967) has called them. In order to compare the loading of athletes, these spheres should be established with reference to a fixed point and should be clearly delineated. For exercises to develop maximum strength, speed, elastic strength, etc., the highest possible individual intensity of stimulation is taken as the point of reference, maximum loading being equal to 100% (tables 39, 40 and 41). In the growing years, with strength development, '10 reps maximum' should be used as the reference point for 100%.

A standard scale of intensity would be most useful. It would establish a basic frame of reference and help in the evaluation of training theory. It is, after all, at the comparative level that the real meaning of loading becomes apparent. For too long there has been no marketplace to exchange the various currencies in which each coach transacts the business of relating unit to athlete. Table 41 is offered as a basis for such an intensity scale.

Best 150 m					% of best time					
100	65	66.7	73	75	80	83	87.5	90	95	97
18.3	27.9	–	25.0	–	–	22.1	20.8	20.1	19.2	18.8
18.5	–	27.4	25.1	24.6	23.1	22.4	21.1	20.5	19.5	18.9
18.8	28.4	27.9	25.57	25.0	23.4	22.7	21.4	20.8	19.7	19.2
18.9	28.9	–	–	25.1	23.8	–	21.7	21.1	20.0	19.5
19.2	–	28.4	26.0	–	24.2	23.1	22.1	21.4	20.3	19.7
19.5	30.0	28.9	26.4	25.5	–	23.4	22.3.	21.7	20.5	20.0
19.7	30.6	–	26.9	26.0	24.6	23.8	22.7	22.1	20.8	20.1
20.0	–	30.0	–	26.4	25.0	24.2	–	–	21.1	20.5
20.3	31.3	30.6	27.4	–	25.4	24.6	23.1	22.4	21.4	20.8
20.5	31.9	–	27.9	26.9	25.9	–	23.4	22.7	21.7	21.1
20.8	–	31.3	–	27.4	–	25.0	23.8	23.1	22.1	21.4
21.1	32.6	31.9	28.4	27.9	26.3	25.1	24.2	23.4	22.4	21.7
(Best 200 m)										
20.0	30.7	29.4	27.3	26.6	25.0	24.0	22.7	22.2	21.0	20.6
20.2	31.2	30.3	27.7	27.0	25.3	24.3	22.9	22.4	21.2	20.8
20.4	–	30.7	–	–	–	24.6	23.2	22.7	21.5	21.0
20.6	31.7	–	28.1	27.3	25.6	–	23.5	22.9	21.7	21.2
20.8	32.2	31.2	28.5	27.7	25.9	25.0	23.8	23.2	21.9	21.5
21.0	–	31.7	28.9	28.1	26.3	25.3	24.0	o	22.2	21.7
21.2	32.7	–	–	–	26.6	25.6	24.3	23.5	22.4	21.9
21.5	33.3	32.2	29.4	28.5	27.0	25.9	24.6	23.8	22.7	22.2

TABLE 39 Example of possible table for percentage intensity to be used for track running. The spheres of intensity are then derived from this. A problem arises where authorities offer varying spheres of intensity (see table 40).

Best 200 m					% of best time					
21.7	–	32.7	29.9	28.9	–	26.3	–	24.0	22.9	22.4
21.9	33.8	–	30.3	29.4	27.3	–	25.0	24.3	23.2	22.7
22.2	–	33.3	–	–	27.7	26.6	25.3	24.6	–	22.9
22.4	34.4	33.8	30.7	29.8	28.1	27.0	25.6	25.0	23.5	23.2
22.7	35.0	–	31.2	30.3	28.5	27.3	25.9	25.3	23.8	23.5

TABLE 39 Continued

Myer	designation of intensity	carl*
	slight	30–50%
	light	50–70%
65–73%	middle	70–80%
75–83%	high	
87.5–97%	submaximum	80–90%
	maximum	90–100%

TABLE 40 Comparison of terms used in describing loading as % max. intensity
* Suggested spheres of intensity in weight training

scale of intensity	percentage of maximum
low	30–49%
light	50–64%
medium	65–74%
high	75–84%
submaximum	85–94%
maximum	95–100%

TABLE 41 Suggested standard intensity scale

When training for endurance events, intensity is ideally evaluated against the best performances over the training distance, or against the average competition speed at the moment. However, in passing, it should be noted that since training at given intensities of VO2 maximum have great relevance to the energy system involved, the measure of intensity may well be 'read' from the working heart rate and against the percentage of VO2 maximum (table 14, p. 99). The extent of loading at certain percentages.

Density in loading

The density or frequency of stimulus in loading is determined by the objective of the unit, the stimulus being controlled both by its intensity and duration. Knowing this, an optimal density can be established which will allow an evaluation of the number of consecutive occasions per unit when the athlete is exposed to the stimulus, and also the amount of time between these occasions. In pursuit of specificity of loading effect, numbers of repetitions and sets are married to the interval of time between them to create an optimal density. From these precepts, crude formulae have evolved for the development of specific endurance capacities (table 42).

In strength and speed work at sub-maximum to maximum intensities, 2–5 minutes are necessary between successive loadings.

characteristic	loading:recovery	intensity
heart endurance	continuous	light
heart endurance	2:1–1:1	high
speed endurance	1:3–1:6	submaximum

TABLE 42 Suggested intra-unit training ratios according to endurance characteristic to be developed

Duration of stimulus in loading

The duration of stimulus is the period of influence of a single stimulus. A difference then exists between this, the relative intensity, and the highest intensity recorded in a particular unit, or cycle. In this case, the value is known as absolute intensity, the distance covered in a repetition, or the total time to complete all loading in a unit. Just as there appear to be thresholds of intensity, so also for duration. Thus, Gundlach (1968) suggests at least 20–30% of maximum holding time is essential for the improvement of isometric strength. Endemann (1973) used this information in his 'auxotonic training' where resistances were consciously controlled in their speed of movement (e.g. five seconds lowering, five seconds raising bar in bench press). Hollmann (1962) determined that at least 30 minutes duration of stimulus was required at a given intensity for significant improvement in aerobic endurance. Moreover, it seems clear from figure 35, p. 105, that a minimum of two minutes duration at a relatively high intensity of stimulus is necessary to adapt the athlete to the acid base imbalance of competition in short and medium duration endurance disciplines. Obviously, the duration of work in maximum and elastic strength, mobility and speed development must not be so long that fatigue reduces the ability to perform efficiently.

Finally, in pursuit of strength endurance, the duration of loading must be such that considerable effort of will is required to complete the unit.

Extent of loading

The extent of loading is the sum of duration (time or distance) and the repetitions of all stimuli in a training unit. Consequently it will be expressed in kilometres in endurance training, in kilograms in strength training (the sum of loadings), and in the number of repetitions in strength endurance, etc. It is necessary, of course, to divide the extent of loadings into various spheres of intensity, or, if it is agreed, to divide the loadings according to the suggested scale in table 41.

The unit, then, is a complex of intensity, extent, duration and density of loading. For optimal value to be derived from each unit, no athlete should arrive at the start of one unit while still fatigued from the previous unit. A full understanding of the unit complex, and the effect each unit has upon the athlete, is essential to the coach. From here the microcycle begins to evolve with an understanding of what should constitute a unit of loading for an athlete and the frequency of exposure of the athlete to that unit.

Extent of training is, therefore, the sum total of hours, kilograms or kilometres of training, calculated from the cumulation of units and their frequency – the whole being expressed over a unit, microcycle, mesocycle, macrocycle, or, indeed, annual cycle (fig. 90).

Progressive loading

'Progression of loading in pursuit of progression of performance improvement' might, in a nutshell, represent the whole purpose of training. From the above discussion of adaptation and loading, 'progression of loading' will be seen as greater extent, higher intensity, longer duration, greater density or increased frequency, or a combination of some or all of these. Loading must always bear a particular relationship to the athlete's present loading capacity. Consequently, no 'absolutes' can be given in terms of loading progression. However, as outlined on pages 329–332, certain general principles do operate to guide the coach when increasing loading.

(1) In technical and tactical training, loading is increased by imposing greater demands on the coordination required of a technique. This can be achieved by:

- demanding greater speed in execution and/or selecting correct technical solution
- requiring technical exactness in an endurance situation

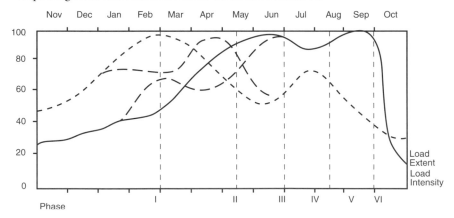

FIG. 90 The suggested relationship between extent and intensity of loading in the annual cycle of single and double periodised years (from Matveyev, 1965)

- combining various elements of practice
- changing external conditions
- learning more complex technical variations
- offering competition pressure.

Not only do such practices develop technical efficiency, but they also develop specific physical capacities such as mobility and the ability to make rapid and correct adjustment when a loss of balance threatens technical precision.

(2) For endurance, strength, speed, elastic strength, etc., the structure of loading must be altered. The main problem here is to decide exactly the alteration of ratio of intensity and extent from mesocycle to mesocycle, or, for that matter, from athlete to athlete, in the whole range from the beginner to the elite. The problem does not end there, however, because great thought must be given to the question of which components (endurance, strength, etc.) should be stressed in the increase of loading. To say simply that this varies according to athlete and event, and that herein lies the art and mastery of coaching, is quite an indictment of coaches' progress in establishing firm training principles. It is true that to date the state of knowledge in this field is most unsatisfactory, yet it is equally true that the roots of such knowledge lie with coaches and athletes. However, until knowledge in this area becomes more specialised, it is clear that, in general, when the athlete's degree of adaptation has been raised, loading must then become more comprehensive and more intensive. This means that the athlete must be exposed to raised loadings specific to all facets of his sport and, that such an increase is not one of extent, but of intensity. This generalisation must be applied to specific sports. Consequently the coach must evaluate both sport and athlete and be able to apply this information to improve the athlete's status of adaptation.

(3) For the beginner in sport, another general principle is 'Fit the sport to the athlete – then fit the athlete to the sport'. Once this introductory stage is past, these athletes will achieve more stable adaptation and, ultimately, a greater improvement in performance if intensity is raised cautiously and loading progression is primarily via more extensive training. According to Harre (1973), the progression is:

- raise the frequency of training (e.g. number of consecutive units, say, from twice weekly to daily training)
- raise the extent of loading per training unit, while keeping frequency constant
- raise the density of loading within the training unit.

This progression can only be applied given stable technical quality. As a rule, it is not acceptable to the athlete to bring about these three stages simultaneously. At first an optimal frequency is sought and only when time is limited should the coach consider increasing the load.

(4) Analysis of individual athletes' training has shown that a linear gradual increase of loading is not as effective as increases by 'jumps' spaced at given intervals. It would appear that increasing loading in such jumps suddenly taxes the status of the athlete's capacities and 'disturbs the physical-psychological balance' (Harre, 1973).

This then forces the athlete's total organism to establish new physical-psychological processes of regulation and adaptation. The most obvious examples of this are seen at the start of mesocycle 1 where extent is advanced by jumps (compared with mesocycles 4 and 6 of the previous cycle), thus affecting rapid strength endurance and aerobic status, and at the start of mesocycle 3 where intensity is advanced due to severe competition specific loadings and is accompanied by rapid improvements in performance. The time interval between such jumps is, again, arrived at individually, but several coaches now tie these in with 4–6 week mesocycles. Chronobiology will almost certainly offer a great contribution to understanding such time intervals. Obviously, the athlete will require some time to adapt to the sudden increase in loading and stabilise his training level, but adaptation of processes and stability do not necessarily advance together.

(5) The 'jumps' of increased loading may be formalised by maintaining a six-weekly programme review where progress follows a 'sigmoid' shape (fig. 91).

(6) The next question is how much to increase loading with each jump, or from year to year. Again, there is little to use as a basis for absolutes, but Matveyev (1965) determined an increase of 20–50% in extent from one year to the next through the developing years. With elite, older athletes there is less increase and sometimes even reduction. This of course will vary from sport to sport and will depend on conditions and time available for training. The progressions then will grow from an educated appraisal by the coach of conditions and time, using a logical progression based upon the foregoing general principles. The hardest area of judgement for the coach is when to maintain rather than increase extent or intensity.

On the subject of increasing intensity, personal observation suggests a maximum increment of 2.5–5% per mesocycle where a particular unit or its derivative runs throughout a year. This policy is only altered for testing sessions, or when the very high intensity demanded of mesocycles 3_1, 3, or 3_2 implies work to maximum (see below).

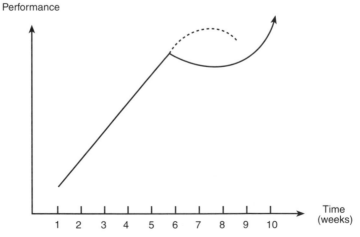

FIG. 91 Although the athlete continues to adapt to the aggregated stressors of a training mesocycle up to around eight weeks, it ensures optimal cumulative training effect when a new mesocycle is introduced at six-weekly (max) intervals.

Repetition runs over 300 m – female long jumper (100% taken as previous best):

Mesocycle 1: 3 x 75% (4 mins) → 5 x 75% (4 mins)
      Test to establish new 100%
4 x 80% (4 mins) → 5 x 80% (4 mins)
      Test to establish new 100%

Mesocycle 2: 4 x 85% (7.5 mins) → 5 x 85% (7.5 mins)
      Test to establish new 100%
3 x 90% (10 mins)
      Test to establish new 100%

Mesocycle 3: 2 x 90% (15 mins)
1–2 x 100% with full recovery
(figures in brackets are recovery times)

(7) Within training units, at the exercise level, there can be considerable confusion over the available avenues for progression. There are only three:

- perform the exercise more often (or for greater duration) (endurance factor)
- perform the exercise against increased resistance (strength factor)
- perform the exercise faster (speed factor).

Progression may only be considered when the athlete's performance of the exercise is technically sound. If the performance breaks down to a comfortable compromise, then clearly there is no basis for progression.

(8) It is important that the coach fully understands that the athlete experiences three separate effects of training. They are: the immediate effect; the residual effect; the cumulative effect. Each contributes to the pattern of events which have been represented in figures 88 and 89 as described on p. 322 & 323.

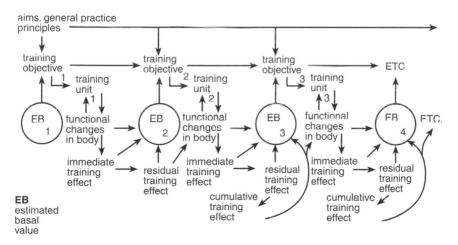

FIG. 92 Summary of the effects of training

TRAINING PHASE PLAN Name (Athlete/Team).

Phase No: _2_

Commencing: _18 . X . 87_

Ending: _28 . XI . 87_

No. of Weeks: _6_

Objectives: 1. SPECIFIC RUNNING ENDURANCE

2. SPECIAL STRENGTH - THROWS - JUMPS

3. TECHNIQUE

Cycle of 7 Days   Registered 6 Times

Day	Unit 1	Unit 2	Unit 3	Unit 4	Unit 5	Unit 6
1.	T4	HURDLES DRILLS		GENERAL JUMPS	DRILLS	STRENGTH B
2.	T3⑭	HURDLES DRILLS	JAVELIN		HIGH	STRENGTH A
3.	T1⑭		SHOT DRILLS	DISCUS	POLE	STRENGTH B
4.	T2	HURDLES ENDURANCE	JAVELIN DRILLS	DISCUS DRILLS	LONG	STRENGTH B
5.	T4		SHOT	DISCUS DRILLS	POLE	STRENGTH B
6.	T1⑥	HURDLES DRILLS	JAVELIN DRILLS		HIGH	STRENGTH C
7.	T3⑥		GENERAL THROWS	DRILLS		
8.						
9.						
10.						
11.						
12.						
13.						
14.						

FIG. 93 Example of a microcycle for a decathlete, and progression through a mesocycle

- the immediate effect is a breaking down or depleting of the adaptation energy reserve – so it is the catabolic effect of training (fig. 88a)
- the residual effect is the regenerating and overcompensating process – so it is anabolic (fig. 88b and c)
- the cumulative effect is the continuing process of capitalising on the advantage which the overcompensation phase (fig. 88d) affords and is represented by (fig. 89)

The overall picture is summarised in figure 92 (see p. 337).

This is all very straightforward when the training objective is singular, for example in progressing leg strength through a weight-training programme. The situation becomes more complex when several training objectives are being pursued. Figure 93 represents the weekly microcycle of a decathlete, and shows how pursuit of the stated objectives will proceed over a six week mesocycle. The proposed progressions for individual units are sound as they stand – but they may not be if the aggregate cumulative effect of all training units is such that the aggregate residual effect cannot reach the level of overcompensation. At this point the overall training load will damage rather than benefit the athlete. The importance of responsible interpretation by coach and athlete of the athlete's subjective evaluation of training effect is clearly highlighted here, and there must be a flexibility built into the programme for adjustment to progressions within the mesocycle. Clearly, progressions in pursuit of all objectives cannot proceed at the same rate.

SUMMARY

To conclude this discussion of adaptation to loading, the basic guiding principle should be:

- step 1 – preparation for training
- step 2 – training for competition.

Without doubt, the most rapid development of performance will come from high intensity specific loadings, but where these are used to too great an extent, they quickly wear out the physical and psychological potential of the athlete. The more thorough and extensive step 1, the longer will be the amount of time before such 'wearing out'. Nevertheless, there are occasions when the athlete appears to.have gone 'stale' for reasons that are not always apparent. This phenomenon has critical implications for coach and athlete and may be examined in the following chapter.

The defining of optimal loading for an athlete is critical to progression of his fitness and maintenance of his health. It demands fine judgements on the part of the coach. The cycle of adaptation, application and regeneration must be followed at all levels. This emphasises the importance of a thorough and extensive preparation part of the cycle and of viewing *stimulus plus recovery* as a total process.

23 TRAINING V STRAINING

Our capacity to adapt protects us from threats to our wellbeing and also enables us to realise our performance potential. At the one extreme it equips us to survive when our very existence is in peril; at the other, it may be applied to enable us to go beyond our present performance limits when challenged to do so. Adaptation is as essential to the effectiveness of our immune system as it is in preparing to raise our game to perform better in progressively tougher arenas. It is an inbuilt auto-regulative feature of our physiology which operates without us realising it, yet can be constructively manipulated and managed in pursuit of performance objectives.

Training programmes based on the performance-related sciences, training theory and coaching methods aim to bring about the adaptations necessary to improve the athlete's performance advantage. However, training is only one of several stressors that persistently and cumulatively bombard the athlete each day (see fig. 68, p. 223). They include studying, domestic and social life, relationships, health, general lifestyle, cultural demands and so on. Where the total load of these stressors is in keeping with the athlete's ability to deal with them, training will progress normally and performance will improve. This demands that the athlete is at the overcompensation phase as illustrated in fig. 88.

Fatigue induced by training should be overcome relatively quickly, depending on the nature of loading; even after very heavy loadings, the athlete should be at the overcompensation phase within 24-48 hours. This sort of fatigue is normal. The athlete will be ready to tackle normal physical, mental and emotional challenges after the training loads and should feel well rested and fully recovered the morning after.

On the other hand, the cumulative stressors may be too much for the athlete and this will be referred to as overstressing the athlete. Short of complete and regular bioprofiles on athletes, which demands access to physiological testing laboratories, the coach has very little with which to assess the contribution of training to the sum total of stressors. This said, in some countries it has become an accepted feature of the National Performance Programme that athletes will undergo periodic 'stress' monitoring to reduce the risks of over-stressing the athlete. In Finland, at Vierumakki, athletes present themselves for such monitoring on the following basis:

| Stress level | Chronic long-term training stress-disturbances at hormonal level. | Acute short-term training stress-disturbances in muscle membranes and in energy production. |

Relevant measurement Measuring the ratio of testosterone:cortisol levels in blood serum. Measuring urea/creatinine/creatinekinase concentration in blood serum.

Timing of measurement Four times per year; twice during the main preparation phase, once during the competition preparation phase, once one month before the main competition. During hard training micro cycles (e.g. training camps) samples taken each morning. Also 2–3 hours post-unit. (Grosser 1986: overstressing if serum urea >8 mmol/litre.)

Clues which the coach might pick up on are shown in table 43.

	optimal loading	excessive loading	recovery after excessive loading
Skin colour	flushed	very flushed	paleness for several days
Sweating	heavy sweat in upper body	sweating throughout body	night sweats
Co-ordination	slight loss of precision as unit proceeds	loss of precision, distressing confusion, increased reaction time	reduced precision beyond 48 hrs or in extreme cases beyond 72 hrs
Concentration	reducing span of attention; reducing capacity to solve technical problems; reducing power of identifying irrelevant cues	inability to concentrate for even relatively short periods; forgets instructions	unable to correct technical errors for more than 48 or even 72 hrs; unable to concentrate on academic work
General health	progressive muscular weakness, reduced efficiency	possible muscle and joint pain, light-headedness and stomach upset. General feeling of malasie, even headaches	difficulty in sleeping; pulse remains higher than normal for up to 24 hrs. continued physical inefficiency and discomfort

TABLE 43 Symptoms of tiring after optimal and excessive loading

	optimal loading	*excessive loading*	*recovery after excessive loading*
Approach to training	desire for longer recoveries but eager to train	desire for complete rest; doubts on value of training; fear of further loading	disinclined to train next day; negative attitude to coach perhaps even inventing excuses for avoiding training

TABLE 43 Continued

A low white cell count is also an indicator of the onset of chronic stress – specifically a low quantity of natural killer cells (NK cells), which are the leukocytes that assist in destruction of foreign substances in the body. More recently, S-1gA (secretory immunoglobin A) levels and the ratio of anti-ageing hormone, DHEA (dehydroepiandrosterone):cortisol are considered key indicators of physiological stress.

Clearly, the failure to ensure adequate recovery and regeneration should not be dismissed as being a little more tired than usual. It can lead to the weakening of the immune system.

It is critical, then, that coaches consider the full implication of figure 88. Planned regeneration recovery is an essential feature of the stimulus of bringing about the intended adaptation. Understanding and managing the loading aspect is only part of the story. Without the same level of understanding and management of recovery, the adaptation objectives are, at least, compromised. The adaptation process occurs because the athlete's physiology recovers into overcompensation. This will happen when, on the one hand, the training load is consistent with the athlete's capacity to accept its challenge against the background of his total stressor profile, and on the other, their recovery is carefully designed and effectively delivered.

This brings training ratio (loading:recovery) into finer focus. It is the failure to ensure effective recovery that leads to subsequent loadings being introduced before entry into overcompensation. This in turn means exposing the athlete to the risk of failure to meet training and competition targets and, if continued over an extended period, to breakdown and burnout.

Overstressing causes progressive fatigue. Capacity is not restored after training in this situation and will continue to deteriorate until the causes of overstressing are removed. If they are not, the athlete may become ill.

Israel (1963) points out that overstressing can produce either of two extremes of response: over-excitement of the system (over-stimulation), or over-depression (over-inhibition). He refers to the former as *basedovoid* overstressing and suggests that, within the training context, this occurs chiefly as a result of suddenly increasing the density of sub-maximum intensity loadings in the training programme, or of making the excessive demands on the power of concentration. He refers to the latter as *addisonoid* overstressing, and this is brought about by very comprehensive endurance programmes with persistent over-emphasis in the extent of loading.

While there is general agreement among coaches and training theorists with Israel's observations, these broad causes of overstressing are seldom exclusively so. In fact they should be viewed more as major contributors to the syndrome. The fact is that the phenomenon of overstressing arises from the cumulative effect of many stressors – which leaves the individual exposed to a reduced threshold of stress tolerance; reduced capacity to adapt to stressors or cope with stress; and, in extreme cases, may contribute to chronic fatigue syndrome and other clear warning signs that the immune system is under threat. Other stressors include the following:

(1) Principal faults in the training process: recovery is neglected (mistakes in the build-up of micro and mesocycles, and inadequate use of general exercise sessions for recovery); demands increased too quickly so that adaptation cannot be con-solidated; too rapid an increase of loading after forced breaks (injuries, illness); too great an extent of loadings of maximum and sub-maximum intensity; too high an intensity of duration loadings in endurance training; excessive and forced technical schooling in complicated courses of movement without adequate re-covery; excess of competitions with maximum demands, combined with frequent disturbance of the daily routine and insufficient training; excessive bias of train-ing methods and units; lack of trust in the coach; repeated setbacks as a result of coach setting sights too high; inability of athlete or coach to maintain adaptation: application: regeneration balance.

(2) Factors reducing performance:

- lifestyle   inadequate sleep; irregular daily routine; dissolute behaviour; use of alcohol and tobacco; excess of caffeine; distracting company; lack of free time or inability to relax; nutritional deficiencies ('empty calorie' foods, lack of vita-mins or antioxidants, low water intake, etc.); frequent necessity to adjust body weight; accepting more stressors when already at capacity
- environment – poor living conditions (overcrowding, etc.); excessive family duties and tensions; difficulties in personal relationships; dissatisfaction with career, studies, school; poor marks in school, studies, etc; conflict with attitudes hostile to sports (family, superiors); excess of stimuli (TV, cinema); temporary upsurge of anxiety (e.g. exams)
- health upsets – feverish colds; stomach or intestinal upsets; glandular fever; chronic infections (e.g. of tonsils, teeth, ovaries, sinuses); after-effects of infectious illnesses (e.g. sore throats, lingering cough, etc.); injury; neglected infections (e.g. athlete's foot, rashes, etc.).

Management of the athlete's lifestyle outside the sporting context, while finally resting with the athlete, requires knowledge and skill in areas including time man-agement; personal health and hygiene; control of interpersonal communication and relationships with people in social and business situations; and direction in pursuit of career. There is no single 'educator' here. Learning resources include parents, family, teachers, friends, and coaches. Because of this, it is often wrongly assumed that 'someone else' is taking care of such matters. The truth is that all of the athlete's potential 'educators' must accept responsibility for relevant input. Ideally they all should work in partnership as a support team. Before anyone loads the athlete with yet another stressor, the existing stressor profile should be known, and help afforded in ensuring that the athlete's tolerance to stress is not overloaded.

It is the coach who must coordinate such input and lead the team of 'educators'. This role will be discussed further in chapter 24.

Within the sporting context, there is much the coach can do in the area of preventing overstressing. With careful planning, means and methods to encourage recovery or regeneration can be included in the training programme. This will ensure that the aggregate effect of the training programme does not constitute a stressor which will tip the athlete into the overstress situation.

The means and methods may be considered at three levels: intra-unit, inter-unit and inter-micro/mesocycle.

Intra-unit (between repetitions and/or sets)

The period of time involved here is measured in seconds or minutes. During this period the athlete must recover to a level which permits the objective of the training unit to be met. For example, if the unit is interval training, the degree of recovery, monitored by noting heart rate, must allow the athlete's heart rate to fall to around the midpoint of the total range. If resting heart rate is 60 and maximum is 180, then the athlete's heart rate should be around 120–130 before he performs the next repetition.

If maximum quality of performance is required over a number of repetitions, say for speed, recovery must be complete between runs. A unit of 3 x 60 m then, will require at least 10 minutes between repetitions.

If incomplete recovery is required to guarantee cumulative fatigue for development of anaerobic tolerance, time periods are chosen to ensure that the athlete can perform sufficient repetitions to guarantee a training effect. This effect may or may not require that the athlete maintains a minimum quality of performance in each repetition. If it does, then clearly the time periods are larger and the quality of performance is submaximum.

Recovery activities include:

- lying down
- walking
- jogging
- doing a related activity
- doing an unrelated activity
- massage

- changing footwear
- warming up
- sipping water or glucose/mineral replacement drinks.

Intra-unit recovery is, by definition, part of the training load. However, it may also be considered part of the stimulus in certain types of training. For example, in some special strength work, where the objective is to accelerate strength levels, instead of:

$$load = stimulus + recovery$$

it becomes

$$load = stimulus\,(1) + stimulus\,(2)$$

So, in leg work, the training unit might become:
stimulus 1–5 x 85% max 1⁄2 squat
stimulus 2–5 x rebounds over 8 hurdles at 90 cm.

Immediately on completing stimulus 2, the athlete starts again with stimulus 1. The total unit is 3–5 x (stimulus 1 + stimulus 2).

Inter-unit (between units on a given day or from day to day)

The period of time involved here is measured in hours or days. Few athletes outside the endurance group pursue the same training objectives in successive units. Having said this, many endurance athletes follow a pattern of 'hard unit'–'easy unit' alternation. In-built to most training programmes then, is a form of recovery from the *stressor of specific training loads*.

Coaches must learn to feel comfortable not only at including rest days and rest units in the microcycle, but also at introducing periods of up to several days recovery when necessary. The flexibility of programme design, as suggested in chapter 22 in connection with the aggregate cumulative effect of training, should allow for this.

Recovery activities include:

- special diets, lying down, sleeping, massage, Jacuzzi, sauna, change of venue, work/study, going out to a show, watching TV, listening to music, etc.
- doing another event/sport at recreational level, e.g. swimming, golf, cycling, etc.
- variety – in the training objective; the level of athlete involvement in decision-making; routine; between training and competition
- general activity units
- warm-up units
- 'feel good' sessions
- 'finding space' sessions
- relaxation units – dynamic/passive
- dance, aesthetic expression.

Although it seems common sense to include such activities, both athletes and coaches can occasionally abandon common sense under pressure. For example, it is not unknown for programmes to be made harder rather than easier when performance in training does not come up to expectation. For athletes who are achievement-orientated, lack of commitment or hard work is not an acceptable explanation for performance problems. Motivation is not the problem but avoiding demotivation can be. It is more likely that the athlete has been over-committing and over-working, or that the work has been inappropriate. Whatever the explanation may be, the coach must ensure that units for recovery or regeneration not only appear in the programme, but are also carried through.

Inter-micro/mesocycle (normally at transition or regeneration macrocycle)

The period of time involved here is measured in days or weeks, and suggests that such training cycles should be considered and introduced to the programme at the same time as the year plan itself is set out. This is not to say, of course, that given certain circumstances, such a training cycle may not be introduced in pursuit of a specific regenerative objective, at any time in the year.

The 'early planned' regeneration mesocycle is normally between conclusion of the competition macrocycle and commencement of the introductory mesocycle of the year plan. It should be planned in such a way that the athlete returns to training highly motivated and fully prepared to commit himself to the rigours and discipline of training. This is best achieved quite simply by taking a vacation. This suggests:

- a different climate
- different surroundings
- different routine
- different social environment
- different physical activities
- different diet
- different emotional and mental demands.

The 'introduced' regeneration mesocycle is normally associated with recovery from crises. Unexpected and critical defeat; selection for a major championship; serious injury/illness; all represent possible crises which may require a regeneration mesocycle to help bring things back into focus. However, it should be said that the crisis situation seldom arrives out of the blue. It can often be spotted early. Timely regeneration will help avoid the situation becoming virtually irretrievable.

We have established that coaches have, over time and through experience, created a reasonable reference framework for the design and delivery of effective recovery. But can we expand this?

A mixture of Eastern and Western influences has now opened our minds to a host of possibilities that focus on a holistic approach to regeneration – often with the sense of sanctuary offered by spas. Such measures are variously described as treatments or therapies which enhance or restore wellbeing. They focus for the most part on rest, recovery, recuperation, relaxation, recreation, rehabilitation and regeneration; some are rooted in oriental and alternative medicine, others in the cosmetic industry.

Within this world, it is certain there are areas of practice which, if understood and founded on sound principle, must surely enrich the training process when thoughtfully applied.

It is beyond the scope of this book to list all such therapies and treatments. But it may be worth outlining the general bases of some, to encourage further thought and study of effective recovery and regeneration management. For example:

The exteroceptors

(1) Electro magnetic waves

The *eyes* are sensitive to light, dark and colour. We may respond to how we see or interpret what we see in movies, pictures, what we witness etc. with a range of emotions.

The *skin* is sensitive to touch, pressure, light, heat, cold and pain. (We use the effect of electro magnetic waves via skin in magnetic resonance, electrical stimulation of muscle, light therapies including ultraviolet and infrared etc.).

(2) Mechanical vibration

The *skin* again. (We use such in massage, Jacuzzis, ice therapies, bathing in salts or essences, soothing the skin with various substances, and so on).

The *ears* are sensitive to sounds and via the labyrinth apparatus, balance/head movement. We use music and sounds to stimulate or relax, emotionally, intellectually and physically.

(3) Chemical changes

The *nose* is sensitive to smell and we have a most sophisticated memory bank for aromas. Once experienced, a smell, even years later, will conjure up the original experience. Aromatherapy uses this sense to advantage.

The *tongue* is sensitive to taste. We use this sense in food and drink flavourings and via digestion to stimulate, soothe etc.

(4) The propriocetors

Propriocetors respond to stretch, tension or pressure in the locomotor system. They provide information about movement, position, balance and coordination. They are located in muscles, tendons, joints and the labyrinth apparatus in the ear. We use this knowledge in a range of therapies including reflexology, and the work of chiropractors, osteopaths, manipulation masseurs and so on.

(5) The interoceptors

The interoceptors are located in the viscera and monitor the internal environment; they are sensitive to distension in the hollow organs. Most therapies here involve preventing situations which lead to distension.

The senses are also involved in creating emotional, physical and intellectual changes as a consequence of how we personally interpret the conduits referred to above. That said, there is much we don't know or understand of why certain treatments or therapies are effective. For example, acupuncture has eluded satisfactory scientific explanation, yet, clearly, it works. Some medical practices now offer both conventional and alternative medicines, including acupuncture, and have been included in athlete's performance services resources. Coaches must work closely with the research areas of sports science in making responsible decisions in the interest of an athlete's wellbeing, development and performance. This is now even more important in the context of regeneration strategies.

But what if the athlete becomes overstressed?

The coach should be aware of the following.

(1) Psychological symptoms: increased irritability; obstinacy; increased argumentativeness; 'flying off the handle'; complaining about trivial things; defiance; anxiety; melancholy; avoidance of contact with coach and colleagues; oversensitivity to criticism; blaming everyone else for problems; laziness; fullness; 'imagining things'; depression; insecurity.

(2) Performance symptoms:

- techniques – increased incidence of disturbance in the basic technical model, e.g. reappearance of old faults; cramps; inhibitions; loss of confidence; disturbance in the rhythm and flow of the movement; reduced ability to differentiate between right and wrong movement
- condition – diminishing endurance, strength, speed; longer recovery times needed; loss of 'bounce' in training – becoming almost a 'slog'; loss of personal effervescence on and off track
- competitive qualities – reduced readiness for competition 'action'; fear of competition (or rather of losing); giving up under pressure; confusion in competition such as departure from competition plan or inability to respond correctly to the strategy of the opposition; easily demoralised; loss of belief in self and abilities; talks about lack of point in continuing the struggle; wants out!

(3) Somatic functional symptoms: sleeping difficulties; lack of appetite; loss of weight; 'addictive' eating; increase in weight; disturbance in digestive function; longer recovery of pulse to resting rate, increased resting heart rate; dizzy spells; night sweating; increased susceptibility to injury/infection; loss of vitality.

Should such symptoms arise, especially if there are several symptoms, the coach should:

- have the athlete check with his doctor
- put the athlete immediately on a regeneration programme.

Selection of components to be included in the regenerative programme vary according to whether the athlete's reaction is basedovoid or addisonoid. Israel identified examples of such variance and these have been divided into three sections.

Basedovoid

Diet: encourage the athlete to eat more; choose basic foods such as milk, vegetables, fruit, and organic foods; eliminate foods with preservatives and/or artificial colourings; avoid spicy or greasy sauces/dressings; avoid coffee, tea, chocolate and soft drinks containing caffeine; reduce protein consumption, especially red meat; take a concentrated course of vitamins, especially B complex plus the antioxidants; take small quantity of alcohol e.g. a glass of sherry prior to sleeping; take tonics and nutritional drinks which are approved by anti-doping bodies.

Physical therapy: swim outdoors; bathe in the evening for 15–20 minutes (at water temperature 33–37°C) with additives such as Radox, Badedas, extract of pine needles, etc; take Jacuzzis; in the morning, take a cold shower followed by a brisk towelling; take soothing massage and relevant aromatherapy; do soothing slow pace aerobics/exercises to music with emphasis on slow stretching.

Climate: move to a quiet area, e.g. forest or mountains; avoid intense ultraviolet radiation; live in moderate temperature of 18°C–24°C.

Addisonoid

Diet: encourage maintaining a strict three meals a day routine; increase protein intake, e.g. meat, cheese, eggs, cereals; prioritise organic foods and eliminate foods with preservatives and artificial colourings; take a concentrated course of vitamins, especially B12 plus the antioxidants; avoid alcohol; take occasional caffeine-based drinks with meals.

Physical therapy: take alternate hot/cold showers in the morning and in the evening; take saunas in the middle or high range of temperatures; take vigorous massage using approved rubbing lotions; do vigorous fast pace aerobics/exercises to music, with emphasis on elasticity.

Climate: move to a bracing climate – windy seaside location is ideal; look for moderate ultraviolet radiation; seaside in a warm climate allows benefits of hot sun and high temperatures to be alternated with plunges in the sea; live in moderate to high temperatures of 22°C-28°C.

Because several people may be involved in an athlete's development and lifestyle, they should all understand the complex business of overstressing. Consequently, there should be regular communication through the 'support team', to help establish that balance of stressors which will not harm the athlete.

SUMMARY

The effect of training may become negative if the athlete's lifestyle outside sport is poorly managed, so the total content of that lifestyle must be known. The coach must accept a responsibility to help ensure sound management in this direction, and also to develop an understanding of the unique aggregate of stressors represented by the athlete's lifestyle.

Both the structure of loading and the training ratio must be carefully planned if negative training effects are to be avoided. More specifically, the coach must ensure adequate recovery before the athlete is exposed to subsequent loadings.

Means of accelerating recovery in normal training and in the event of possible over-stressing, should be understood and applied.

Close observation of the athlete for early identification of symptoms of over-stressing may help eliminate any serious damage to the athlete's fitness status in the long term.

24 COMPETITION PERIOD

COMPETITION

The purpose of a competitive athlete's training programme is to produce optimal performance in competition. After all, there are no awards offered for world records in training! This point must be emphasised. The coach is preparing the athlete to improve his competition performance, and therefore all training is in pursuit of this end. The concept of periodisation implies producing or reproducing the high point of performance in a particular competition.

Training competitions

Bridging mesocycles 2 and 3 is a 'grey area' where specific training is mainly composed of competitions themselves. These competitions have immense importance in the development of the athlete's training status and his competition performance. Moreover, they are a means of evaluating status and stability of performance. These competitions are seldom used to evaluate status relative to other athletes. Instead, they may evaluate the athlete's status relative to his own previous competition performance, or those at the same time last year, etc. It seems reasonable to refer to all such competitions as 'training competitions'. These may be simple competitions to assess training status, or progressively sophisticated in terms of objective (and frequently referred to as 'build-up competitions'). It is worth pointing out that these competitions may well include events other than the athlete's own. For example, a 400 m hurdler may run 500 m to assess speed endurance, or a breaststroke swimmer may swim medleys to assess strength endurance, and so on.

Principal competitions

Apart from these training competitions, one should also distinguish principal competitions. These competitions dictate the patterns of mesocycles in the competition macrocycle, just as the pattern of the complete annual cycle is dictated by the climax of the competition macrocycle. The mesocycles must be so arranged that the best possible performance can be produced in each principal competition. The principal competitions should be seen as including the 'main' and the 'major' competitions. These main competitions are the final preparations for the major competition or the 'competition climax'. According to the nature of the sport, Matveyev (1965) believes two or more peaks (including the competition climax) are possible. However, from practical experience, it is most unusual for an athlete to produce more than four peaks even in the explosive sports where the technical component is high.

By way of summary of these points, the competition programme for a long jump athlete is set out in figure 94.

Competition v training

But why should competitions have anything more to offer training than, say, a trial in a training session? In training, one can only simulate competition situations. In competition, the athlete, due to the experience of competition and its

Date	Level event	Meso-cycle	Mesocycle content	Mesocycle objective
April 5		II	Progression into optimal competition frequency: loading extent reducing: training itself reduced but loading not yet at optimal intensity. Probably one mesocycle only.	Rapid increase in competition performance. Training competition 'hardness'. Evaluation of technical performance and training status. Stabilising competition performance: putting together competition experience.
12				
	(a) 200 m: 110H: 4 X 100			
19				
	(a) LONG: TRIPLE: HIGH			
26				
	(a) LONG: 100 m: 4 X 400			
May 3				
10	(b) LONG: 100 m			
			Emphasis on training: correction of technical faults found in previous mesocycle: intensity progressing steadily.	Correction of technical faults: preparation for III/III₂ based on above evaluations: commencement of main competitions.
17	(a) 200H: 200 m			
	(b) 100 m: LONG			
24	(a) 100 m			
31	(c) LONG: 4 x 100			
June 7			Main competitions with gradual reduction of extent as loading now moves to optimal intensity, but structure of loading is still inkeeping with event requirements. There will be several mesocycles here.	Stabilising optimal competition performances. Recording these in main competitions. Collection of all relevant data on behaviour in all competition situations.
14	(a) LONG: 100 m: 4 x 100	III or III₂		
21	(d) LONG: 4 x 100			
28				
	(a) 100 m			
July 5	(c) LONG: 200 m			
12	(d) LONG: 4 x 100			
	(a) 4 x 100: 4 x 400			
19			Period of special preparation. Extent of loading rises for 3 wks then decreases as intensity reaches opitmal – and highest in the annual cycle. The whole of this phase is a complete mesocycle.	Special preparation for major competitions based on analysis of III/III₂.
26	(b) 100 m: 200 m	IV		
Aug 2	(b) LONG			
9				
16	(d) LONG			
23		V		
30				

Note: (a) Simple training, (b) build-up, (c) main competition, (d) peaks.

FIG. 94 Possible distribution of competitions for an athlete whose main discipline is long jump. Note that from approximately April 12th–May 21st there is almost a 'grey area' where mesocycles II and III are bridged.

emotional demands, emerges more completely exhausted than in training. Consequently the stimulus for adaptation to high or maximum loading is more effective than that which can be reproduced in training. Just as important, however, is that competition is the most specific training that exists to master emotional excitement, and in such a way that it helps the athlete surpass present limits of performance. It is not unusual to hear of an athlete producing superb achievements in training, yet experiencing disasters in competition. He has failed to master himself in competition, reacting negatively to the threat of insecurity of living life on the edge of challenge. Once back in the quietness and security of the training situation, all is well again. Competition is the only means of adapting to the stressor of competition and to avoid its particular stress simply increases the stress potential of the next one.

It is essential that the level of competition is perceived by the athlete as a challenge relevant to the stage of preparation. So preceding a major competition with 'soft' competition is pointless. There is no adrenaline and, consequently, there is no rehearsal of competition intensity sharpness – intellectually, physically or emotionally.

In addition to this factor which validates competition as a training means, exposing the athlete to a wide variety of competition situations lessens the likelihood of him being confronted with the unfamiliar. Every competition has a character of its own, determined not only by the physical environment of stadium, wind, humidity, and so on, but also by the group of athletes involved. Athletes must be encouraged to seek out opposition, especially if the opposition is known to be better. By competing with the same opponents, a system of stereotyped, albeit efficient, reactions will evolve. Varied opposition and environment develops the capacity to adapt more readily to varying competition conditions.

Competition frequency

Frequency of competition is determined by athlete preference and relevant competition availability at one extreme, and the structure of sports competitions at the other. Weather conditions also play a part in the UK!

Time is needed for recovery from the physical and emotional stress of a main or build-up competition, and also to correct training deficiencies. Consequently, the 'build-up' and principal competitions will be 7-10 in number. Any additional competitions should be low key, at the level of 'simple training' status. Against this background, speed and elastic strength events in track and field can amount to one or two per week, while strength endurance and the longer track events can be separated by up to 14 days.

Occasionally there are instances where athletes saturate part of the competition season with a concentration of quality performances. In 1965, Ron Clarke raced 21 times in 56 days, lowering the 5000 m record twice, and the 10 mile record once. Moreover, in the month preceding this period, he set a world record for three miles; and three months after this period, in the space of 40 days he set world marks on three occasions: 3 miles/5000 m, 3 miles, and 6 miles/10,000 m. In 1980, Sebastian Coe established three world records again over a very brief timescale:

July 3	Oslo – 800 m	1 min 42.33 secs.
July 17	Oslo – 1 mile	3 mins 48.95 secs.
August 15	Zurich – 1500 m	3 mins 32.03 secs.

Only after several years preparation can such a programme be contemplated – and it certainly cannot be repeated over 2-3 successive years. At this level, the concept of using a year to regenerate is not uncommon. On the other hand, at the lower end of the scale, it has already been suggested that the young and developing athlete seems to be quite uninhibited in his appetite for competition. In fact, according to Thiess (1967), improvement in performance is directly proportional to competition frequency. He recommended, following the 1966 Spartakiad, taking part in 20–30 competitions in the period cycle leading up to the major competition.

Before moving on to competition preparation, and by way of summary, the following points should be noted:

- the athlete must compete as often as is necessary to achieve and stabilise a good competition performance
- the better opponent must not be avoided without good reason
- the athlete should only compete when he is physically and emotionally prepared for it
- too many competitions (especially when they are close together or involve considerable travel) not only interfere with training progression, but cause cumulative psychological fatigue
- competitions should be in ascending order of difficulty, building up towards a major competition with all competitions subordinate to it.

Long season sports

A team at the top of the FA Premier League may, due to the success of the club, have roughly 60 competitions in the course of approximately 270 days. Some of the players will also have international duties, and no allowance is made here for any replays. It still means, however, that for 75% of the year, players are potentially in line for one competition every 3½–4½ days!

In such cases, competition frequently becomes a central factor in maintaining a player's level of conditioning. It also, of course, saps the player's physical and emotional energies establishing a climate for the negative effects of stress.

Managers and coaches must, then, create a rotating cycle of development for *each* player, where regeneration is ensured and conditioning status is updated to give consistent high performance and motivation. It should not be injury or illness which determine when a player is rested, but value judgements related to an individual player's conditioning and motivational status. A system of player rotation must be understood by players and coaches, and fitted into the year phase in a way which allows the club to meet team and player development objectives. For the non-competitive 25% of the year it becomes essential that all players build the greatest possible conditioning base and regenerate fully from the competition season, so that the 'player rotation' approach can be effected with minimal difference to team performance.

Competition preparation

Specific competition preparation assumes a given status of training in the athlete for a given sport. This understood, the coach must carefully prepare units, etc., leading up to the competition itself. The following points should then be taken into account:

(1) The specific objective of the competition must be known by, and discussed with, the athlete. If it is not known, there is no means of evaluating success or failure, nor is there any distinct purpose to training. The objective may fall into one of two categories, or be a combination of both:

- competition with the athlete himself. These contests are to advance training status, improve performance, etc. Here, the opposition is used to aid pursuit of the objective. This is about performance.
- competition with an opponent. These contests are to win a point for the club/country, qualify for the next round, eliminate opposition, win a title, etc. Here the opposition is to be defeated. This is about results.

(2) An athlete's or team's game plan for a given competition must be constructed to his or its strengths. The opposition should be obliged to address that game plan. These may be a plan A and B, but it is negative thinking to enter the arena with the primary objective of countering the opponents' game plan. The opposition are always better at their game plan than yours; and less equipped to play yours! That said, the opposition must be clearly identified and known to the athlete, as not all athletes in a contest may be opponents. Information on each opponent should include previous best performance, recent history of competition, and behaviour in competition (e.g. how effective they are in aspects of play which may challenge your game plan).

(3) It is difficult to adapt quickly to unfamiliar conditions (a strange surface, humidity, altitude, temperature, etc.). Where possible, training should involve similar conditions to those at the competition venue.

(4) The chronobiologist encourages the coach to understand the peak and trough of human performance in terms of body rhythms of daily and longer cycles. The athlete must be able to compete at specific times and the coach should make allowances for adjustments in body rhythms. For instance, if travel has meant an

East/West time shift, the athlete should arrive at his destination with enough time to spare to 'reset' his body clock. If this is impossible, the athlete's normal day must be 'shifted' in training.

(5) The athlete should be educated towards complete independence and the capacity to act 'executively' in the competition situation, and must take his opposition seriously yet concentrate upon the task in hand. The athlete must never be afraid of the opposition and certainly never be encouraged to avoid opponents equal, or superior, to himself. In fact, the athlete should be hungry for such opposition, looking forward to these encounters with a positive anticipation. After all, this level of opponent represents the highest stimulus to increased adaptation levels and higher performance (see also chapter 10).

(6) Despite the athlete's physical and emotional concentration on the forthcoming competition, anxiety should be discouraged. The contest must not be seen as some kind of threatening monster. In the last few days, the coach should stimulate the athlete's belief in success, aid relaxation via recreation and reading, avoid boredom between training units by organising interesting but relaxing outings, and so on. Autogenic training, as formulated by Schultz (1956), or by the variation advanced by Machak (1964) may have something to offer in the control of 'pre-start reaction'. The athletes are originally 'trained' to relax by the coach, but eventually may induce the same state of relaxation themselves. Hypnotherapy is also very effective in affording a deeper state of relaxation. Hypnosis, of course, does not allow an athlete to adjust his behaviour to an unexpected situation that might occur in competition (see also chapter 10).

(7) Athletes naturally vary in their behaviour immediately prior to competition. Puni (1961) refers to this as 'pre-start reaction' and tabulated variations of this are shown in table 44. If the athlete shows start-fever, warm-up should be relaxed, while for those with start-apathy the warm-up should be vigorous and lively. According to Vanek and Cratty (1970), both extremes should benefit from autogenic training. Athletes also vary in their degree of sociability during warm-up, and over the last few days before a competition. A stronger feeling of security can sometimes come from being in a group, but this is not always the case. Many athletes seek to isolate themselves in order to concentrate a tighter focus on the forthcoming challenge (see also chapter 10).

(8) The younger athlete will especially benefit from observing other events prior to his own. The more mature athlete may learn something of the atmosphere of the stadium, the temperature, variations in wind, and so on. There is always the morale boost, of course, when witnessing a successful performance by a colleague. On the other hand, morale can slide with an early defeat. While this can be turned to advantage as a spur to other team members, the athletes who are yet to compete should not be exposed to the demoralising effect of discussing the defeat with the unfortunate athlete. There will be time for this after the day's competitions

are over. The coach should ensure that there is careful management of the pre-competition environment to the athlete's advantage.

(9) It is the athlete's responsibility to check his personal equipment, but it is the coach's responsibility to ensure that the athlete knows what is the specific equipment required.

(10) In the construction of the special competition preparation cycle, the following should be noted:

- a decision must be made by the coach whether to programme for improved performance or stabilisation of existing performance level. There are times when to demand increased levels of intensity will 'burst the bubble'
- the athlete's own status, that of his opposition, and the competition environment must be evaluated
- microcycles must allow complete recovery between units
- any additional competition must not itself be a peak but rather a build-up. Errors here will deplete reserves of emotional and physical energy. At least one such competition should be at, or near, the venue of the major competition, especially if the athlete must travel East/West, to altitude, to extreme humidity, and so on.
- the coach must develop the athlete's emotional focus and his appreciation of the need for complete preparation for the forthcoming contest. Too often an Olympic qualifying mark is reached, an athlete selected, and apathy follows. Or, again, a player who has gained international selection may lose his edge in the next game for his club. It is as if gaining selection was the major objective. Once targets have been reached, *new* targets must be set or qualifying targets should be higher than is necessary
- the first week of the special mesocycle leading up to the major contest should emphasise general development, relaxation and the recharging of batteries before the concentrated four weeks of build-up are started. This will be interpreted variously according to the patterns of performance in the previous mesocycle
- no technical variations should be attempted
- a thorough check by a physiotherapist or sports medicine specialist should be sought in the first week of this five-week mesocycle
- rules and regulations specific to the forthcoming competition should be clearly understood by the athlete. Moreover, commands and instructions in a foreign language should be rehearsed, where applicable.

(11) While the content and composition of units, microcycles and mesocycles vary between individual athletes, all are focused on ensuring that the athlete is intellectually, emotionally and physically prepared to compete with distinction in pursuit of the agreed goal.

state of readiness for competition	start-fever (nervous anticipation)	start-apathy (listlessness/inhibition)
All physiological processes proceed normally.	The athlete radiates great excitement; acute physiological changes (considerable increase in pulse rate, trembling in the limbs, feeling of weakness in lower extremities, etc.).	Listless, completely inhibited movements, yawning.
Slight excitement, enjoyable and rather impatient anticipation of the coming challenge, optimal power of concentration in complete control of own behaviour, radiating energy.	Great nervousness, uncontrolled movements, forgetfulness, absent mindedness, uncertainty of action, haste, unnecessary activity.	Limp, lazy, apathetic, anxious; low spirits; desire to 'cry off' from competition, tired, 'sour', unable to get going.
The athlete enters into competition in a highly organised way and exactly according to plan, sees the way ahead clearly, masters the situation, all forces at his disposal are brought into use in a tactically correct way; the anticipated result is achieved or surpassed.	Athlete's activity is disturbed, partially disorganised, he competes rashly, departs from his usual tactical line, loses the feeling for tempo, exhausts himself prematurely; movements are uncontrolled, accumulation of mistakes in face of high technical demands; very cramped.	He does not compete energetically, will-power soon abates, the athlete is incapable of mobilising the strength he possesses, action does not flow; after competition he is not exhausted because all reactions were on a low level.

TABLE 44 Principal forms of pre-start reaction from Harre (1973) according to Puni (1961)

On the day, only one person can bring the hours of work to a successful conclusion. The athlete's own will to coordinate all that has been learned and worked on, and to bring character, through his personality, to fruition within the opportunity represented by the challenge of the arena, are the most vital qualities of the successful athlete. He takes the risk of winning.

When the competition is over, the athlete will have a post-event reaction. This will be coloured by whether or not the acknowledged objectives of the competition have been met. Those who have not met the objective need not be reminded of it! Those who have been successful need little encouragement to be aware of this! The coach should encourage a state of normality and relaxation for the rest of the day of competition. Certainly there must be no criticism unless the athlete has for some reason misinterpreted the result relative to the objective. Review of the competition, evaluation of performance and clarification of lessons learned, should be pursued in the hours immediately after competition, or at the latest the next day. Such evaluation and modification is part of the athlete's preparation for the next competition and must not be neglected, whether the competition outcome was excellent or fell short of excellent.

SUMMARY

It is in the competition period that the objectives of the periodised year are met. Each competition should be seen as fulfilling several roles. It serves as training for future competition, is a test situation for evaluation status, and is the *raison d'être* of training. The athlete's objectives in competition will vary and they must be identified prior to a given competition. The coach, in planning and distribution and frequency of competitions, and in identifying competition objectives, must have detailed knowledge of the competition programme available and the level of each competition. Only then can he bring the athlete to each competition prepared to meet the identified objectives.

25 COACHWORKS: PRINCIPLES IN PRACTICE

PERFORMANCE

The coach's purpose is to improve an athlete's or team's performance in competition. This means guiding their endeavours to do things differently and better, or to do different things to ensure that they fully realise their competition performance potential.

On the one hand this is about technical development, on the other, behavioural development. Together, it is about preparing the athlete or team to deliver their best performance under increasing and changing pressures of competition. It is not only what they do but how they do it, according to the agreed core values and within the framework of the sport's laws.

When this process is effectively carried through, the athlete or team not only achieves personal performance excellence in their chosen areas, but each athlete or team member is prepared, through the experience, for their role in society and to enrich the quality of life for those whose society and culture they share.

DEVELOPMENT

So the coach contributes to the athlete's overall personal development by applying a holistic approach throughout the process. In this role, he is a member of a development 'team' which includes parents, teachers, other coaches, other support people, partner (where there is one), and, in some cases, a manager or agent. It is important that all members of this 'team' share the same core values and ensure that the athlete is supported in adhering to those values.

RESULTS

But what of results? The coach and athlete or team agree the result/goal that they are aiming for; it is the coach's task to prepare them to deliver the performance necessary to achieve it. It is the athlete's or team's task to commit to the work required and to deliver the performance. But, of course, there is opposition. The opposing athlete or team have also prepared to deliver a performance to get the result. Whatever the nature of the competition, the central focus is to think of each moment as the most important in the struggle and to push the boundaries of personal and/or collective performance persistently to turn the moment to advantage, or, in some cases to the opponents' disadvantage so that their performance is compromised. It demands the commitment of mind, body and emotion. When it is over, no matter what the result is, this has to be the best performance of the athlete or team on the day. If the competition was the main one of the year, the performance must be at least a season's best – or even a lifetime best.

Ideally, first place is what any athlete or team aspires to: if that is not possible, second; if not second, then third; if not third, then the best placing achievable. But, whatever the position, performance must be delivered, or how can the athlete, team or coach be considered to have performed their roles effectively and with distinction?

The point is that each competition produces its own uncertainties, so results are not always things over which you will have total control, despite excellent preparation and outstanding performance. For example, in the Christchurch (New Zealand) Commonwealth Games of 1974, John Walker (New Zealand) was prepared for and produced a world record beating performance in the 1500m. Unfortunately, Filbert Bayi (Tanzania) beat the world record by more! John's preparation and performance were excellent and he competed with distinction – even if the medal was not the colour he wanted.

So what is winning? It is being better today than yesterday – every day. It is doing the very best you can do with what you have: to be the very best that you can be with who you are.

Coaching is about more than sport. The dedicated coach sees preparation for achievement in sport not only as a mission in itself but also as a catalyst to prepare the athlete for a purposeful life. So he operates a holistic approach, keeping vision and values front and centre. The great coaches develop their own philosophy off

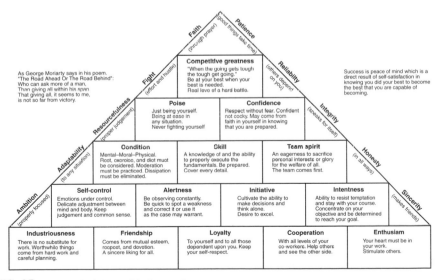

FIG. 95 John Wooden's 'pyramid of success'

this. For example, the legendary John Wooden, who coached the University of California, Los Angeles (UCLA) Bruins basketball team to 10 NCAA championship titles in 12 years, designed a 'pyramid of success' that would hold true as a kind of development code in most fields of endeavour – inside or outside sport (fig. 95, see previous page).

SYSTEMS

The process of performance improvement is approached through one of three systems which are described as follows:

(1) Escort system
Where the coach and athlete are together from the earliest days through to the conclusion of the athlete's competitive career. This is more consistent with individual rather than team sports. It has been the most popular system with UK-based trainers. To be effective it demands that the coach is competent to deal with progressive levels of athlete development.

(2) Transfer system
Where the athlete or team moves from coach to coach as they progress from one level of performance to the next. Each new coach is expert at working with athletes or teams at a specific performance or age level, similar to how we transferred from one teacher or tutor to another as we went through school or university. The transfer system was very popular with former Eastern European trainers. For team coaches it requires skills of adapting to different teams; preparing players for the next level where they will often play with different players, building on their previous levels of development; and being in clear and regular communication with other coaches working at different levels of athlete development. This all must be achieved as one seamless process from beginner to elite.

(3) Partnership system
Where the process is athlete- or team-centred; coach led; and performance services supported. Figs 96 and 97 illustrate the personal coach and team coach versions respectively. As the athlete or team moves towards high performance/elite performance status, this model becomes necessary to ensure that the performer's needs are met at the level demanded of such status. The athlete or team is at the centre of the model; the coach works to lead the process of athlete development and to lead the partnership of a performance services team. People in this team will change according to the athlete's or team's changing development and performance needs. This model may also be applied to the role of chief coach to a national sport (fig. 98).

Whatever the system, the coach will base his planning, decision-making and practical coaching on a sound foundation of performance- and learning-related sciences and arts. Providing such a base is the purpose of coach education and certification programmes provided by various national all sports coach programmes, national sports specific programmes, federations, coaches associations, university programmes and international sports bodies. The dedicated coach soon shifts from prescribed learning to self-managed learning as a life long commitment.

Generally, the coach who works with starter- and development-level athletes via escort or transfer systems runs a solo show and so his role is simply to lead the athlete's or team's development process, while advancing his learning through personal coaching knowledge and experience. For the most part, there is ready access to advice and guidelines on transferring cumulative multi-disciplinary knowledge and expanding experience into athlete and/or team development

Personal Coach

Leading the Players Performance Development and Delivery Process

C2 (Technical Specialist(s))

Performance Analyst

Doctor

C1

Biomechanist

Conditioning Specialist

A

Physiotherapist

Technical/Tactical Analyst

Manager

Physiologist

Psychologist

Nutritionist

Career Advisor

FIG. 96 Coaching model for coordinating input of a personal performance resource team

Team Coach

Co-ordinating the best fit of individual player performance contribution within the team, to develop and deliver optimal team performance.

Team Manager

Team Coaching Technical Specialists

Personal Coaches

Team Physiotherapist

C1

Tournament/Championships Analyst

Team Conditioning Coach

A / T

Team Psychologist

Team Nutritionist

Opposition Analyst

Team Doctor

Team Physiologist

Team Notational Analyst

FIG. 97 Coaching model for coordinating input of a team performance resource team

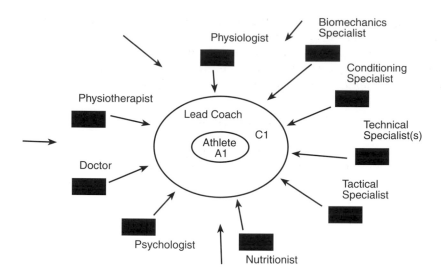

FIG. 98 Coaching model for coordinating input of a chief coach performance resource team

and performance advantage. However, coaches must apply a learning through experience-sharing ethos for this to raise coaching standards. This should become a component of every sport's coach education resource through an interactive online service.

Once coaches move to the high performance end of the development continuum (national/international potential and above), the coach is now the focus of input from experts in performance-related specialisms. Each expert has a very important contribution – advising on those small changes which are the difference between gold or silver, winning or losing, performance improvement or stagnation. Such contribution individually and collectively must produce the intended outcome of athlete or team competitive advantage. Moreover, the athlete/team, performance-related experts, other support people and coaches must be led by the coach to be what athlete and team need it to be.

Harmonising people and process

The partnership system of coaching is quite a different picture to that former image of the coach as a maverick, entrepreneurial character battling away to achieve against the odds and despite the perceived establishment! Now it is similar to an orchestra conductor, where a soloist (athlete or team) is accompanied and supported by the orchestra (the experts) under the leadership of the conductor (the coach). It is the soloist who must produce the virtuoso performance, but this is impossible without the musicians performing with excellence individually and collectively. The conductor cannot play any of the instruments in the orchestra as well as the musicians. Most of the instruments he cannot play at all. Yet he must understand what each brings to the performance; then harmonise the contribution of each instrument and section to ensure that the soloist's performance is supported to the full. Most importantly, he is the only person in that 'team' who hears the overall performance and can adjust the balance of things to ensure excellence is achieved by the entire 'team' in producing an outstanding soloist performance.

Changing coaching competencies

The problem is that at this level, access to synthesis skills development and leadership skills development, essential to the partnership system is often not readily available to coaches. Synthesis skills are those required by the coach to synthesise input from experts in science, technology and other performance-related specialist fields. This is essential for the creation of a programme appropriate to the athlete's needs. Lack of accesss leads to fractured relationships within the 'team'.

Awareness of this situation has led to some initiatives for change in coach development. For example, the Canadian Association of Coaches through its Sports Leadership Program is continuously researching innovative processes for developing coaching synthesis skills. The International Association of Athletics Federations has, through its Academy, built into the elite coach and chief coach programmes, blocks of modules which focus on leadership, behavioural change strategies, relationship management and culture change programmes to ensure that coaches are supported in their role.

Once a given coaching model is in place, there must be a serious commitment from all parties to make it work effectively. So, from the outset there must be a clear definition and understanding of everyone's roles and responsibilities. More than this, each person must be prepared to deliver their role and to adopt the vision and values of the 'team'. A strategy must also be in place where, continuously:

- the coach learns the skills necessary to lead the team of experts and the skills of synthesis necessary to customising input to the athlete's or team's development
- coach, athlete and experts learn to work together to ensure an effective outcome to the coaching process
- the learning generates effective action that leads to athlete or team achievement.

Cyclical planning

The process of designing the athlete's or team's performance plan is illustrated in figs 99a and b, and the framework within which the process is set as described by Arbeit (2000), is shown in fig. 100.

It is important to understand that the Arbeit framework involves continuous monitoring of **athlete, plan and coach** in order to have an inbuilt agility to create, adapt and learn, ideally at six week intervals (see fig. 100) eight weeks at the latest (see note 6, p. 330).

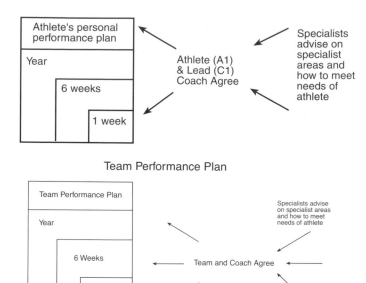

Team Performance Plan

FIG. 99a and b Process for designing an athlete's personal performance plan and team performance plan

FIG. 100. Framework of continuous planning-delivery-review adapted from Arbeit (European Athletics Coaches Conference, Warsaw, 2000)

In any given coaching environment, there should be commitment on the part of all coaches to build the performance and development database.

As the athlete's development needs change, the coach will adapt his coaching style accordingly (see chapter 10 pages 155–182).

```
┌──────────────────────────────────────────────────────────────────────┐
│          Daley Thompson's Decathlon Technical Team 1982–88             │
│                                                                        │
│          100   400    1500   110H  S     D     J     H     L     P      │
│  Coach   C1    CI     CI     C1    C2    C2    A2    C1    A3    C3      │
│                                                                        │
│  A2 – David Ottley          Silver – Javelin 1984 Olympics             │
│  A3 – Greg Richards         1988 Olympian Decathlon; Coach to Dean Macey│
│                             Silver – Decathlon 1999 World Championships │
│                                                                        │
│  C1 – Frank Dick                                                       │
│  C2 – Art Vanegus           UCLA Throws Coach & Coach to several Olympic│
│                             & World Throws Champions                    │
│  C3 – Paul Brooke           Pole Vault Coach                           │
└──────────────────────────────────────────────────────────────────────┘
```

FIG. 101. A coaching team approach in practice
   KEY:
   a = Directing
   b = Coaching
   c = Supporting
   d – Counselling

Daley Thompson was Olympic, World, European and Commonwealth Champion and Record Holder during this period. Fig. 101 illustrates how a partnership system can operate and affords example of possible coaching style selected at a particular phase of Daley Thompson's development.

A process of learning and changing

Coaches believe that winners are made not born: their view is that it doesn't matter what we come into life with, it is what we do with it that matters. The coach accepts that there are certain things which are *given*; certain things there are certain things which the coach will work to *adapt* and *change*: and certain things which will give the athlete *focus* and which will help the athlete realise his potential and goal. (See table 45).

Given	Nature and nurture start pack. Talent and aptitudes, early learning experience, early motivation framework
Adapt and change	Technical and tactical skills, behaviours and attitudes, relationships, interpersonal and intrapersonal skills = what to do and how to do it
Focus and realise	Pursuit of shared vision within shared values framework. Avoiding demotivation

TABLE 45 Components in pursuit of competitive achievement

The coaching process, through one or several coaches, leads the athlete or team from being dependent to being independent. From a position where the coach has ownership of the development and performance delivery process to where the athlete has ownership. In that journey, the athlete learns that:

'Probably the only sustainable competitive advantage you have is the ability to learn faster than the opposition.'

Arie De Geuss (presentation to Shell Oil 1998).

That advantage is gained more by sharing what is learned than by restricting education exclusively to personal experience. Consequently, although athletes are coached to take personal ownership of their destiny in the arena, they must be interdependent in learning faster how to achieve their goals in that arena.

There are three Rs (responsibilities) that should be addressed when learning interdependence.

R1. Responsibility for personal performance. In individual sports, performance is solely the athlete's responsibility. In a team endeavour, it is the athletes' collective responsibility.

R2. Responsibility for personal performance development. The coach can achieve nothing without the athlete's commitment to living this responsibility.

R3. Responsibility to learn from every experience and share it. Passing experience on to others – whether the coach, the performance services experts, or even other athletes – accurately reflects the interdependence necessary for continuous learning for athlete, coach and team. The athlete is as critical to the learning of those who coach and support him as they are to him. Such personal investment of learning will, for all but the irresponsible, find reciprocation.

The three Rs are as relevant to the coach and all members of the performance services support team, as to the athlete.

Double vision

The coach also has 20:20 double vision! (fig. 102)

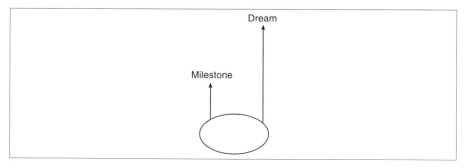

FIG. 102 The coach has 20:20 double vision relating to the 'dream' and the milestone

The 'dream'

There must be a very clear picture of where the athlete or team is trying to get to in the long term.

'If you can't imagine it you can't do it.'

(John F. Kennedy)

That 'dream' may be a four-year Olympic cycle away and will require the pursuit of all the technical and behavioural adjustments demanded for that challenge, when the athlete will be in his peak performance years and when performance standards will have progressed.

The milestone

The milestone is any moment where the coach, athlete or support team can influence the outcome of their collective endeavour. This means hitting the immediate training targets through to their week's or month's competition targets. But how can you hit immediate milestone targets and prepare for the different and tougher challenge of tomorrow's 'dream'? This goes back to the three Rs! (see fig. 103)

FIG. 103 The three Rs!

A discipline

Coaches do not plan forwards; they plan backwards – from the 'dream'. If the target competition is four years away, where do you have to be three months before that? Then three months before that? Work your way back to the present. Coaches start with the end in mind, and there is a 10-step discipline to this.

(1) What result defines the dream?
     Agree the result being sought, e.g. Olympic Gold – 2012 – men's 400m track.
(2) What performance is needed to make this a realistic probability:
     (given current progressions, this will be around 43.25 secs.)
(3) What level of quality consistency in training, lifestyle and performance
     is required to deliver 43.25 secs on the day?
(4) What technical, tactical and fitness conditions would give this consistency?
(5) What is the athlete's current status relative to (4), (3) and (2) above, and what
     do performance potential indicators suggest for the athlete?
(6) What are the timescales and intermediate challenges?
(7) Review your (the coach's) level of competence to lead the process and
     the competencies required of the performance services support team.
     What do you and/or they have to do to improve?
(8) Select, build and develop a dedicated performance services support team
     to take the athlete from here (where the athlete/team is now) to there
     (where he/they need to get to).
(9) Design a plan from strategic level through to unit level and include a tight
     review process.
(10) Execute to the highest standards of professional quality excellence.

Performance build

There is an order to building performance of athlete and team.

(1) Learn and persistently practice quality of technique or techniques

The very precious resource that the athlete represents must be given the very best coaching in establishing the technical model or models. If the athlete does not get this right it will waste time, energy and even economics to put it right. Faulty basic technique leads to one compensation after another. Once established, technical review and realignment must be built cyclically into the year plan. Jack Nicklaus spent two weeks out of every year realigning his golf swing right through to retirement! Why? The pressures of competition, compensatory adjustments due to muscle imbalance, injury, fatigue and so on, can compromise technical quality, so regular technical 'realignment' is essential. Sound, robust, effective technique is basic to performance development and performance quality. Get it right then keep it right.

(2) Develop fitness to be technically effective

Once the model is sound, the athlete must develop the general, related and specific strengths to get the most out of it, plus the endurances necessary to produce technical excellence even in the presence of fatigue induced stressors. So fitness here is about excellence every moment of every training and competition challenge.

(3) Develop maximum speed without compromising technical effectiveness

Speed of movement, decision-making and so on cannot be pursued at the expense of technical quality. In team sports there should be a harmonious and synchronised approach to speed development or there will be breakdown in quality and consistency of the team's rhythm. For example, in passing a ball, the player passing it must know that the ball the person receiving can be used, so he must know the player's movement and speed potential so the ball is not passed too late or too early. Speed work is as demanding on the mind as the body and requires patient but exacting practice otherwise individual segments of overall technique become asynchronous. In some instances, new technical detail must be learned to make the speed increases possible. For example, the sprinter's propulsion dynamics at maximum speed are not the same as in accelerating from the blocks.

(4) Develop optimal cruising pace

Once maximum speed levels are established, fitness must be maintained to allow the athlete to perform ever closer to his maximum speed. This allows pace in a race or rhythm of play in a game, where the opposition fatigue mentally and/or physically because they cannot operate at that same pace or rhythm. It is a climate of fatigue where speed or power is a key determinant of performance. Tactically, an athlete or team, equipped to perform at a higher speed or rhythm than the opposition, makes the opposition play to that level. To drop speed or rhythm to that of the opposition, makes you vulnerable.

(5) Release extremes and change of pace

There are no certainties in any competitive arena. Anything – weather, light, sound, inconsistent refereeing decisions, or even opponent or colleague behaviour – changes the conditions of the contest and nature of the challenge. Given the previous four stages of performance build, now is the time to introduce practices to produce performance excellence while dealing with the uncertain and unusual. Competitive challenge is seldom plain sailing. Sometimes there are white water situations, yet the fight still has to be won. Practice can be virtual, such as mentally taking on a tough set of variables and working out how to adjust physically, emotionally and mentally to cope with them and win. Or it can be real, as in seeking out or modelling conditions in training and competition to learn to fight through them to win. The opposition will also change the pace of things to disrupt personal or team rhythm. Athletes or teams must be given the opportunity in training or in specially-structured competitions to learn how to turn the situation around to get back into their own winning rhythm.

(6) Read the game and respond faster and more effectively that the opposition

The reason why the coaching process leads the athlete towards controlling performance in the arena is because the athlete must read each moment of the game and respond with action that will give him or the team, competitive advantage. The coach can influence things off the field, outside the arena, but the athlete and team must control each moment on the field, inside the arena. If an athlete gets a stone in their shoe in the first mile of the marathon, does he wait until he sees the coach to take it out? If the game plan is not working after 10 minutes of play, does the team wait until half time for instruction to change things? The coach prepares the athlete or team to read the game or contest; to have technical options they can deliver with quality; to choose the best option; to execute it at speed; and to learn from the experience. In team situations the coach also prepares every athlete to communicate how they are reading the game and build other athletes into an effective solution.

(7) **Win, and win again, and again**

The purpose of competing is to win. After every competition, there is immediate review to understand what happened and why. It is as important to know why we win as it is to know why we lose. If we don't know why we win, it is an accident. The best athletes learn how to win then keep practising how to win! There is a ruthlessness to it, but it is the reward we have fought to have for the price we have paid in sweat and toil and pain and personal sacrifice. The ruthlessness turns a winner into a champion who keeps on winning!

The right climate to grow

Against the backdrop of chapter 10, coaches live the truism:

'People who feel good about themselves, perform better.'

(Anon)

Coaches create and maintain a positive motivational climate for athletes, for coaching colleagues and for all other performance services people. They are aware that the task is not only about motivating people, but also avoiding de-motivating them. They work constantly to weighing the scales of motivation in favour of the will to win rather than on the fear of failure: this means for athlete, coaching colleagues, services people and management performance:

* giving people the right size of mountain to climb – reasonable, yet stretching goals
* using only positive statements in discussion
* helping people rationalise and understand poor or disappointing performance
* helping people plan intelligently for the challenge of the arena
* being continuously more knowledgeable in all performance-related areas
* being strong-willed, resolute and unwavering whatever the pressure
* demonstrating passion, yet keeping emotions robustly stable before, during, and after competitions
* prioritising the development of people's strengths, focusing on weaknesses only if they compromise delivery of their strengths or delivery of other team members' strengths
* living the notion that coaches inspire people. Coaches are not indispensable; their job is to create self-reliant athletes and self-reliant members of the performance team
* teaching people how to win, how to behave when they win, and how to behave if they don't.

So, the coach makes everyone involved feel they are an important and contributing member of the team. By demonstrating appreciation and recognition when it is merited, that message is conveyed. The coach must display genuine interest in each person, addressing them directly by name, talking about their interests and concerns, and exercising best endeavours in meeting their needs. He also shares responsibility when things do not go as intended. He encourages people to rationalise both why things have not worked out and why success has been theirs. Finally, the coach makes a point of not proving people wrong.

Qualities

So what characteristics do the best coaches share?

(1) Keep vision and values front and centre
The coach is visionary and lives life by adhering to core values. He should have very real strength of character and commitment to personal integrity and honesty. Winning at any point should never come at the expense of values.

(2) Think deeply about and pursue holistic education
The coach sees himself preparing people not only for achievement in sport, but through sport for a life of personal fulfilment and for the enrichment of community.

(3) Dedicated to life-long personal development and professionalism
The coach tirelessly pursues personal education, formally and informally, both in the performance-related sciences and in liberal arts. He sees the journey to coaching excellence as a never-ending story; seen not only in terms of a chosen sport and coaching theory and practice, but in understanding how to successfully live a balanced and full life, while facing tougher and tougher challenges in the chosen field of endeavour.

(4) Mentally tough
The coach is focussed, determined, tenacious, hard – even ruthless – but never cruel. His resolve to overcome all obstacles and challenges in pursuit of the agreed goal is unshakeable. No matter how many setbacks, he has the resilience to keep coming back, to keep fighting. He always has heart for the fight. He persistently seeks for the advantage and no matter how small that is, he will seize it and maximise its value. He is devoted to passing these qualities on to everyone he influences as coach. That means driving them to go beyond what they think they are capable of, even when this means tears and pain.

(5) Meticulous in preparation
The coach takes the advice of Abraham Lincoln:

'If I had eight hours to chop down a tree; I'd spend six of them sharpening the axe.'

He is a master of strategic thinking and quality control, and is guardian of good order throughout the coaching process. He is thorough in briefing and preparing his athlete, team, coaching colleagues, management and performance services experts for the specifics of a given competition or campaign; he constantly seeks new and better ways of doing so. In this aspect of his role, he is thoroughly disciplined to system and method. His approach to preparation includes anticipation and coping with uncertainty.

(6) Excellent communication skills

The coach makes the complex simple and ensures that what is heard, seen, understood and translated into action is exactly the intended response to his verbal, visual and kinaesthetic messages. He communicates as much through the emotions as the intellect, and leans as heavily on anecdote, metaphor and simile as on data and drawing board.

(7) Relationship management

The coach exercises excellence in initialising social interaction and persistently applies best endeavours to ensure that relationships work effectively for the individuals concerned and for the collective purpose. This means taking time to understand each person in their sphere of influence; what they need from the relationship; what they bring to it; and how they can connect in learning, in performance, and in delivering the strength of interdependence. The coach is always visible, accessible, and approachable.

(8) Decision-making

The coach has exceptional decision-making abilities. These range from decisions which determine the route to achieving long-term goals, to resolving situations under pressure and at speed, selecting the right course of action in a crisis. So he is very competent in making the judgement to change direction from an agreed game plan in order to seize the opportunity of success for the enterprise. He knows his most important decisions are selection of his team, from athlete to support staff. His operational network to facilitate this is part of such selection. He is well aware of his areas of strength and recruits people to make these even stronger. He is equally aware of his areas of weakness and brings in those who will compensate for these. While challenging each person in the team to raise their game, he also expects to be challenged to raise his. He creates a culture where correct decisions are based on what needs to be heard, which may not always be what is wanted to be heard.

(9) Self-knowledge and awareness

The coach knows himself. He never underestimates his leadership role, responsibilities and accountabilities, yet he may understate his leadership value. He is acutely aware of his limitations and measures himself persistently and more harshly than he measures others; 99% of his best he considers failure, even when in others he would see 51% of their best as a win. He is true to himself and naturally to those professional standards of excellence for which he is known. In being true to himself, he knows that, being human, he is imperfect and even fallible! Achievement, for him, is only in part reflected in performance and results in the competition arena. Rather, it is in what he did and how he did it in his leadership and coaching roles, and, in the longer term, in his legacy to those whose life he touches, to the sport, and to his community.

(10) Belief, faith and trust
The coach radiates self-belief, belief in his people and belief that the agreed goals will be successfully achieved. Those around him respond to this by believing in themselves and in him more. A shared sense of personal value grows, fuelled by his passion, pride, patience, persistence and powers of persuasion. Yet he has personal humility and an inbuilt sense of belonging to a great scheme of things. He sees trust as pivotal in that scheme: his trust in others sharing the struggle to reach the goal, and their trust in him. It is a trust where each knows the other will do the right thing, and, whatever the outcome, all will learn to be even better in meeting challenges that will follow. He has great personal strength of spiritual faith according to his beliefs. And, finally, he has an unshakeable conviction that even in those ruthless arenas of life where facts and figures conspire to set limits to human performance, it is the intangible but irrepressible power of the human spirit to go beyond those limits, that is the winning difference. The great coach fans the flame of that human spirit.

(11) Passion
The coach is passionate about life, people and coaching. It is this that is at the root of his capacity to motivate.

'You won't sweep anyone off their feet if you can't be swept off your own.'

(Anon)

That passion is infectious; however, he is also instinctively compassionate when occasion requires.

SUMMARY

Knowledge and understanding of information and resource central to the delivery of the coach's purpose is a never-ending story. The broad framework of sports training principles within which a coach pursues that purpose is continually evolving. The detail within that framework changes constantly, and in many aspects the rate of change is increasing through the creativity and adaptability of people. The coach, then, must become master not only of the general and specific technical business of the science of his work, but also of the people business of the art. His own continuous learning is as critical in delivering milestones and dreams as is the athlete's.

Coaches invest their learning and experience in people. Some of the great coaches in history have done so not only in the sense of their work with athletes and/or teams, but as a legacy for future generations of coaches and for the community outside sport. John Wooden was such a coach. Another was 'Woody' Hayes (Head Coach, Ohio State Football 1951–1978). He built his approach to investing in people through his interpretation of some lines from the essays of Ralph Waldo Emerson.

'. . . In the order of nature, we cannot render benefits to those from whom we receive them, or only seldom, but the benefit we receive must be rendered again line for line, deed for deed, cent for cent to somebody. Beware of too much good staying in your hand . . . pay it away quickly in some sort.

Woody Hayes took this to mean,

'We cannot pay back all those who have helped us, so we have to pay forward.'
(Gary M. Walton. Beyond Winning. Leisure Press, 1992)

Coaches commit themselves through a life of continuous learning and relentless practice to exercising their passion for creating personal excellence in others. Investment in people of the unique expertise this represents is their *raison d'être*.

They pay forward.

That is what coaches do.

SUMMARY OF PART 5

When planning the athlete's annual training programme, the coach must have access to a considerable volume of information and also have the ability to interpret this in the light of current training theory. The structure of this programme begins to take its final shape during the transition macrocycle at the conclusion of the previous competition season. However, this is not to say that the programme is inflexible. The coach must appreciate the dynamic nature of his work and be prepared, where appropriate, to make any necessary adjustment within the structure. Information required by the coach is as follows:

(1) He should know the programme of competition available to the athlete or team and the precise nature of each competition.

(2) He should know how to plan the year to accommodate the best competition programme for the athlete's development and/or the team's.

(3) He should know the theoretical distribution of general, related and specific training in each mesocycle of the year.

(4) He should know the number of training units and the training environment available to the athlete or team.

(5) He should know the relevant training practices, structures of loading and training ratios for development of specific fitness each athlete requires to meet his training objectives.

(6) He should know the principles of unit, microcycle, mesocycle and macrocycle construction, and their variations according to its position in the annual cycle.

(7) He should apply the 10-step approach on page 355.

The final product should reflect the coach's interpretation of training theory and application of experience in a programme designed to meet the unique needs of an athlete to persistently perform better than before.

The athlete's fundamental objective in sport is pursuit of competitive advantage. It represents a serious commitment of time and effort, but is nevertheless undertaken for the pleasure which that commitment brings. To be invited to direct the athlete's growth and development in sport is a great honour; to accept that invitation is to acknowledge an immense responsibility. The coach must know that his work with the athlete will provide a systematic progression towards his fundamental objective, while contributing to his total wellbeing. Such knowledge is born of an understanding of those areas of study which feed into the science of sport as outlined in parts 1, 2 and 3, and of an appreciation of how these relate to the athlete via training theory, as presented in parts 4 and 5. It is my belief that when the coach thoughtfully weaves this knowledge into the fabric of practical experience, the athlete must certainly achieve his fundamental objective. The athlete's life in sport will, then, be a purposeful and enjoyable experience which will add a lasting richness to his life outside sport. Moreover, the visionary coach will not only contribute to the athlete's or team's lifetime achievements, but will learn through the experience to contribute to establishing a dynasty of excellence.

REFERENCES FOR PART 5

Bauersfeld, M. & Voss, G. Neue wege im schnelligkeitsteaincing. Munster: Philippka 1992. In *Trainer Bibliotek*, Vol. 28

Bellotti, P. (March 1991) A few aspects of the theory and practice of speed development. In *New Studies in Athletics, Vol. 6*, No. 1

Bonov, P. (2001) *2nd International Scientific Congress Report: Sport, Stress, Adaptation*. National Sports Academy, Sofia, Bulgaria

Bosco, C. Eine neue methodic zur eimschatzung und programmierung des trainings. In L*eistungssport*, Munster 22 (1992), No. 5, pp 21–28

Carl, G. (1967) *Gewichtheben*. Sportverlag, Berlin

Craig, T. (1973) *Analysis of Female Athletic Injury Frequency*. lVth Coaches' Convention Report

Dick, F. W. (1993) *Foundation of Jumps Development and Initial Conditioning*. Proceedings of E.A.C.A. Congress, Berlin

Donati, A. (March 1995) The development of stride length frequency in sprinting. In *New Studies in Athletics, Vol. 10*, No. 1

Endemann, F. (1973) *Throws Conditioning*. IVth Annual Coaches' Convention Report

Gladwell, Malcolm (2006) *Blink*. Penguin Books, UK

Gundlach, H. (1968) Zur Trainierbarkeit der Kraft und Schnelligkeitsfahigkeiten Im Prozess der Korperlichen Vervollkommnung. In *Theorie Und Praxis Der Korperkultur* 17

Harre, D. (1973) *Trainingslehre*. Sportverlag, Berlin

Hettinger, T. (1968) *Isometric Muskelkrafttraining*. Thieme-Verlag, Stuttgart

Hettinger, T. & Müller, E. A. (1953) Muskelleistung und Muskeltraining. *Arbeitsphysiologie*, 15 111–126

Hollmann, N. & Venrath, H. (1962) Experimentelle Untersuchungen zur Bedeutung Eines Trainings Unterhalb Und Oberhalb Der Dauerbelastunsgrenze. In *W.u.a.*, '*Carl Diem Festschrift*', Frankfurt

Israel, S. (1963) Das Akute Entlastungssyndrom. In *Theorie Und Praxis Der Korperkultur* 12

Karvonen, M. J., Kentala, E. & Mustala, O. (1957) The effects of training on heart rate. In *Annales Medicinae experimentalis et Biologae Fenniag*, Vol. 35

Kruger, A. (1973) Periodisation or peaking at the right time. *Track Technique*, December

Machak, M. (1964) Relaxacne–Aktivacni, Autoregulacni Zasah, Metoda Nacviku a Psychologicka Charackteristika. *Czechoslovakian Psychology*, 3

Matveyev, L. P. (1962) Die Dynamic Der Belastungun Im Sportlichen Training. In *Theorie Und Praxis Der Korperkultur* 11

Matveyev, L. P. (1966) *Periodisation of Sports Training*. Fiskultura i Sport

Osolin,

N. G. & Markov, D. P. (1972) *Distribution of Training* (part translation from Russian). Lehka Atletika, Moscow

Puni, A. Z. (1961) *Abriss Der Sportspsychologie*. Sportverlag, Berlin

Schiffer, J. (September 1994) Overtraining. In New Studies in Athletics, Vol. 9, No. 3

Schmolinksy, G. (1974) *Leichtathletic*. 7th Edn. Sportverlag, Berlin

Schultz, H. H. (1956) *Das Autogene Training*. Konzentrative Selbstentspannung, Stuttgart

Sinkkonen, K. (1975) *The Programming of Distance Running*. Paper to E.L.L.V. Congress Budapest

Ter-Ovanesyan, I. (1965) 'Ter-Ovanesyan on the Long jump', *Modern Athlete and Coach*, Vol 4 No 4. (Translation from Russian – Lehka Atletika, Moscow)

Thiess, G. (1967) Wettkampfhaufigkeit Im Nachwuchstraining. In *Theorie Und Praxis Der Korperkultur* 16

Vanek, M. & Cratty, B. J. (1970) *Psychology and the Superior Athlete*. MacMillan Co., Toronto

Walton, Gary M. (1992) *Beyond winning*, Leisure Press, Champaign, Illinois

Zhelyazkon, Tsvetan, Dasheva, Daniele (2001) *Training and Adaption in Sport*, Digital-The Document Co., Sofia, Bulgaria

I have also received personal communications from Erkki Oikarrinen (Finland), Peter Tschiene (Germany), Helmar Hommel (Germany), Dr Ekkart Arbeit (Germany), and Elio Locatelli (Italy), and am grateful for their exchange of views.

INDEX